Doing Better and Feeling Worse

Essays by

Ivan L. Bennett, Jr.
Philip Berger
Daniel Callahan
Merlin K. DuVal
Robert H. Ebert
Leon Eisenberg
Renée C. Fox
Donald S. Fredrickson
Eli Ginzberg
Beatrix Hamburg
David Hamburg
Herbert E. Klarman
John H. Knowles
Walsh McDermott
Stanley Joel Reiser
Julius B. Richmond
David E. Rogers
Ernest W. Saward
Lewis Thomas
Aaron Wildavsky

Doing Better and Feeling Worse
Health in the United States

Edited by JOHN H. KNOWLES, M.D.

W · W · NORTON & COMPANY · INC · *New York*

Library of Congress Cataloging in Publication Data
Main entry under title:
Doing better and feeling worse.
   Includes index.
   1. Medicine—United States.   2. Medical care—United
States.   3. Public health—United States.   I. Knowles,
John H.
R152.D64   1977   362.1'0973   77-3382

ISBN   0   393   06419   0
ISBN   0   393   06423   9 pbk

   5 6 7 8 9 0

Contents

Preface

"DOING BETTER AND FEELING WORSE"—is this a fair appraisal of the "health system" that now prevails in the United States? Those who are openly skeptical of many features of health care in late-twentieth-century America will ask whether it makes any sense even to speak of a "health care system" in a country where services are so fractionated, largely controlled by private physicians who appear almost indifferent to demands for certain kinds of attention. While the cost of medical service continues to rise dramatically—in most instances galloping ahead even more rapidly than the price of other goods in this inflationary era—new evidences of fraud and malpractice are discovered in federal programs as well as in the private sector. These revelations only provide additional fuel for the already widespread opinion that in health—as in education, justice, and welfare—things have recently gone strangely awry and that only substantial reforms will set them right.

Not the least of this volume's accomplishments is the agreement among many of its authors that it is impossible to be sanguine about certain of the medical practices that now obtain. Some are troubled, indeed incensed, by such conditions as the inaccessibility of services, unnecessary surgery, excessive prescription of drugs, unexplained hospital bills, which are adversely affecting the health, well-being, and confidence of many individuals in America. These complaints, however justified, cannot diminish the very real and widely expressed satisfaction with the many tangible medical accomplishments of recent years; it would be wrong to ignore them—any balance sheet purporting to give a fair accounting of the system must acknowledge advances no less than shortcomings. Because the health-care industry is so variegated and complex, the elaboration of a viable alternative health policy can only be predicated on an understanding of those complexities.

Is this book a subtle apologia, then, for existing medical practices and priorities? Not at all. Indeed, it ought to be read as a detailed inquiry into many of the conditions that prevail in American health care today, touching institutions as various as hospitals, insurance companies, medical schools, research laboratories, health-care centers, and governmental agencies. If certain practices are clearly indefensible and merit criticism, others are less obviously pernicious, and some are without doubt beneficial. Abuses, where they exist, will not necessarily be remedied by some sweeping legislative act, whether a national health-insurance program or some other major institutional reform. Care must be taken not to create false optimism about the likely benefits of any one measure for reform. The American "health-care system" is so complex, composed of so many parts, reaches out into, and is influenced by, so many non-medical institutions that it is unlikely to be substantially altered by a single act of Congress, however bold or venturesome.

The choices are many; they involve so many bodies, public and private, and call for so many different kinds of calculations that only a thorough inquiry into the politics, economics, and sociology of health care will suggest all the public (and private) dilemmas that exist. But to solve even the problems that are widely perceived calls for a sensitivity about professional, public, and patient interests that goes beyond the rigid cost-accounting calculus of those who concentrate solely on price. It is not only because the health-care industry has grown so large or so expensive (it is expected, by some estimates, to consume well over $130 billion in 1977) that it has become the object of such intense scrutiny. Medicine touches intimately on the physical and emotional lives of most Americans, eliciting strong reactions, whether of approval or disapproval. It provides an almost infallible measure of public sentiment about the efficiency of government, the vitality of the medical professions, and the justice of new moral perceptions and demands that modern medical practices have elicited.

This volume is intended to be a first, quite tentative, step toward redefining the health-care problems of the country. In showing how these relate to specific social conditions that appear almost endemic in contemporary American society, how they depend on numerous political decisions—and not only those made by legislators in Washington—and how they reflect widespread values, beliefs, and preferences that are not susceptible to quick or easy change, our authors stress the role of certain cultural components heretofore all too frequently ignored or denied. In a labor-intensive industry such as health care, the views and opinions of both professionals and workers weigh heavily. So, also, do the opinions of those who seek medical help, who, in one way or another, express concern about its availability, quality, humanity, and cost. Then, of course, there is the whole other agenda of preventive medicine, a subject that concerns many Americans somewhat less than professional health workers would wish. Both problems—health care and the prevention of disease—can only be dealt with in the context of a medical research program, very largely federally financed, that is now somewhat curtailed, but is still thought by many to be without peer in the world today.

An expression must be made of the great debt owed to Dr. John H. Knowles, president of the Rockefeller Foundation. He assumed all the burdens of guest editor of this issue, giving unstintingly of his time in every kind of editorial chore, and always showing great patience, judgment, and humor. We are much beholden to him.

We wish also to thank Nelson Rockefeller, who, in his capacity as chairman of the Commission on Critical Choices for Americans, first invited Dr. Knowles to organize a group to study problems of health care; a good number of the essays in this volume originated as drafts prepared for the Commission. Thanks are due as well to the Robert Wood Johnson Foundation and the Rockefeller Foundation for funds that made possible the commissioning of additional papers, the extensive revision of almost all of them, and the preparation of a volume that we believe merits wide circulation. Our hope is that this volume will encourage a dialogue in the United States on a wide range of subjects in the health-care field, and that specific policy recommendations will result from this more deliberate study and discussion. Few subjects are more interesting or more important; few could profit more from greater scrutiny.

Stephen R. Graubard

Doing Better and Feeling Worse

JOHN H. KNOWLES, M.D.

Introduction

> One of the troubles of our age is that habits of thought cannot change as quickly as techniques, with the result that as skill increases, wisdom fades.
>
> Bertrand Russell, 1962

> With technological advance, more things are possible, but social and technical organization is increasingly necessary to bring them off. In effect then, the sense of potency—the idea of the possible—increases in scope, but the artificer of the possible is now society rather than the individual.
>
> Jerome Bruner, 1962

> In America the passion for physical well-being . . . is general.
>
> Alexis de Tocqueville, 1835

IN THE MID-NINETEEN-FIFTIES, the United States became the first country in the world to shift from a predominantly blue-collar society of industrial workers to a predominantly white-collar society of service workers. By 1970, over 62 per cent of the labor force was employed in services such as communications, transportation, public utilities, trade, finance, education, health, police, public administration, and research. Scientific and technological advances resulted in the transition from a rural-agricultural to an urban-industrial society, a society committed to improving the quality of life through the development of services to meet human needs. In every discussion of human services, issues of cost, quality, and accessibility immediately become paramount.

These problems are particularly pressing in the field of health. The economic and emotional devastation visited upon individuals and families as a result of unexpected and unanticipated disease, disability, or death appears to be, at least in our culture, more important than crises that recur in other aspects of American life. Consequently, there exists a profound national concern that, despite a massive increase in health expenditures together with a marked expansion in health workers over the past decade, the nation's health has improved less than was promised or expected. The benefits have not appeared to justify the costs. To make matters worse, broad indicators of social pathology, including drug abuse, illegitimate births, divorce rates, crime and violent behavior, learning difficulties, and psychological problems—the last most frequently found in the uncertainty of adolescence or the loneliness of old age— tell us that the nation is not as healthy as it should be. While some of these problems result from ignorance, poverty, suppression of civil rights, and unequal opportunities for employment and education—all major societal maladies—it is thought that

1

medicine can, and should, assume at least part of the responsibility for preventing, curbing, or curing these conditions.

Although it is often claimed that the United States has no national health policy and that a crisis exists in the American health system, neither statement is quite true. A "health policy" *has* evolved, and though it cannot be called a "system" in any sense, it has very specific characteristics. Thus, for example, public responsibility has been assumed for financing services—and, in specific instances, facilities—for the care of certain groups; these include the indigent sick (through Medicaid, which is left to individual states for implementation), the elderly (through Medicare, which is part of the federal Social Security System), the mentally ill, members of the armed forces and veterans, and indigent American Indians and migrant workers. Health care, however, remains largely a private, pluralistic system: 60 per cent of the total expenditure comes from private sources. Because of inflation, improvement in the quality and quantity of services, and of accessibility to them, not to speak of wholly new services, health expenditures have markedly increased. They have risen three-fold from $39 billion (5.9 per cent of the gross national product) in 1965 to $119 billion (8.3 per cent of the gross national product) in 1975. It is estimated that $134 billion will be spent in 1976. Much of this will go to cover hospital bills, physicians' fees, and drug costs.

We have developed an acute, curative, hospital-based system which favors older people, particularly those over 65 who represent 10 per cent of the population and consume about a quarter of all health expenditures. In 1975, hospitals took in $47 billion, physicians' services came to $22 billion, and drugs costs, $11 billion. There is evidence of gross over-use of all three—they consumed 67 per cent of the total national health expenditure—but no one knows quite how to deal with the problem. The situation is made all the more serious by the lack of emphasis on the detection and prevention of disease. Health education (including school health services and counseling on nutrition), rehabilitation services, and lower-cost chronic-hospital extended care, including nursing home facilities, are all slighted. There is a serious deficiency in the numbers of accessible community health centers. We have empha-sized high-cost, hospital-based technologies to the neglect of other services where the benefits are much greater relative to costs incurred, such as those involved in rehabilitation. It is significant that legislation for renal dialysis was passed long before legislation was enacted to stimulate the detection and treatment of hypertension.

Health insurance has generally emphasized hospital and surgical expenses. Cov-erage has been less extensive, in order of decreasing magnitude, for regular medical expenses, ambulatory care, dental care, drugs, psychiatric care, home health services, preventive care, and family-planning services. As of 1975, about 90 per cent of all hospital-care expenditures was paid by third-party payers (37 per cent was covered by private health insurance; 53 per cent was paid for by the government); 60 per cent of payments for physicians' services came from third parties, leaving 40 per cent to direct payment by consumers; only 14 per cent of drug and dental expenses were covered by insurance of any kind.

There has been increasing specialization in medical (and postgraduate) education; over 70 per cent of all American physicians are specialists. While there is one medical doctor for every 645 people, there is only one general or primary-care physician for every 4,771 people. Unfortunately, we depend on the "free market" and on foreign medical graduates for the rational distribution of manpower. This has resulted in serious imbalances, both within specific geographic areas and among the various specialties. Between 1963 and 1973, the number of foreign-trained physicians practicing in the United States increased from 11.2 to 19.5 per cent of the total. Between 1962 and 1971, 75,639 foreign medical graduates entered the United States and 77,867 physicians were graduated from American medical schools. Because of problems of access, discontinuity, and high cost of specialized care, not to speak of depersonalization, a renewed interest in general or family practice ("primary care") has recently developed.

The prevailing American medical system is based on solo, fee-for-service practice—sometimes in the form of self-incorporated groups of physicians. Salaried physicians, pledged to deliver comprehensive service under contract with specific consumer groups on a prepaid, per capita basis, are rare. The delivery systems are sometimes well planned, as, for example, is the Kaiser-Permanente Foundation in California, but they are more often haphazard. Over 90 per cent of all active physicians are directly involved in patient care, with some 62 per cent of them committed to office-based practice.

The labor market in the health-care industry is changing rapidly. Between 1950 and 1970, the numbers employed in health services rose from 1.7 million (2.96 per cent of those totally employed) to 4.3 million (5.6 per cent); the number of women rose from 65 to 75 per cent of the total; of the 4.3 million employed, 2.7 worked in hospitals (this is 65 per cent of all health workers and 3.5 per cent of the total labor force). While less than 3 per cent of physicians and surgeons are black, over 20 per cent of dieticians and practical nurses are black. There is considerable evidence to suggest that the work ethic among health workers, doctors included, has also changed: collective bargaining among all health workers, including hospital interns, residents, and even practicing physicians, is increasingly common.

Public health interests have been, and continue to be, isolated from American medical education and practice. Issues that influence health, such as nutrition, family size, population density, environmental mobility, poverty, racism, sexual practices, unemployment, housing, transportation, and the like, are rarely taken into account in any overall calculation of the health needs of the nation. At the same time, there is a trend toward what one critic has described as "medicalizing everything." Thus, certain conditions, such as criminal behavior and juvenile delinquency, alcoholism, and heroin addiction, once thought to be examples of personal irresponsibility requiring punishment (including imprisonment) are now thought to be socially induced conditions, for which society as well as the individual is held responsible. Very substantial efforts are being made to determine where medical and psychiatric treatment, rather than incarceration, may better serve both the individual and the community interest.

Governmental support for medical research has increased markedly, although it is now leveling off. Between 1950 and 1975, expenditures for health research and development in this country increased from $160 million to over $4.7 billion; the federal government provided over two-thirds of this amount. More recently, expenditures have not grown so markedly, and most of them have involved categorical and contractual arrangements. Government sources provide 34 per cent of the funds for the construction of research and medical facilities; private sources provide the rest.

Biological research and technological development are heavily favored over proposals for improved health services and social-science research.

The ethics of medicine is also receiving new emphasis, exemplified in "right-to-die" and "patient bill-of-rights" manifestoes and in the development of specific requirements for ethical guidelines in human experimentation. The courts have also been actively involved: increased litigation, larger awards to plaintiffs, and the consequential rise in the cost of malpractice insurance make the issue of the rights and responsibilities of patients—as well as of physicians—a very compelling one. Complex ethical problems attendant upon organ transplant, sickle-cell detection, renal dialysis, and amniocentesis to detect mongolism are also being discussed, along with the more emotionally charged issues—the "right to die," abortion, and the like.

Many argue that greater attention must be given to the training of health professionals (including physician's assistants and nurse practitioners) and to a change in the locus of training (e.g., baccalaureate programs for nurses) and problems of licensing and re-licensing physicians.

The interest in national health insurance remains high. Twenty-five million Americans have no medical insurance whatsoever; fewer than half of those under 65 (90 million people) and virtually none over 65 (21 million people) are covered against the ruinous cost of "catastrophic" illness. Partly because of this, there is increasing consumer unrest, although the majority of Americans today still place crime, drugs, and the high cost of living, inflation, housing, schools, unemployment, and corruption in government above health care when they list their major grievances. Those that express dissatisfaction with the health-care system cite high costs, particularly those attendant upon catastrophic illness, as their principal complaint. They also worry about the quality of health care, the accessibility of services, and the impersonality and frequent lack of continuity often associated with the "medical encounter."

Over the past eighteen months, a group which was formed at the request of the Commission on Critical Choices for Americans, a national body established by Nelson Rockefeller, met periodically to attempt to find new insights into the problems confronting the United States and to consider what a viable health policy should be. So that its views might become known to a larger public, the decision was made to publish essays on those issues that this group found central to any consideration of America's health dilemma. The essays that resulted comprise this volume. They are intended principally for persons outside the health professions, for it is hoped that the dissemination of information grounded in reality and stressing the complexities of the existing "system" will bring more reason and less emotion to bear on the discussion of the nation's health-care problems. Our initial enthusiasm for detailing every aspect of a national health policy gave way to the more sober hope that we might be able to delineate certain of the major areas of concern, thereby casting new light on the subjects chosen and offering some help in resolving issues of priority and purpose in a field where there are ambiguities about both. The reader will note opposing views among the authors; no effort has been made to create an artificial agreement where agreement did not in fact exist.

The American people have clearly come to expect much from medicine, especially in recent years, but they have matched these rapidly rising expectations with rising anxieties over the cost, quality, and accessibility of health services. Many within the profession believe that both the expectations and the anxieties are the result of a definition of health that has become much too broad and that certain limits on the responsibility to society of the medical profession need to be established. At a time when the relations between health, illness, and medicine are being viewed in wholly new ways and are acquiring new meanings in our culture, some talk of too much "medicalization," and argue for "demedicalization"—a return to a simpler set of health practices—even as others call for greater efforts toward realizing the advantages that only an improved science and technology can provide. They say that we are only at the beginning of a "scientific revolution" in the health field, although, if that is so, it becomes all the more incumbent upon us to develop effective ways of assessing the economic, social, ethical, and medical impact of new technologies before they are generally introduced into practice. Medicine ought not to be berated for the high cost of "halfway" technologies when definitive technologies are not available. And unless more support for fundamental research is forthcoming, definitive (i.e., curative or preventive) technologies will not be developed that can markedly reduce the cost of disease.

The evolution of and support for the American biomedical-research effort and the present subdivision of responsibility—whether in the National Institutes of Health or in other agencies—were developed at a time when sustained growth and stability of funding were taken for granted. New approaches are needed, if only because these assumptions are now in jeopardy. Medical knowledge and scientific technologies have raised profound moral and ethical questions that must be addressed. The assessment of the quality of care rendered by physicians involves not only a delineation of the "samaritan" function, but also an understanding of all that derives from technological advances, for the physician is required to choose from among the technologies available to him. The complexities of assessing "quality" in an era when chronic and degenerative diseases have replaced acute infectious ones as the primary health problem demand long-term study. They call for an understanding of the interaction between the multiple variables in both the causation and the course of a disease, if therapy is to be evaluated effectively (this is, incidentally, an area where computers have much to offer).

The pressing need for more primary-care practitioners, recognized by the profession and the public alike, and the need to delineate more clearly the functions and responsibilities of the university and the teaching hospital are already producing substantial changes in medical education and in health-care delivery. The evolution of the various professional, governmental, and consumer groups interested in, and responsible for, health—now viewed by most American citizens as a fundamental "right"—represents a typical American response. The health industry is pluralistic, competitive, and essentially committed to the tenets of a laissez-faire ethos. It involves sharing by public and private interests with diverse power centers; it is based upon multiple decision-making mechanisms; it tolerates multiple conflicts (although they are increasingly frustrating to all concerned). Any discussion of financing mechanisms and national health insurance brings with it certain hopes for cost controls, for improvements in the quality of health care, and for accessibility to services for all. It presumes a more rational utilization of services (requiring definitive changes in the behavior of both providers and consumers) and an improved organization of delivery systems. Sober reflection reveals the complexity of the subject—what may and may not be expected—and the unknowns that indicate the need for further research. The current debate is taking place in an intellectual vacuum of ideological bias and self-fulfilling prophecies. The individual's responsibility for his own health is supposed to be self-evident; how the rights of the individual relate to the social good of the community and of the nation that are required to bear the costs of his irresponsibility and poor health habits is less obvious. Changes in behavior are notoriously difficult to achieve; add to this the problems resulting from the steadily expanding array of drugs, unnatural food additives, and environmental contaminants that also influence health and the full dimensions of the problem become apparent. They call for a more rigorous legislative effort which in turn presumes a citizenry sufficiently enlightened to know its interests and civic-minded enough to participate actively in the democratic process.

The health of children determines the future strength of the nation, so statistics on this score are particularly dispiriting. To improve the situation, comprehensive efforts in integrated local service systems directly related to the schools must be introduced. These will stress the application of what is known, while seeking to lessen those recalcitrant social forces—ignorance and poverty—that condition the health of children. Mental illness is another of the country's major health problems. A scientific revolution has taken place with the advent of modern psychopharmacologic research; these advances, together with others that stem from recent research in human behavior, offer new hope in the care and cure of those afflicted with mental illness, but much remains to be done, particularly on the social and cultural level. Physicians have always performed a vital social function in responding to distress; the relief of apprehension has profoundly beneficial psychic as well as somatic effects on the patient and on his level of ease or dis-ease. The understanding physician is able to influence the patient's behavior, whether in his compliance with therapeutic regimens, his willingness to improve his health habits, or in his capacity to cope with death and dying.

The authors represented in this volume, concerned with values, attentive to the growing preoccupations of many in society who are not at all satisfied with the way things seem to be moving, view the problems in historical perspective and try to relate them to a whole series of long-range considerations that must be taken into account in any consideration of national health policy: medicalization and demedicalization; both the promise *and* the problems of medical science and technology; the quality of care; the political pathology of health policy; the financing and organization of health services; the ethical imperatives that are known to be critical and the moral dilemmas that they create; the need for primary-care physicians; the redirection of teaching-hospital and medical-school functions; the evolution of critical public and private institutions, power centers, and decision-making mechanisms; the special problems of children and of the mentally ill; the individual's responsibility for maintaining his own health and for participating as a citizen in efforts to control environmentally induced maladies; the continuing search for support, and the special qualities of the caring physician.

There is reason for optimism. We know that the infant-mortality rate is once again declining after a period of stability; deaths from heart disease have dropped below one million for the first time since 1967, and deaths from heart attack are 7 per cent below the level of 1970; over the past 25 years, death rates for practically all major diseases have decreased in the age group 45 to 64 (notable exceptions are cancer, cirrhosis of the liver, bronchitis, and emphysema); overall death rates have declined and the life expectancy has increased; and the gap between rich and poor, black and white has continued to narrow. We have developed the finest biomedical research effort in the world, and our medical technology is second to none. The poor have both gained greater access to health services and are using the services gained. Medicare has benefited the elderly. Medical education is improving, and increasing numbers of women and blacks are gaining entry into medical schools. Delivery systems are also improving and primary-care physicians are once again being trained. National programs to reduce smoking and to detect and treat hypertension have been remarkably successful. New knowledge is being generated about the hazards of drugs, faulty diets, and environmental contaminants, and the nation has shown its willingness to ban the production and use of certain toxic substances.

And yet we feel dis-eased. We find intolerable the levels of deprivation and ill health suffered by significant numbers of the American people, and not only among the elderly. While trying to balance public and private interests, maintaining the ideal of individual freedom even as we assert the imperatives of social responsibility and justice, we know that we are confronted with complexities that call for ways of thinking that are not bound to the old and exhausted ideologies of an earlier day. It is a new kind of pragmatism that is needed, one that admits that truth is plural and contingent, but that takes into account the strengths and weaknesses that exist without being overwhelmed by either the exaggerated hopes of science and technology or the despair of poverty and ignorance. The challenge to the United States is to estimate correctly what reason, confronted by irrefutable facts, can accomplish, particularly at a time when something more than a reputation for humanity is called for.

RENÉE C. FOX

The Medicalization and Demedicalization
of American Society

THE STATEMENT THAT AMERICAN SOCIETY has become "medicalized" is increasingly heard these days. During the past decade or so, the allegation has been made by social scientists, jurists, politicians, social critics, medical scientists, and physicians. In many instances, it has been accompanied by the claim that the society is now "overmedicalized," and that some degree of "demedicalization" would be desirable. There are those who not only espouse "demedicalizing the society," but who also predict that, in fact, it will progressively come to pass.

One of the most extreme statements of this kind is Ivan Illich's monograph, *Medical Nemesis*, which opens with the assertion that "the medical establishment has become a threat to health," and goes on to develop the many damaging ways in which the author considers modern medicine to be responsible for "social" as well as "clinical" and "structural" iatrogenesis:

> The technical and non-technical consequences of institutional medicine coalesce and generate a new kind of suffering: anesthetized, impotent and solitary survival in a world turned into a hospital ward. . . . The need for specialized, professional health care beyond a certain point can be taken as an indication of the unhealthy goals pursued by society . . . . The level of public health corresponds to the degree to which the means and responsibility for coping with illness are distributed amongst the total population. This ability to cope can be enhanced but never replaced by medical intervention in the lives of people or by the hygienic characteristics of the environment. The society which can reduce professional intervention to the minimum will provide the best conditions for health. . . . Healthy people are those who live in healthy homes on a healthy diet; in an environment equally fit for birth, growth, work, healing and dying: sustained by a culture which enhances the conscious acceptance of limits to population, of aging, of incomplete recovery and ever imminent death. . . . Man's consciously lived fragility, individuality and relatedness make the experience of pain, of sickness and of death an integral part of his life. The ability to cope with this trio autonomously is fundamental to his health. As he becomes dependent on the management of his intimacy, he renounces his autonomy and his health *must* decline. The true miracle of modern medicine is diabolical. It consists not only of making individuals but whole populations survive on inhumanly low levels of personal health. That health should decline with increasing health service delivery is unforeseen only by the health managers, precisely because their strategies are the result of their blindness to the inalienability of life.[1]

There are numerous grounds on which Illich's thesis can be criticized. He minimizes the advances in the prevention, diagnosis, and treatment of disease that have been made since the advent of the bacteriological era in medicine, and he attributes totally to non-medical agencies all progress in health that has ensued. He implies that modern Western, urban, industrialized, capitalist societies, of which the United States is the prototype, are more preoccupied with pain, sickness, and death, and less able to come to terms with these integral parts of a human life, than other types of society. Although his volume appears to be well documented, a disturbing discrepancy exists between the data presented in many of the works that Illich cites in his copious footnotes and the interpretive liberties that he takes with them. Perhaps most insidious of all is the sophistry that Illich uses in presenting a traditional, orthodox, Christian-Catholic point of view in the guise of a vulgar Marxist argument. For he repeatedly claims that "when dependence on the professional management of pain, sickness and death grows beyond a certain point, the healing power in sickness, patience in suffering, and fortitude in the face of death must decline."[2] In Illich's view, this state is not only morally dubious, but also spiritually dangerous. Because it entails the "hubris" of what he deems arrogant and excessive medical intervention, it invites "nemesis": the retribution of the gods.

But whatever its shortcomings, Illich's essay is a kind of lightning rod, picking up and conducting the twin themes of medicalization and demedicalization which have become prominent in the United States and a number of other modern Western societies. These themes will concern us here. We shall begin by identifying the constellation of factors involved in what has been termed "medicalization," offer an interpretation of these phenomena, and consider and evaluate certain signs of demedicalization. Finally, some speculative predictions about the probable evolution of the medicalization-demedicalization process in American society will be offered.

One indication of the scope that the "health-illness-medicine complex" has acquired in American society is the diffuse definition of health that has increasingly come to be advocated: "a state of complete physical, mental, and social well-being," to borrow the World Health Organization's phrase. This conception of health extends beyond biological and psychological phenomena relevant to the functioning, equilibrium, and fulfillment of individuals, to include social and cultural conditions of communal as well as personal import. Such an inclusive perspective on health is reflected in the range of difficulties that persons now bring to physicians for their consideration and help. As Leon Kass picturesquely phrased it:

> All kinds of problems now roll to the doctor's door, from sagging anatomies to suicides, from unwanted childlessness to unwanted pregnancy, from marital difficulties to learning difficulties, from genetic counseling to drug addiction, from laziness to crime. . . .[3]

A new term has even been coined by medical practitioners to refer to those clients who seem to have some legitimate need of their therapeutic services, but who technically cannot be considered to be ill. With discernible ambivalence, such persons are often called "the worried well."

Accompanying the increasingly comprehensive idea of what constitutes health and what is appropriate for medical professionals to deal with is the growing conviction that health and health care are rights rather than privileges, signs of grace, or lucky, chance happenings. In turn, these developments are connected with higher expectations on the part of the public about what medicine ideally ought to be able to accomplish and to prevent. To some extent, for example, the rise in the number of malpractice suits in the United States seems not only to be a reaction to the errors and abuses that physicians can commit, but also a reflection of the degree to which the profession is being held personally responsible for the scientific and technical uncertainties and limitations of their discipline. The vision of an iatrogenesis-free furthering of health, which social critics such as Illich hold forth, is also an indicator of such rising expectations.

One significant form that the process of medicalization has taken is the increase in the numbers and kinds of attitudes and behaviors that have come to be defined as illnesses and treatment of which is regarded as belonging within the jurisdiction of medicine and its practitioners. In an earlier, more religiously oriented era of a modern Western society like our own, some of these same kinds of attitudes and behaviors were considered sinful rather than sick, and they fell under the aegis of religious authorities for a different kind of diagnosis, treatment, and control. In a more secular, but less scientifically and medically oriented, stage of the society than the current one, certain of these ways of thinking, feeling, and behaving were viewed and dealt with as criminal. Although sin, crime, and sickness are not related in a simple, invariant way, there has been a general tendency in the society to move from sin to crime to sickness in categorizing a number of aberrant or deviant states to the degree that the concept of the "medicalization of deviance" has taken root in social-science writings. The sin-to-crime-to-sickness evolution has been most apparent with respect to the conditions that are now considered to be mental illnesses, or associated with serious psychological and/or social disturbances.[4] These include, for example, states of hallucination and delusion that once would have been interpreted as signs of possession by the Devil, certain forms of physical violence, such as the type of child abuse that results in what is termed the "battered child syndrome," the set of behaviors in children which are alternatively called hyperactivity, hyperkinesis, or minimal brain dysfunction, and so-called addictive disorders, such as alcoholism, drug addiction, compulsive over-eating, and compulsive gambling.

This "continuing process of divestment"[5] away from sin and crime as categories for abnormality, dysfunction, and deviance and toward illness as the explanatory concept has entailed what Peter Sedgwick calls "the progressive annexation of not-illness into illness." "The future belongs to illness," he proclaims, predicting that "we . . . are going to get more and more diseases, since our expectations of health are going to become more expansive and sophisticated."[6] If we include into what is considered to be sickness or, at least, non-health in the United States, disorders manifested by subjective symptoms which are not brought to the medical profession for diagnosis and treatment, but which do not differ significantly from those that are, then almost everyone in the society can be regarded as in some way "sick."

> At least two . . . studies have noted that as much as 90 percent of their apparently healthy sample had some physical aberration or clinical disorder. . . . It seems that the more intensive the investigation, the higher the prevalence of clinically serious but previously undiagnosed and untreated disorders. Such data as these give an unexpected statistical picture of illness. Instead of it being a relatively infrequent or abnormal phenomenon, the empirical reality may be that illness, defined as the presence of clinically serious symptoms, is the statistical *norm*.[7]

Such a global conception of illness acutely raises the question of the extent to which illness is an objective reality, a subjective state, or a societal construct that exists chiefly in the minds of its social "beholders," a question that will be considered in greater detail below.

The great "power" that the American medical profession, particularly the physician, is assumed to possess and jealously and effectively to guard is another component of the society's medicalization. In the many allusions to this medical "power" that are currently made, the organized "autonomy" and "dominance" of the profession are frequently cited, and, in some of the more critical statements about the physician, these attributes are described as constituting a virtual "monopoly" or "expropriation" of health and illness. The "mystique" that surrounds the medical profession is part of what is felt to be its power: a mystique that is not only spontaneously conferred on its practitioners by the public but, as some observers contend, is also cultivated by physicians themselves through their claim that they command knowledge and skills that are too esoteric to be freely and fully shared with lay persons.

However, it is to the biotechnological capacities of modern medicine that its greatest power is usually attributed: both its huge battery of established drugs and procedures and its new and continually increasing medical and surgical techniques. Among the actual or incipient developments that are most frequently mentioned are the implantation of cadaveric, live, or mechanical organs, genetic and other micro-cellular forms of "engineering," and *in vitro* fertilization, as well as various chemical, surgical, and psychophysiological methods of thought and behavior control. The potentials of medicine not only to prevent and to heal, but also to subjugate, modify, and harm are implicated in such references.

The high and rapidly growing cost of medical and health care is still another measure of increased medicalization. In 1975, Americans spent $547 per person for health care and related activities such as medical education and research. This represented 8.3 per cent of the GNP. In 1950, 4.6 per cent and in 1970, 7.2 per cent of the GNP was spent. From 1963 to the present, health expenditures have risen at a rate exceeding 10 per cent annually while the rest of the economy as reflected in the GNP has been growing at a rate between 6 and 7 per cent.

In addition to allocating an ever increasing proportion of society's economic resources for health care, greater amounts of political and legal energy are also being invested in health, illness, and medical concerns. The pros and cons of national health insurance, which continue to be vigorously debated in various arenas, are as much political, ideological, and legal issues, as they are economic ones. The volume of legislation relevant to health care has grown impressively. In 1974, for example, more than 1,300 health-care bills were introduced in the Congress, and more than 900 such bills in the state legislature in New York alone. The health subcommittees of the Senate and the House of Representatives are particularly active, and they have become prestigious as well. Furthermore, partly as a consequence of various congressional investigations and hearings, the federal government is now significantly involved in bioethical questions (especially those bearing on human experimentation) in addition to their more traditional interests in medical economic and health-care-delivery problems.

During the past few years, a number of medico-legal decisions have been made that are of far-reaching cultural importance, affecting the society's fundamental conceptions of life, death, the body, individuality, and humanity. These include: the

Supreme Court's decisions in favor of the legal right of women to decide upon and undergo abortion; the Court's ruling against the involuntary, purely custodial confinement of untreated, mentally ill persons; the Uniform Anatomical Gift Act, adopted in fifty-one jurisdictions, which permits persons to donate all or parts of their bodies to be used for medical purposes after their death; death statutes passed in various states which add the new, "irreversible coma" criterion of "brain death" to the traditional criteria for pronouncing death, based on the cessation of respiratory and cardiac function; and, in the case of Karen Ann Quinlan, the New Jersey Supreme Court's extension of "the individual's right of privacy" to encompass a patient's decision to decline or terminate life-saving treatment, under certain circumstances.

One other, quite different, way in which medical phenomena have acquired central importance in the legal system is through the dramatic escalation of malpractice suits against physicians. An estimated 20,000 or more malpractice claims are brought against doctors each year, and the number seems to be rising steadily. In New York, for example, the number of suits filed against physicians rose from 564 in 1970 to 1,200 in 1974; in the past decade, the average award for a malpractice claim grew from $6,000 to $23,400, with far more very large awards being made than in the past.[8]

Increasing preoccupation with bioethical issues seems also to be a concomitant of the medicalization process. Basic societal questions concerning values, beliefs, and meaning are being debated principally in terms of the dilemmas and dangers associated with biomedical advances. Consideration of particular medical developments such as genetic engineering, life-support systems, birth technology, organ implants, and population and behavior control have opened up far-reaching ethical and existential concerns. Problems of life, death, chance, "necessity," scarcity, equity, individuality, community, the "gift relationship," and the "heroic" worldview are being widely discussed in medical, scientific, political, legal, journalistic, philosophical, and religious circles. A bioethics "subculture" with certain characteristics of a social movement has crystallized around such issues.

The unprecedented number of young people who are attempting to embark on medical careers is also contributing to the medicalization process. In this country, on the average, more than three persons apply for each medical-school place available to entering first-year students, and there is as yet no sign of a leveling off. Paradoxically, this is happening during a period when medicine and the medical profession are being subjected to increased scrutiny and criticism.

Complex, and by no means consistent, the process of medicalization is not an easy one to analyze. Several preliminary *caveats* seem in order. In part, they are prompted by two sorts of assumptions made by critics of medicalization in America: one is that the central and pervasive position of health, illness, and medicine in present-day American society is historically and culturally unique, and the other, that it is primarily a result of the self-interested maneuvers of the medical profession. Neither of these assumptions is true without qualification.

To begin with, in all societies, health, illness, and medicine constitute a nexus of great symbolic as well as structural importance, involving and interconnecting biological, social, psychological, and cultural systems of action. In every society, health, illness, and medicine are related to the physical and psychic integrity of individuals, their ability to establish and maintain solidary relations with others, their capacities to perform social roles, their birth, survival, and death, and to the ultimate kinds of "human condition" questions that are associated with these concerns. As such, health, illness, and medicine also involve and affect every major institution of a society, and its basic cultural grounding. The family, for example, is profoundly involved in the health and illness of its members, and, especially in non-modern societies, the kinship system is as responsible for health and illness as are specialized medical practitioners. The institutions of science, magic, and religion are the major media through which the "hows" and "whys" of health and illness, life and death are addressed in a society, and through which culturally appropriate action for dealing with them is taken. The economy is also involved in several ways: the allocation of resources that health, illness, and medicine entail; the occupational division of labor relevant to diagnosis and therapy; and the bearing of health and illness on the individual's capacity and motivation for work. The deviance and social-control aspects of illness have important implications for the polity which, in turn, is responsible for the organized enforcement of health measures that pertain to the community or public welfare. And in all societies, the influence, power, and prestige that accrue to medical practitioners implicate the magico-religious and stratification systems as well as the polity.[9]

As the foregoing implies, there are certain respects in which health, illness, and medicine are imbued with a more diffuse and sacred kind of significance in non-modern than in modern societies. For example, in traditional and neo-traditional Central African societies, the meaning of health and illness, the diagnosis and treatment of sickness, and the wisdom, efficacy, and power of medical practitioners are not only more closely linked with the institutions of kinship, religion, and magic than in American society; they are also more closely connected with the overarching cosmic view through which the whole society defines and orients itself. One indication of the larger matrix into which health, illness, and medicine fit in such a society is that in numerous Central African languages the same words can mean medicine, magico-religious charms, and metaphysically important qualities such as strength, fecundity, and invulnerability, which are believed to be supernaturally conferred.

In the light of the multi-institutional and the cultural significance of health, illness, and medicine in all societies it is both illogical and unlikely to believe that the current process of medicalization in American society has been engineered and maintained primarily by one group, namely, the physicians. What the manifestations of medicalization that we have identified do suggest, however, is that the health-illness-medical sector has progressively acquired a more general cultural meaning in American society than it had in the past.[10]

Within this framework, the medicalization process entails the assertion of various individual and collective rights to which members of the society feel entitled and which they express as "health," "quality of life," and "quality of death." The process also involves heightened awareness of a whole range of imperfections, injustices, dangers, and afflictions that are perceived to exist in the society, a protest against them, and a resolve to take action that is more therapeutic than punitive. Medicalization represents an exploration and affirmation of values and beliefs that not only pertain to the ultimate grounding of the society, but also to the human condition, more encompassingly and existentially conceived.

Thus, in American society, health and illness have come to symbolize many positively and negatively valued biological, physical, social, cultural, and metaphysical phenomena. Increasingly, health has become a coded way of referring to an individually, socially, or cosmically ideal state of affairs. Conversely, the concept of illness has increasingly been applied to modes of thinking, feeling, and behaving that are considered undesirably variant or deviant, as well as to more forms of suffering and disability. In turn, this medicalization of deviance and suffering has had a network of consequences.

Talcott Parsons's well-known formulation of the "sick role" provides important insights into what these effects have been. According to him,[11] the sick role consists of two interrelated sets of exemptions and obligations. A person who is defined as ill is exonerated from certain kinds of responsibility for his illness. He is not held morally accountable for the fact that he is sick (it is not considered to be his "fault"), and he is not expected to make himself better by "good motivation" or high resolve without the help of others. In addition, he is viewed as someone whose capacity to function normally is impaired, and who is therefore relieved of some of his usual familial, occupational, and civic activities and responsibilities. In exchange for these exemptions which are conditionally granted, the sick individual is expected to define the state of being ill as aberrant and undesirable, and to do everything possible to facilitate his recovery from it. In the case of illness of any moment, the responsibility to try to get well also entails the obligation to seek professionally competent help. In a modern Western society, such as the United States, this obligation involves a willingness to confer with a medically trained person, usually a physician, and to undergo the modes of diagnosis and treatment that are recommended, including the ministrations of other medical professionals and hospitalization. Upon entering this relationship with institutionalized medicine and its professional practitioners, an individual with a health problem becomes a patient. By cooperating and collaborating with the medical professionals caring for him, the patient is expected to work toward recovery, or, at least, toward the more effective management of his illness.

The fact that the exemptions and the obligations of sickness have been extended to people with a widening arc of attitudes, experiences, and behaviors in American society means primarily that what is regarded as "conditionally legitimate deviance" has increased. Although illness is defined as deviance from the desirable and the normal, it is not viewed as reprehensible in the way that either sin or crime is. The sick person is neither blamed nor punished as those considered sinful or criminal are. So long as he does not abandon himself to illness or eagerly embrace it, but works actively on his own and with medical professionals to improve his condition, he is considered to be responding appropriately, even admirably, to an unfortunate occurrence. Under these conditions, illness is accepted as legitimate deviance. But this also implies that medical professionals have acquired an increasingly important social-control function in the society. They are the principal agents responsible for certifying, diagnosing, treating, and preventing illness. Because a greater proportion of deviance in American society is now seen as illness, the medical profession plays a vastly more important role than it once did in defining and regulating deviance and in trying to forestall and remedy it.

The economic, political, and legal indicators of a progressive medicalization cited above also have complex origins and implications. For example, the fact that activities connected with health, illness, and medicine represent a rising percentage of the gross national product in the United States is a consequence of the fee-for-service system under which American health-care delivery is organized; the central importance of the modern hospital in medical care; the mounting personnel, equipment, and maintenance costs that the operation of the hospital entails; and the development of new medical and surgical procedures and of new drugs, most of which are as expensive as they are efficacious. Some of this increase in costs results from the desire for profits that medical professionals, hospital administrators, and members of the pharmaceutical industry share to varying degrees. But how much is difficult to ascertain, though radical ideological criticisms and defensive conservative statements on the point are both rife at present.

In addition to such political and economic factors, the heightened commitment to health as a right and the medicalization of deviance have also contributed to the growth of health expenditures. Because health is both more coveted and more inclusively defined, and because a greater amount of medical therapeutic activity is applied to deviance-defined-as-illness, increasing economic resources are being invested in the health-illness-medicine sector of the society.

The political and legal prominence of questions of health care and medicine in American society at the present time reflects in part a widespread national discontent with the way medical care is organized, financed, and delivered, and with some of the attitudes and behaviors of physicians. The inequities that exist in access to care, and in its technical and interpersonal excellence, are among the primary foci of political and legal activities. Another major area of current political and legal action concerns the internal and external regulation of the medical profession better to insure that it uses its knowledge and skill in a socially as well as medically responsible way, and that it is adequately accountable both to patients and to the public at large. Various new measures, which represent a mixture of controls from within the medical profession and from outside it, have been set into motion. For example, in 1972, the Professional Standards Review Organization was established through the passage of amendments to the Social Security Act which were designed to provide quality assessment and assurance, utilization review, and cost control, primarily for Medicare and Medicaid patients. Over the course of the years 1966 through 1971, a series of government regulations were passed which mandate peer review for all biomedical research involving human subjects, supported by the Department of Health, Education, and Welfare (and its subunits, the National Institutes of Health and the Public Health Service), as well as by the Food and Drug Administration. In 1975, the American College of Surgeons and the American Surgical Association set forth a plan for systematically decreasing the number of newly graduated doctors entering surgical training. In part, this plan represented an organized, intraprofessional attempt to deal with what appears to be an oversupply of surgeons in the United States, and thereby to reduce the possibility that federal health manpower legislation would have to be passed to remedy this maldistribution.

The fact that an extraordinary number of young people are opting for careers in health, particularly as physicians, is the final concomitant of medicalization previously mentioned. Reliable and valid data are not available to explain the mounting wave of young persons who have been attracted to medicine since the nineteen-sixties. We do not know as much as we should about how they resemble their predecessors, or differ from them. We are aware that more women, blacks, and members of other minority groups are being admitted to medical school than in the past, partly because of "affirmative action" legislation. But we do not have overall information about the characteristics of those who are accepted as compared with those who are not. Only sketchy materials are available on the impact of those changes in medical-school curricula during the past decade that were designed to make students more aware of the social and ethical dimensions of their commitment to medicine. We do not know whether their attitudes, their professional decisions, or their medical practice actually changed. More data are needed before we can interpret the short- and long-term implications of the rush of college youth toward medicine. As pre-medical and medical students themselves are first to testify, the prestige, authority, "power," autonomy, and financial rewards of medicine attract them and their peers to medicine, along with scientific interests, clinical impulses, and humanitarian concerns. But there is also evidence to suggest that even among those who readily contend that their reasons for choosing medicine are self-interested, a "new" medical-student orientation has been emerging. In fact, the very candor that medical students exhibit—and in some cases flaunt—when they insist that, regrettably, like their predecessors, their competitiveness, desire for achievement, and need for security have drawn them into medicine is part of this new orientation. Activist and meditative, as well as critical and self-critical, the "new medical student" not only wants to bring about change in the medical profession, but to do so in a way that affects other aspects of the society as well. The structural and symbolic meaning acquired by health, illness, and medicine has led such students to hope that their influence will be far-reaching as well as meliorative. How many students with this ostensibly "new" orientation will maintain it throughout their medical training and whether their entrance into the profession will significantly alter the future course of medicalization in American society remain to be seen.[12]

Along with progressive medicalization, a process of demedicalization seems also to be taking place in the society. To some extent the signs of demedicalization are reactions to what is felt by various individuals and groups to be a state of "over-medicalization." One of the most significant manifestations of this counter-trend is the mounting concern over implications that have arisen from the continuously expanding conception of "sickness" in the society. Commentators on this process would not necessarily agree with Peter Sedgwick that it will continue to "the point where everybody has become so luxuriantly ill" that perhaps sickness will no longer be "in" and a "backlash" will be set in motion;[13] they may not envision such an engulfing state of societally defined illness. But many observers from diverse professional backgrounds have published works in which they express concern about the "coercive" aspects of the "label" illness and the treatment of illness by medical professionals in medical institutions.[14] The admonitory perspectives on the enlarged domain of illness and medicine that these works of social science and social criticism represent appear to have gained the attention of young physicians- and nurses-in-training interested in change, and various consumer and civil-rights groups interested in health care.

This emerging view emphasizes the degree to which what is defined as health and illness, normality and abnormality, sanity and insanity varies from one society, culture, and historical period to another. Thus, it is contended, medical diagnostic categories such as "sick," "abnormal," and "insane" are not universal, objective, or necessarily reliable. Rather, they are culture-, class-, and time-bound, often ethnocentric, and as much artifacts of the preconceptions of socially biased observers as they are valid summaries of the characteristics of the observed. In this view, illness (especially mental illness) is largely a mythical construct, created and enforced by the society. The hospitals to which seriously ill persons are confined are portrayed as "total institutions": segregated, encompassing, depersonalizing organizations, "dominated" by physicians who are disinclined to convey information to patients about their conditions, or to encourage paramedical personnel to do so. These "oppressive" and "counter-therapeutic" attributes of the hospital environment are seen as emanating from the professional ideology of physicians and the kind of hierarchical relationships that they establish with patients and other medical professionals partly as a consequence of this ideology, as well as from the bureaucratic and technological features of the hospital itself. Whatever their source, the argument continues, the characteristics of the hospital and of the doctor-patient relationship increase the "powerlessness" of the sick person, "maintain his uncertainty," and systematically "mortify" and "curtail" the "self" with which he enters the sick role and arrives at the hospital door.

This critical perspective links the labeling of illness, the "imperialist" outlook and capitalist behavior of physicians, the "stigmatizing" and "dehumanizing" experiences of patients, and the problems of the health-care system more generally to imperfections and injustices in the society as a whole. Thus, for example, the various forms of social inequality, prejudice, discrimination, and acquisitive self-interest that persist in capitalistic American society are held responsible for causing illness, as well as for contributing to the undesirable attitudes and actions of physicians and other medical professionals. Casting persons in the sick role is regarded as a powerful, latent way for the society to exact conformity and maintain the status quo. For it allows a semi-approved form of deviance to occur which siphons off potential for insurgent protest and which can be controlled through the supervision or, in some cases, the "enforced therapy" of the medical profession. Thus, however permissive and merciful it may be to expand the category of illness, these observers point out, there is always the danger that the society will become a "therapeutic state" that excessively restricts the "right to be different" and the right to dissent. They feel that this danger may already have reached serious proportions in this society through its progressive medicalization.

The criticism of medicalization and the advocacy of demedicalization have not been confined to rhetoric. Concrete steps have been taken to declassify certain conditions as illness. Most notable among these is the American Psychiatric Association's decision to remove homosexuality from its official catalogue ("Nomenclature") of mental disorders. In addition, serious efforts have been made to heighten physicians' awareness of the fact that because they share certain prejudiced, often unconscious assumptions about women, they tend to over-attribute psychological conditions to their female patients. Thus, for example, distinguished medical publications such as the *New England Journal of Medicine* have featured articles and editorials on the excessive readiness with which medical specialists and textbook authors accept the undocumented belief that dysmenorrhea, nausea of pregnancy, pain in labor, and infantile colic are all psychogenic disorders, caused or aggravated by women's emotional problems. Another related development is feminist protest against what is felt to be a too great tendency to define pregnancy as an illness, and childbirth as a "technologized" medical-surgical event, prevailed over by the obstetrician-gynecologist. These sentiments have contributed to the preference that many middle-class couples have shown for natural childbirth in recent years, and to the revival of midwifery. The last example also illustrates an allied movement, namely a growing tendency to shift some responsibility for medical care and authority over it from the physician, the medical team, and hospital to the patient, the family, and the home.

A number of attempts to "destratify" the doctor's relationships with patients and with other medical professionals and to make them more open and egalitarian have developed. "Patients' rights" are being asserted and codified, and, in some states, drafted into law. Greater emphasis is being placed, for example, on the patient's "right to treatment," right to information (relevant to diagnosis, therapy, prognosis, or to the giving of knowledgeable consent for any procedure), right to privacy and confidentiality, and right to be "allowed to die," rather than being "kept alive by artificial means or heroic measures . . . if the situation should arise in which there is no reasonable expectation of . . . recovery from physical or mental disability."[15]

In some medical milieux (for example, community health centers and health maintenance organizations), and in critical and self-consciously progressive writings about medicine, the term "client" or "consumer" is being substituted for "patient." This change in terminology is intended to underline the importance of preventing illness while stressing the desirability of a non-supine, non-subordinate relationship for those who seek care to those who provide it. The emergence of nurse-practitioners and physician's assistants on the American scene is perhaps the most significant sign that some blurring of the physician's supremacy vis-à-vis other medical professionals may also be taking place. For some of the responsibilities for diagnosis, treatment, and patient management that were formerly prerogatives of physicians have been incorporated into these new, essentially marginal roles.[16]

Enjoinders to patients to care for themselves rather than to rely so heavily on the services of medical professionals and institutions are more frequently heard. Much attention is being given to studies such as the one conducted by Lester Breslow and his colleagues at the University of California at Los Angeles which suggest that good health and longevity are as much related to a self-enforced regimen of sufficient sleep, regular, well-balanced meals, moderate exercise and weight, no smoking, and little or no drinking, as they are to professionally administered medical care. Groups such as those involved in the Women's Liberation Movement are advocating the social and psychic as well as the medical value of knowing, examining, and caring for one's own body. Self-therapy techniques and programs have been developed for conditions as complicated and grave as terminal renal disease and hemophilia A and B. Proponents of such regimens affirm that many aspects of managing even serious chronic illnesses can be handled safely at home by the patient and his family, who will, in turn, benefit both financially and emotionally. In addition, they claim that in many cases the biomedical results obtained seem superior to those of the traditional physician-administered, health-care-delivery system.

The underlying assumption in these instances is that, if self-care is collectivized and reinforced by mutual aid, not only will persons with a medical problem be freed from some of the exigencies of the sick role, but both personal and public health will thereby improve, all with considerable savings in cost. This point of view is based on the moral supposition that greater autonomy from the medical profession coupled with greater responsibility for self and others in the realm of health and illness is an ethically and societally superior state.

We have the medicine we deserve. We freely choose to live the way we do. We choose to live recklessly, to abuse our bodies with what we consume, to expose ourselves to environmental insults, to rush frantically from place to place, and to sit on our spreading bottoms and watch paid professionals exercise for us. . . . Today few patients have the confidence to care for themselves. The inexorable professionalization of medicine, together with reverence for the scientific method, have invested practitioners with sacrosanct powers, and correspondingly vitiated the responsibility of the rest of us for health. . . . What is tragic is not what has happened to the revered professions, but what has happened to us as a result of professional dominance. In times of inordinate complexity and stress we have been made a profoundly dependent people. Most of us have lost the ability to care for ourselves. . . . I have tried to demonstrate three propositions. First, medical care has less impact on health than is generally assumed. Second, medical care has less impact on health than have social and environmental factors. And third, given the way in which society is evolving and the evolutionary imperatives of the medical care system, medical care in the future will have even less impact on health than it has now. . . . We have not understood what health is. . . . But in the next few decades our understanding will deepen. The pursuit of health and of well-being will then be possible, but only if our environment is made safe for us to live in and our social order is transformed to foster health, rather than suppress joy. If not, we shall remain a sick and dependent people. . . . The end of medicine is not the end of health but the beginning. . . .[17]

The foregoing passage (excerpted from Rick Carlson's book, *The End of Medicine*) touches upon many of the demedicalization themes that have been discussed. It proclaims the desirability of demedicalizing American society, predicting that, if we do so, we can overcome the "harm" that excessive medicalization has brought in its wake and progress beyond the "limits" that it has set. Like most critics of medicalization on the American scene, Carlson inveighs against the way that medical care is currently organized and implemented, but he attaches exceptional importance to the health-illness-medical sector of the society. In common with other commentators, he views health, illness, and medicine as inextricably associated with values and beliefs of American tradition that are both critical and desirable. It is primarily for this reason that in spite of the numerous signs that certain *structural* changes in the delivery of care will have occurred by the time we reach the year 2000, American society is not likely to undergo a significant process of *cultural* demedicalization.

Dissatisfaction with the distribution of professional medical care in the United States, its costs, and its accessibility has become sufficiently acute and generalized to make the enactment of a national health-insurance system in the foreseeable future likely. Exactly what form that system should take still evokes heated debate about free enterprise and socialism, public and private regulation, national and local government, tax rates, deductibles and co-insurance, the right to health care, the equality principle, and the principle of distributive justice. But the institutionalization of a national system that will provide more extensive and equitable health-insurance protection now seems necessary as well as inevitable even to those who do not approve of it.

There is still another change in the health-illness-medicine area of the society that seems to be forthcoming and that, like national health insurance, would alter the structure within which care is delivered. This is the movement toward effecting greater equality, collegiality, and accountability in the relationship of physicians to patients and their families, to other medical professionals, and to the lay public. Attempts to reduce the hierarchical dimension in the physician's role, as well as the increased insistence on patient's rights, self-therapy, mutual medical aid, community medical services and care by non-physician health professionals, and the growth of legislative and judicial participation in health and medicine by both federal and local government are all part of this movement. There is reason to believe that, as a consequence of pressure from both outside and inside the medical profession, the doctor will become less "dominant" and "autonomous," and will be subject to more controls.

This evolution in the direction of greater egalitarianism and regulation notwithstanding, it seems unlikely that all elements of hierarchy and autonomy will, or even can, be eliminated from the physician's role. For that to occur, the medical knowledge, skill, experience, and responsibility of patients and paramedical professionals would have to equal, if not replicate, the physician's. In addition, the social and psychic meaning of health and illness would have to become trivial in order to remove all vestiges of institutionalized charisma from the physician's role. Health, illness, and medicine have never been viewed casually in any society and, as indicated, they seem to be gaining rather than losing importance in American society.

It is significant that often the discussions and developments relevant to the destratification and control of the physician's role and to the enactment of national health insurance are accompanied by reaffirmations of traditional American values: equality, independence, self-reliance, universalism, distributive justice, solidarity, reciprocity, and individual and community responsibility. What seems to be involved here is not so much a change in values as the initiation of action intended to modify certain structural features of American medicine, so that it will more fully realize long-standing societal values.

In contrast, the new emphasis on health as a right, along with the emerging perspective on illness as medically and socially engendered, seems to entail major conceptual rather than structural shifts in the health-illness-medical matrix of the society. These shifts are indicative of a less fatalistic and individualistic attitude toward illness, increased personal and communal espousal of health, and a spreading conviction that health is as much a consequence of the good life and the good society as it is of professional medical care. The strongest impetus for demedicalization comes from this altered point of view. It will probably contribute to the decategorization of certain conditions as illness, greater appreciation and utilization of non-physician medical professionals, the institutionalization of more preventive medicine and personal and public health measures, and, perhaps, to the undertaking of non-medical reforms (such as full employment, improved transportation, or adequate recreation) in the name of the ultimate goal of health.

However, none of these trends implies that what we have called *cultural* demedicalization will take place. The shifts in emphasis from illness to health, from therapeutic to preventive medicine, and from the dominance and autonomy of the doctor to patient's rights and greater control of the medical profession do not alter the fact that health, illness, and medicine are central preoccupations in the society which have diffuse symbolic as well as practical meaning. All signs suggest that they will maintain the social, ethical, and existential significance they have acquired, even though by the year 2000 some structural aspects of the way that medicine and care are organized and delivered may have changed. In fact, if the issues now being considered under the rubric of bioethics are predictive of what lies ahead, we can expect that in the future, health, illness, and medicine will acquire even greater importance as one of the primary symbolic media through which American society will grapple with fundamental questions of value and belief. What social mechanisms we will develop to come to terms with these "collective conscience" issues, and exactly what role physicians, health professionals, biologists, jurists, politicians, philosophers, theologians, social scientists, and the public at large will play in their resolution remains to be seen. But it is a distinctive characteristic of an advanced modern society like our own that scientific, technical, clinical, social, ethical, and religious concerns should be joined in this way.

REFERENCES

[1]Ivan Illich, *Medical Nemesis: The Expropriation of Health* (London, 1975), pp. 165-69.

[2]Illich, *Medical Nemesis, passim.*

[3]Leon R. Kass, "Regarding the End of Medicine and the Pursuit of Health," *The Public Interest*, 40 (Summer, 1975), p. 11.

[4]In his novel *Erewhon*, written in 1872, Samuel Butler satirized this evolution, and the degree to which what is defined as illness is contingent on social factors. In Erewhon (the fictitious country that Butler created by imagining late nineteenth- and early twentieth-century England stood on its head), persons afflicted with what physicians would call tuberculosis are found guilty in a court of law and sentenced to life imprisonment, whereas persons who forge checks, set houses on fire, steal, and commit acts of violence are diagnosed as suffering from a "severe fit of immorality" and are cared for at public expense in hospitals.

[5]Nicholas N. Kittrie, *The Right To Be Different: Deviance and Enforced Therapy* (Baltimore, 1971). See especially chapter 1, "The Divestment of Criminal Justice and the Coming of the Therapeutic State," pp. 1-49.

[6]Peter Sedgwick, "Illness—Mental and Otherwise," *The Hastings Center Studies*, 1:3 (1973), p. 37.

[7]Irving Kenneth Zola, "Culture and Symptoms—An Analysis of Patients' Presenting Complaints," *American Sociological Review*, 31:5 (October, 1966), pp. 615-16.

[8]These figures were cited in the June 9, 1976, issue of *Newsweek*, p. 59.

[9]These ideas are presented in more detail in the monograph I am currently writing on "Medical Sociology" which will appear as a volume in the Prentice-Hall *Foundations of Modern Sociology* series.

[10]See article by John H. Knowles, "The Responsibility of the Individual," in this issue.

[11]Talcott Parsons's formulation of the sick role is the most important single concept in the field of the sociology of medicine. For his own elaboration of this concept, see, especially, Talcott Parsons, *The Social System* (Glencoe, Illinois), pp. 428-79, and "The Sick Role and the Role of the Physician Reconsidered," *Milbank Memorial Fund Quarterly, Health and Society* (Summer, 1975), pp. 257-77.

[12]See Renée C. Fox, "The Process of Professional Socialization: Is There a 'New' Medical Student? A Comparative View of Medical Socialization in the 1950's and the 1970's," in Laurence R. Tancredi, ed., *Ethics in Health Care* (Washington, D.C., 1974), pp. 197-227.

[13]Sedgwick, "Illness—Mental and Otherwise," p. 37.

[14]In addition to Illich, *Medical Nemesis*, and Kittrie, *The Right To Be Different*, see, for example, Rick J. Carlson, *The End of Medicine* (New York, 1975); Michael Foucault, *Madness and Civilization* (New York, 1967); Eliot Freidson, *Professional Dominance* (Chicago, 1970); Erving Goffman, *Asylums* (New York, 1961); R. D. Laing, *The Politics of Experience* (New York, 1967); Thomas J. Scheff, *Being Mentally Ill* (Chicago, 1966); Thomas S. Szasz, *The Myth of Mental Illness* (New York, 1961); and Howard D. Waitzkin and Barbara Waterman, *The Exploitation of Illness in Capitalist Society* (Indianapolis, 1974).

[15]This particular way of requesting that one be allowed to die is excerpted from the "Living Will" (revised April, 1974, version), prepared and promoted by the Euthanasia Educational Council.

[16]See the article by David Rogers, "The Challenge of Primary Care," in this issue.

[17]Carlson, *The End of Medicine*, pp. 44, 141, and 203-31.

DANIEL CALLAHAN

Health and Society: Some Ethical Imperatives

WHETHER INDUCED BY INTERNAL OR BY EXTERNAL CIRCUMSTANCES, every major social change in a society forces a confrontation with its values. Nowhere is this more evident than in the changes that have been wrought in medicine. In earlier societies, people were necessarily fatalistic about illness; there was little the physician could offer beyond psychological comfort and minor palliation. Modern medicine, by contrast, commands a powerful arsenal of weapons to forestall death, relieve pain, cure malignancies, and rehabilitate the crippled. But this power, impressive as it is, is nevertheless still less than absolute, and thus it poses particularly difficult questions of a kind which previous generations had no need to consider.

If death can be forestalled, for how long and in what circumstances should it be? At what point does rehabilitation of the crippled cease to be of real benefit to them? At what point does it cease to be of benefit to society? If one malignancy can be cured only to set the stage for death by another, just what, if anything, is gained? Medicine has not conquered death, nor is it likely to. But within that limit its power continues to increase, and it is precisely this increase that compels a reexamination of our basic ethical attitudes and premises toward it.

Consider only some of modern medicine's more obvious powers. Effective contraceptives and safe, legal abortions allow a choice in the number of children a couple will bear, while population pressures force another and perhaps different choice. Advances in amniocentesis and prenatal diagnosis are gradually permitting the avoidance of the birth of children with certain defects. The possibility of controlling both the quantity of children and their genetic quality has obvious and enormous ramifications for traditional sex roles, family life, composition of the work force, and patterns of child-rearing.

If one moves from procreation and birth to the other end of the spectrum, developments have no less important implications. An ability artificially to sustain life by machines compels newer and more precise definitions of "death" (and, for that matter, "life"). A capacity to transplant organs, to cure the diseases of some systems, to keep people alive (but not necessarily happy) demands that one ask what kind of a life is worth living and what kind of death is worth pursuing. That is to ask, in the end, about "death with dignity," about euthanasia, about suicide, about ceasing "useless" medical treatment.

Between the extremes of birth and death, medicine is learning how to manipulate and, in some cases, control human behavior. Psychosurgery, the techniques of depth psychiatry and behavior modification, and psychotropic drugs all offer the promise, and in many cases the reality, of medical intervention in human emotion and cognition. But what could this kind of intervention do to traditional Western notions of autonomy and self-determination? Take aggression in society: Should medicine be made to find alternatives to bankrupt penal systems? Should it become involved in the legal system, for example, by defining "normality" and "deviancy"? In short, what should the role of medical technology be in serving society's broad political and social needs?

As the frontiers of medical research expand, as new things are learned and new treatments are developed, more and more experimentation on human beings becomes necessary. In the move from biomedical theory to clinical practice and application, human beings must necessarily be the final testing ground. Research can be advanced and lives—often large numbers of them—saved by experimentation. But those often anonymous individuals experimented upon can also be harmed, sometimes killed. If research is hampered by a lack of experimental subjects, whether through their own unwillingness or through bureaucratic obstacles, many thousands may be victimized by the failure to utilize promising treatments. On the other hand, if the individual research subject is casually thought to be expendable for the good of future generations, then harm can be done to hard-won values of human dignity and inviolability.

In its power, then, to change the conditions of birth and death, to alter ways of life and behavior, to impose new dilemmas about the relationship between individual and social good, medical research and clinical practice force a new confrontation with some of the oldest of human questions. What do we account as "happiness," and what should medicine's role be in bringing it about? What is a "good life," and how much health is necessary for it? What is a "good death," and what are the possibilities and limitations of medicine in contributing to that? How much sacrifice of individual health can society demand in the name of general health? How far must society go in making use of medical means to satisfy individual and sometimes idiosyncratic desires?

Questions of that kind are ultimately philosophical and ethical. For that very reason, many would say they are inherently speculative and unanswerable. In some final sense, that may well be true. But in the meantime—as history attests when such questions are posed—the way in which societies incline their tentative answers, the provisional ways in which hard dilemmas are resolved in one direction rather than another, the ways in which biases, predilections, and general attitudes develop, all make a very concrete difference in the emergence of mores, policies, laws, and regulations. No one has ever "solved" the problems of abortion, of death, of freedom, of the meaning of health, or of the ideal relationship between the individual and society. Nevertheless, how a society thinks about those old questions, the way it frames the issues, the means by which it acts on its rough-hewn answers can, and usually does, make all the difference in the lives of people.

In a society as diverse as ours it is proving extraordinarily painful to cope in some rational way with ethical issues, although the price of avoiding these questions, of letting them go by default, will no doubt be even more painful in the long run. Developments occur, things are done—but without reflection, without thought for the consequences, without a clear sense of the goals being sought. So long as this continues we, or our children, will spend as much of our time and energy cleaning up our past mistakes as we will in trying to take fruitful steps into the future.

The development of new values as they become necessary to manage modern medicine, the modification of old moral standards, and perhaps the outright jettison-ing of still other traditional norms are the ineluctable consequences of advances in medical research, clinical application, and mass delivery of health care. The creation of a process by which the old and new values can be examined and tentative directions chosen must be in harmony at once with our culture, our politics, and our individual rights. A new "right to health care" has been affirmed, but what it means and just what solutions are possible when there is a scarcity of resources are yet to be determined. Medical technology offers a more efficient and productive medicine. But are productivity and efficiency the only goals of medicine? Are there not, in any case, other areas where the need for better technologies is no less imperative—housing, agriculture, transportation? Some basic moral choices will have to be made; all of them will not be possible. Power and limitation of power, uses and abuses, promises and dangers: that has been the story of modern technology, and a story not yet fully unfolded.

A logical place to begin an examination of the moral choices at stake is with the concept of "health" itself. From there it will be possible to move to the special problems posed by technology, not only in medicine but in the culture more generally. Finally, a direct examination of the increasingly vexing questions of rights and obligations and of decision-making processes can be confronted.

The Concept of "Health"

Like most other very general concepts—"peace," "truth," "justice," "freedom"—that of "health" poses enormous difficulties of definition. We all know experimentally and intuitively what it means to be sick: we hurt, and, to a greater or lesser extent, we cannot function well. That the pain or misery we feel can lead in many cases to death—either socially, by disability or impairment, or literally—only increases the burden; a reminder that we are mortal. Yet even when we attempt to grasp the notion of "health" by looking at what are normally taken to be its opposites—illness, pain, death—complications immediately arise. People can adapt to illness, learn to put up with their "dis-ease," and to cope with the fact that their body is performing in something less than an optimal way. Moreover, as the sociologists of medicine have taught us, people respond to and interpret illness in very different ways; what is considered sick in one culture or group may be considered health in another. Nevertheless, most people in most places have a rough idea of what they mean by "ill"; a recognizable area of human experience is evoked by the term, even if the borderlines can be exceedingly fuzzy.

To move from a definition of "sickness" to one for "health" is, however, not so easy. The term connotes bodily integrity, the absence of pain and infirmity, the state of a well-functioning and thus unremarkable organism. In a curious way, like "goodness," it can seem bland, if only because the alternative states of human affairs are so marked by drama and suffering. However bland the concept, the reality it invokes is regarded as eminently desirable. When one is in "good health" it is not even noticed; when one is not, it is desperately desired.

Whatever the conceptual problems posed by a philosophical attempt to define "health," and they are very real, the attempt to define the term for ethical or policy purposes brings forth even greater ones. Oddly enough, for all the debates about "health," few attempts have ever been made to give the term some substance; it seems to be taken for granted that everyone knows what is being talked about. The most notable, and undoubtedly still the most influential, definition of health was that of the World Health Organization (WHO) in the late forties: ". . . a state of complete physical, mental, and social well-being and not merely the absence of disease or infirmity." The historical origin of that definition was the conviction of the organizers of the WHO that the security of future world peace would lie in the improvement of health, both physical and mental. That no reputable historian of the origins of the Second World War would trace it to bad health is probably beside the point. The great strides made by medicine during the war no doubt encouraged the development of this strain of utopian thinking, and it continues up to the present time.

It is a dangerous definition, and it desperately needs replacement by something more modest. Its emphasis on "complete physical, mental, and social well-being" puts both medicine and society in the untenable position of being required to attain unattainable goals. There is no reason whatever to think that medicine can, for instance, make more than a modest contribution to "complete . . . social well-being," which involves (among others) political, cultural, and economic factors. Health may be, most of the time, a necessary condition for well-being, but it is not a sufficient condition. By even suggesting that medicine can succeed in such a goal—which is tantamount to making medicine the keystone in the search for human happiness— there is posited for it an impossible and illusory task.

The consequences of this definition, or at least of the ambitious spirit which it represents, can be seen all around us. Health so defined can encompass every human state. This bottomless conceptual pit makes it impossible in any practical way to specify the limits of the health enterprise, that is, to distinguish what is a political, or ethical, or cultural problem from what is a "health" problem. It has even permeated our everyday speech: how many of us designate any political or cultural movement or any person we do not like as "sick"? The ground is thus laid for a limitless economic burden on society. If anything and everything from the state of the prisons, the schools, and the economy to the anxieties invoked by life can be called a "health problem," there is no end to the resources that can be expended in the name of medicine to cope with those unpleasantries.

The difficulty legislators have had in trying to determine who, under what circumstances, and with what "medical" conditions should qualify for governmental assistance is direct testimony to the depth of the confusion. Far from clarifying our notions of human health, and thus our systems of care and distribution, the WHO definition has only made matters worse. Our society cannot continue to work with a concept of "health" that is infinite in its scope, and, at the same time, try to carry on a sensible discussion of the "right to health" or the "right to health care." A narrow, limited concept of "health" would make it possible to have a rational discussion of "rights"; a vague and woolly one does not.

Needs, Desires, and Technology

Nothing accounts for the strides and successes of modern medicine so much as the combination of basic biomedical research with ingenious technological application. And nothing accounts for the rising cost of medical care and the exasperation many feel at the gap between the cost of that care and the meager gain in general health so much as that same combination. Perhaps it is beside the point that costs keep rising:

medicine is big business, providing profits, jobs, and social diversion; its practice can thus become an end in itself, quite apart from whether it results in significantly improved health. This has happened with other technologies, and there is no reason to think that medicine should prove the exception. That possibility aside, the place of technology in medicine—and the place of technology more generally in contemporary life—provides the most significant obstacle to the development of a reasonable and limited concept of "health."

How much health do people need? How much and what kind of sickness should be combatted? These are exceedingly difficult questions to answer, in great part, as I noted above, because of the enormous variation among individuals and groups in their tolerance for, and interpretation of, illness. Nonetheless, attempts have been made to find some reasonably objective standards for defining "illness," because without a working definition, there is no way to determine the nation's health needs. These efforts have, on the whole, taken the form of trying to establish a cost in dollars for various illnesses, both in terms of lost wages and in terms of the cost to the economy from illness and disease. Complementary to these calculations are those that employ cost-benefit techniques to determine the net economic gain resulting from investment in research and delivery systems sufficient significantly to reduce the incidence and impact of various diseases. Parallel attempts are made on social grounds: these ordinarily point to the disparities in the incidence of various diseases and disabilities among different groups and classes of people that indicate, not surprisingly, that the downtrodden (whether because of race, age, poverty, or geographic location) bear a disproportionate and thus inequitable burden of poor health.

The advantage of attempts to determine national health needs is that they allow in principle a considerable degree of quantification; reasonably accurate comparisons can be made between alternative health-policy strategies. In practice, however, the objectivity of their figures are frequently more illusory than real. Statistics can only be developed by making a number of arbitrary assumptions, some quantitative, others entailing value judgments. While it may be possible, for instance, to calculate in a rough way the economic cost to society of arthritis, it is by no means as easy to calculate the psychological cost to the afflicted individuals or their families. While unhappiness (even if those afflicted are economically "productive") ought surely to have a place in any full equation, it does not readily lend itself to calculation. In making comparisons between the full costs of different diseases (economic and psychological), is it possible, say, to find any very reasonable way to compare arthritis and hemophilia? Because of the far greater incidence of the former, one might say that the total sum of suffering is greater, but the impact of the latter (not to mention the cost) is probably far greater in terms of individual suffering.

In short, the more involved one becomes in making calculations and comparisons, the more problematic the venture. It is very well to argue that money invested in preventive medicine would, in the long run, produce more health per dollar than any other investment; that may or may not be true. But even if it is true, it could only be acted upon by systematically ignoring the presently ill. They would have to be deprived of help as allocations were shifted away from them to those who would benefit in times to come. The argument can only rest on the highly problematic premise that the value of averting future suffering is greater than the value of relieving present pain.

I am not trying to argue here that techniques for determining health needs should

be abandoned. They at least reveal some interesting and suggestive figures, specula-
tions, and projections providing those responsible for making policy decisions with
something to work on, and something in this case is better than nothing. But they do
evade the most difficult problem: that of determining the positive moral weight to be
given to the pursuit of health in a society and the negative moral weight to be given to
illness and disease. Just what is good about "health" anyway, and just what is evil
about illness, disease, and death? These are nasty questions to ask, because if put too
bluntly they imply a callousness to a major source of human misery and an
indifference to the destructive effect of illness. But if they are not asked, it will be
impossible to reach some decision regarding the limits to be placed on the quest for
health and the priority to be given to societal health needs within those limits.

Two social realities are, at present, bedeviling that necessary task. The first is the
almost total breakdown of the ethical distinction between "need" and "desire" in our
culture. The second, closely related to the first, is the continuing utopian lure of
technology, a lure whose net effect is to thwart any attempt to place limits on medical
aspiration.

I would define "need" as the minimal requirements for a satisfactory life, and
"desire" as those things human beings want and demand as requirements for what
they would consider an optimal life. Working with that kind of distinction, it ought to
be possible for societies to find ways of providing for minimal needs. Once that is
accomplished, if there is a surplus, they can then set about improving the "quality of
life," that is, trying to provide people with some of the things they would like to have
beyond their requirements for survival. But this simple model breaks down immediately in Western technological societies. First, through habit and the requirements of
the economic order, what people think they "need" for a minimally satisfactory life is
set at an extremely high level. What a poor society might consider optimal (plentiful
meat, spacious dwellings, refrigerators, and television sets, for instance), Western
technological societies consider imperative. That many people, both in and out of
government, could seriously contemplate going to war as a means of combating a fuel
crisis which somewhat lowered our standard of living (but posed no possible threat to
survival) is as good an indicator as any of the terms in which "need" is defined, at least
in the United States.

Second, technological societies are committed to economic growth. Despite
occasional discussions of a "steady-state society," most people still believe that a
society which does not continue to grow economically is doomed. The key to
continuous growth is the stimulation of production through increasing consumption;
and the key to increasing consumption is the stimulation of desire. People must be
induced to want more and more. Hence, to bring matters full circle, "needs" and
"desires" become one—the satisfactory life and the optimal life turn out to be one and
the same life; the satisfactory life is defined as one in which the optimal life can be,
and must be, provided. Unless the individual pursues what he desires, and not just
what he needs, the economy cannot continue to give him even what he needs. Desire
becomes king.

The import of this process for medicine may not be so immediately apparent as it
is, say, in the case of the environment. Whatever the weaknesses of the environmental
movement, it has probably succeeded at least in convincing people that there must be
a limit to our utilizing and exploiting natural resources. The globe is a finite resource;
therefore we cannot have everything we desire.

No comparable wisdom is yet apparent in medicine. On the contrary, technological optimism is as vital as ever. It rests on two assumptions: One is that, technologically, something can be done about any medical condition. The "something" may not be much in many cases—perhaps only painkillers, when medicine can do nothing further—but that in itself is taken to be sufficient evidence that even in the most difficult cases medicine is not totally devoid of technological resources. The other is that all physical and mental ills are potentially subject to cure, control, or amelioration. This is a guiding heuristic proposition of biomedical research, fueled by the remarkable, almost unimaginable progress medicine has in fact made in recent decades and, negatively, by the fact that there is no conceivable way to disprove it. Since there is no way of disproving that proposition, a systematic optimum can remain enthroned. There is "hope against hope," if not for this generation then for the next, or the next after that, *ad infinitum*. (The equivalent argument applied to the environment is to say, yes, the resources of the earth are limited, but the ingenuity of technology in finding substitutes and in learning how to recycle resources counteracts the limitation, and is therefore tantamount to having unlimited resources.)

Against that systematic biomedical optimism (which has been no small element in the sharp increases in the funds demanded for biomedical research in recent decades), a curbing of aspiration and desire is now in order. Two strategies, not mutually incompatible, might be tried to achieve it. The first is to allow every person, whether patient, physician, researcher, or special-interest group, to press his case as far as he can. It can be stated in terms either of need or desire (it hardly matters which). The case made, a resolution is then achieved through the political process: the public through its representatives decides to which plea(s) it will respond and to what extent. The allocation of medical resources is left to public decision; public opinion will fight out the conflicting moral and value judgments. To do so, it is not necessary for the public to have uniform theoretical ideas about the nature of health, the limits to health, or the relationship of health to other human goods (education, housing, national defense, etc.). On the contrary, desire can continue to dictate, knowing no theoretical limits at all. Conflicts will be resolved by brokerage politics, pragmatic judgments, and the trading off of relative values.

The trouble is that there is no real reason, other than lack of political power, for people to curb their desires about what they would like medicine to deliver to fulfill their notions of the optimal life. It is a system bound, therefore, to breed injustice, since some groups will have more power than others, if only by virtue of the larger pool of sick people they represent; and the individual will ineluctably ask of medicine more ("complete social well-being") than it can reasonably be expected to provide.

The other strategy (which still lacks a program) centers its attention more directly on philosophical and ethical questions. It would ask just what human beings *should* seek in the name of health and what they should avoid in the name of forestalling sickness and death. It would try to distinguish between what people need (while also trying to establish a reasonable notion of what "need" is) and what they desire. It would emphasize not just the contributions medicine could make with ample research funds, but also the limits to medicine's role in securing human happiness and security. It would encourage answering some fundamental questions about the goals of medicine, assuming that what people desire from medicine is not necessarily what they need. Medicine would be in less trouble today had it long ago promoted such an inquiry. But neither the profession nor the public (for it shares the blame) was willing to face these questions, for they are questions that threaten individualism, easy ethical relativism, and that systematic optimism which has been the stock-in-trade of medical research and technology. And that is so even if the answers might end up supporting the present system.

Rights, Obligations, and Decisions

Two slogans, the "right to health" and the "right to health care," encapsulate the thinking that has recently dominated medicine in this country. The two have arisen in a society that is under great pressure to extend the scope and application of its individual rights, particularly welfare rights, and in the face of rising costs in medical care combined with the fact that an absence of care can now more often make the difference between life and death. A plausible case can be made for asserting that until a half-century or so ago the nation laid the greatest emphasis on the obligations of the individual toward society, while now the emphasis is increasingly upon the obligations of society toward the individual. It is a shift that most find attractive, and nowhere is it more strikingly apparent than in the debate over the methods of medical-care payment. Few public voices would dare support a laissez-faire approach to the cost of medical treatment any longer. Health, it is at least ostensibly agreed, cannot be treated as one more commodity to be sold only to those who have the money to pay the bill.

The slogans about "rights" provide the ideological and political ground on which to lay the foundation for some other solution to the distribution of medical care. But the language of "rights" is notoriously slippery, not only because opinions differ regarding their nature and basis but also because rights that are claimed are not all compatible or consistent with one another. What does it mean to have a "right to health"? It might mean that everyone has a right not to be sick. But that is to enter a claim against the weaknesses of the flesh and against all of those natural processes that lead to disease and bodily decay. That kind of claim could only be entered against God Himself, or nature, or the evolutionary process. Clearly, the claim can be entered; just as clearly, it will not be honored.

The right might mean that society has an obligation to guarantee the health of its members. But even the most superb present and foreseeable medicine cannot guarantee that a person will always be healthy. Then, one might say that, if no society can guarantee the health of its members, the right implies at least an obligation to make the attempt. Even that more modest formulation raises problems: Just why, for instance, is any one person responsible for the health of another, particularly if the one bears no responsibility whatever for the lack of health of the other? More generally, on what basis can it be said that citizens have a mutual obligation for one another's health? Perhaps it can reasonably enough be said that citizens have an obligation not to jeopardize the health of others, but it is an enormous step from there to claiming that the good health of all is the responsibility of all. No plausible argument can be made that would justify that step. The concept of a "right to health" neither makes sense in itself nor provides the basis for any kind of rational social policy.

The "right to health care" is, if properly qualified, a more promising idea. A society can, out of concern for the general welfare, decide to invest in the improvement of its level of health. Our society and many others have already made that decision. Whether a society has an *obligation* to do so—especially vis-à-vis other ways in which it might invest its resources—is a question I will not wrestle with here. I am only asserting that it *may* quite legitimately make that decision. Once it has done so, the question arises as to who has a claim on the resources thus put aside, and under what circumstances. If the "right to health care" is construed to mean, as it commonly is, a right to "equal access" to the general health care which the society has decided to make available, then it is at least in theory possible to conceive of an equitable arrangement for guaranteeing that access. The presumption behind the "equal access" theory is that, whatever the total amount of general resources devoted to health, all should have a chance to avail themselves of some fair portion of it. Occasionally, however, the "right to health care" seems to be construed in a way which differentiates it very little from a more general "right to health." It is seen as a claim to whatever resources are needed, even those as yet undeveloped, to guarantee as much health as possible. This more extreme version consequently entails many of the same theoretical and practical problems as a "right to health" does.

The "right to health care," even in its more modest form, is not without its problems as it competes with other welfare rights. It is possible in the cases of education, nourishment, housing, and income to establish minimal levels of need and (assuming the availability of money) to meet each of them (e.g., the mandatory twelve years of education in this country). This cannot so readily be done in the case of health, primarily because of the great variety of illnesses which can afflict people and the great discrepancies in the expenses attendant upon treating each of them. One person may need penicillin for a few days to save his life; another may need open heart surgery; still another may need an expensive drug for his entire life (as is the case with the hemophiliac).

A strict theory of equity would require that each person get what he needs to save his life. But that means that some will get much more than others, which is in a sense inequitable. Further complications arise when decisions must be made about the magnitude and type of health-care services and facilities to be made available. Using the utilitarian rule of thumb, the "greatest good for the greatest number," it could be argued that the emphasis should be placed on meeting the health needs of the largest number of people. Yet that kind of decision could result in great injustice to those unfortunate enough to be afflicted with statistically rare diseases or with conditions which require unusually expensive or long-term treatment. Still another complication arises when decisions must be made about limits. Should everyone have equal access to health care regardless of age or physical condition? Should an eighty-year-old person have the same free access to open-heart surgery as a child? Should a person who has consumed a great deal of expensive health care over the years have as much right to future treatment as the person who has hitherto required little or none?

What about those whose illnesses can be traced to their poor living and health habits? Evidence is accumulating that many major diseases—lung cancer and heart disease, for instance—often are the direct result of (to use an old term) "abuses" of the body. Why in the world, one might ask, should the public bear any responsibility to provide health care for those who bring their illnesses upon themselves? The question is worth dwelling upon a moment primarily because it can reveal a naiveté about the causal context of disease, and about human nature as well. Take the case of the heavy smoker. In one sense, of course, he could simply stop smoking; if he continues, despite all the known evidence regarding its harmful effects, he has no one to blame but himself. But is that really true? After all, he has been bombarded since youth by high-powered advertising in favor of cigarettes, he has been exposed to their ready availability, and he may have taken up smoking—thus establishing an addiction—well before he was fully aware of what he was getting into. Just how "free," then, is his choice to continue smoking?

It is also by no means clear just why some people smoke and others do not: genetic predisposition, unrecognized psychological demands, the absence of some necessary vitamins or minerals? Unless one is willing to entertain a rather primitively moralistic view of human behavior, it is not so easy to explain why people do undertake, or maintain, harmful habits in life. No one has, at any rate, been able to show that smokers are, as a group, generally less responsible, less moral individuals than non-smokers; nor that the obese, who run a higher risk of heart disease, are less virtuous or poorer citizens than those who are sensibly thin.

Even if it were possible to work through some of these problems, there would still be a final difficulty. While it has been shown that certain ways of life lead to a higher incidence of certain diseases, it has also been shown that those same diseases can appear in the absence of all those causes. For that reason, if for no other, it would be impossible to *prove* that someone's disease was the result of his culpable, willful irresponsibility. Many who smoke do not contract lung cancer or any other disease traceable to smoking; and many who do not smoke do in fact contract those same diseases. Given all of these contradictions, or possibly paradoxes, a public policy based on assigning personal responsibility, and denying health care accordingly, could amount to an exceeding unjust arrangement.

Lurking behind these issues is the abiding problem of the relationship between individual good and common good. American medicine has been based upon the value the society places on the individual; the medical researcher is free to pursue whatever interests and challenges him; the medical patient is free to seek whatever kinds of medical care he thinks he needs, including the freedom to determine what he wants to regard as a medical condition; physicians, patients, and researchers are all free to determine their own value systems and their own ethical codes; everyone is free to get whatever he is willing to pay for, just as everyone is free to live the kind of life he wants, whatever the costs to himself or to society of hazardous living habits. Obviously, a number of practical limitations stand in the way of a full exercise of these freedoms; but there has been, until recently, very little challenge to their abstract validity.

The most important changes which American medicine is likely to witness in the next few decades will come from a systematic questioning of those premises. The beginnings of that challenge can already be seen. Congress is starting to question the right of researchers to pursue whatever happens to interest researchers—at least at public expense. The development of a comprehensive national health insurance program will make it impossible for each to decide for himself when he has become a "patient," to make unlimited demands on medicine in the name of his private desires. Emerging trends regarding the definition of death and the care of dying patients, on human experimentation, on the pursuit of potentially hazardous lines of medical research, all indicate a move away from subjective standards of judgment toward outside control. There are growing objections from the poor that the rich have medical treatment superior to theirs just because they can pay for it, and there is an obvious questioning of the notion that society ought to pay the costs that result from the failure of people to take care of their own good health.

Yet it is by no means clear where these trends will lead. They point toward, if not a theory of medical limits, at least the ingredients for one, toward the establishment of common codes of practice and ethics, and toward requiring more self-discipline and self-restraint (not only in terms of what people do but also in terms of what they desire). The most discussed ethical issues are all likely to reflect the force of these trends, as some new balance is sought between public needs and private desires.

Scarcity—restraint—limit: these are rapidly becoming the slogans of the times, and it is difficult to foresee that they will cease to be so very soon. Curiously enough (I would hold, anyway), these are precisely the conditions under which it becomes possible effectively to examine ethical goals. Medicine is in part a moral enterprise, one that seeks the human good. But excessive affluence combined with excessive individualism discourages our asking just what constitutes this human good; no one need bother with that kind of question. Now we can ask once again about that good which medicine is said to serve, and about what its role in the quest for a larger human good might reasonably be. The question has forced itself upon us whether we are ready for it or not.

The implications of what I propose here are not, for public-policy purposes, immediately evident. For the most part, public policy is based on the assumptions, value judgments, and moral predilections of the day. Legislators and administrators are notorious for avoiding a fundamental questioning of the framework upon which practical judgments have to be made. It is understandable, if deplorable: societies must run, decisions must be made, things must move on. Yet what I propose may now have its attractions, if only because so many problems have emerged from the assumptions now regnant. One can never know how attempts to answer basic questions will turn out. One can only guess, at least in this case, that the resulting changes will be profound.

SUGGESTED READING
    Leon R. Kass, "Regarding the End of Medicine and the Pursuit of Health," *The Public Interest*, 40 (Summer, 1975), pp. 11-42.
    Hans Jonas, *Philosophical Essays: From Ancient Creed to Technological Man* (Englewood Cliffs, N.J., 1974).
    Paul Ramsey, *The Patient as Person* (New Haven, 1970).
    "The Concept of Health," *Hastings Center Studies*, 1:3 (1973).

LEWIS THOMAS, M.D.

On the Science and Technology of Medicine

THE COMMON THEME RUNNING THROUGH ALMOST ALL the criticisms leveled at the American health-care system these days is the charge of inadequacy or insufficiency. There are not enough doctors and nurses, and those around lack sufficient interest and compassion; there are not enough clinics, and those around lack sufficient time to see everyone; there are too few medical schools, medical centers, and specialized hospitals, with inequities in their distribution around the country; most of all, there is not enough money, not enough commitment.

And yet, the system has been expanding with explosive force in the last quarter-century. It has been nothing short of a boom. In 1950, the total national expenditure in health care was estimated at $10 billion. By 1972, it had risen to over $70 billion. In 1974, it was $110 billion. This year it will at least exceed $130 billion, and it will be still larger if a national health-insurance program emerges. According to some more or less official estimates it could exceed $250 billion by the nineteen-eighties.

Whatever the defects, it cannot be claimed that the nation has been failing to react. Any enterprise that amplifies itself over a twenty-five-year period in this exuberant fashion is surely making a try. It is, whatever else, a massive effort to improve.

The question is: What are we improving? What, in fact, have we been trying to accomplish with these vast sums?

An alien historian would think, from a look just at the dollar figures for each of those years, that some sort of tremendous event must have been occurring since 1950. Either (1) the health of the nation had suddenly disintegrated, requiring the laying on of new resources to meet the crisis, or (2) the technology for handling health problems had undergone a major transformation, necessitating the installation of new effective resources to do things that could not be done before, or (3), another possibility, perhaps we had somehow been caught up in the momentum of a huge, collective, ponderous set of errors. If any of these explanations is the right one, we ought at least to become aware of it, since whatever we are improving will involve, in the near future, an even more immense new bureaucracy, an even larger commitment of public funds, regulations that will intervene in every aspect of the citizen's life, and, inevitably, still more expansion. This paper will deal with the arguments around each of these three possible explanations.

The Health of the Nation, 1950-1975

There is, to begin with, no real evidence that health has deteriorated in this country, certainly not to the extent indicated by the new dollars spent each year for health care. On the contrary, we seem to have gotten along reasonably well.

35

There is perhaps more heart disease, but this is to be expected in a generally older population living beyond the life expectancy of fifty years ago. Heart disease is, after all, one of the ways of dying, and death certificates do not usually distinguish between heart failure as the result of time having run out and other forms of heart disease, except by noting age. The total numbers have increased somewhat, and perhaps there are also somewhat more cases of coronary occlusion in middle-aged men, but we have not suddenly been plagued, just since 1950, by new heart disease in anything like frightening numbers.

Cancer, stroke, kidney disease, arthritis, schizophrenia, cirrhosis, multiple sclerosis, senility, asthma, pulmonary fibrosis, and a few other major diseases are still with us, but the change in incidence per capita is not sufficient to account for the move from a $10 billion enterprise to a $130 billion one.

Aging is not in itself a health problem, although a larger number of surviving old people obviously means proportionately more people with the disabling illnesses characteristic of the aged. However, the increased number of such patients since 1950 is not great enough to account for much of the increased investment.

Meanwhile, there has been a general improvement in the public health with respect to certain infectious diseases which were major problems in the twenty-five-year period prior to 1950. Lobar pneumonia, scarlet fever, erysipelas, rheumatic fever, subacute bacterial endocarditis, typhoid fever, poliomyelitis, diphtheria, pertussis, meningococcal meningitis, staphylococcal septicemia, all of which filled the wards of municipal and county hospitals in the earlier period, have become rarities. To be sure, new sorts of bacterial infection have appeared in hospital communities, as complications of other therapy in most instances, but the total number of these is a small figure alongside the infectious diseases of the pre-antibiotic, pre-immunization period.

On balance, then, no case can be made for a wave of new illnesses afflicting our population in the years since 1950. If anything, we are probably a somewhat healthier people because of the sharp decrease in severe infectious disease.

But this is not the general view of things: the public perception of the public health, in 1975, appears to be quite different. There is now a much more acute awareness of the risk of disease than in earlier periods, associated with a greater apprehension that a minor illness may turn suddenly into a killing disease. There is certainly a higher expectation that all kinds of disease can be treated effectively. Finally, personal maladjustments of all varieties—unhappiness, discontent, fear, anxiety, despair, marital discord, even educational problems—have come to be regarded as medical problems, requiring medical attention, imposing new, heavy demands for care. In addition, there are probably many more people in this country requiring specialized rehabilitation services for disabilities resulting from physical trauma (Korea and Vietnam veterans, automobile- and industrial-accident victims, etc.).

Health-Care Technology, 1950-1975

Has the effective technology for medical care changed in the past twenty-five years to a degree sufficient to explain the increased cost? Is there in fact a new high technology of medicine?

Despite the widespread public impression that this is the case, there is little evidence for it. The most spectacular technological change has occurred in the management of infectious disease, but its essential features had been solidly established and put to use well before 1950. The sulfonamides came to medicine in the late nineteen-thirties, penicillin and streptomycin a few years later, and the major advances in the control and cure of infectious disease occurred during the nineteen-forties. There has been no quantum leap in anti-infectious technology since 1950. Several new virus vaccines have been developed. The antibiotics have come into more widespread use (probably with considerable overuse and waste); a multiplicity of new variants of antibiotics and chemotherapeutic agents has appeared on the market, but one would not expect that the rational use of this technology, even allowing for the high cost of development and marketing, would have proven to be anything like the previous cost of hospital care in the absence of such a technology. A typical case of lobar pneumonia, pre-antibiotic, involved three or four weeks of hospitalization; typhoid was a twelve-to-sixteen-week illness; meningitis often required several months of care through convalescence; these and other common infectious diseases can now be aborted promptly, within just a few days. The net result of the anti-infection technology ought to have been a very large decrease in the cost of care.

There have been a few other examples of technology improvement, comparable in decisive effectiveness, since 1950, but the best of these have been for relatively uncommon illnesses. Childhood leukemia and certain solid tumors in children, for example, can now be cured by chemotherapy in a substantial proportion of cases, but there are only a few thousand of these per year in the country. Endocrine-replacement therapy has become highly effective and relatively inexpensive ("relative" considering the cost of caring for untreated endocrine abnormalities) for a variety of disorders involving the adrenals, pituitary, parathyroid, ovary, and thyroid; in particular, the biochemical treatment of thyroid dysfunction has improved markedly. Hematology has offered new and effective replacement treatment for certain anemias. Immunologic prophylaxis now prevents most cases of hemolytic disease of the newborn. Progress in anesthesia, electrolyte physiology, and cardiopulmonary physiology has greatly advanced the field of surgery, so that reparative and other procedures can now be done which formerly were technically impossible.

But the list of decisive new accomplishments is not much longer than the contents of the above paragraph.

We are left with approximately the same roster of common major diseases which confronted the country in 1950, and, although we have accumulated a formidable body of information about some of them in the intervening time, the accumulation is not yet sufficient to permit either the prevention or the outright cure of any of them. This is not to suggest that progress has not been made, or has been made more slowly than should reasonably have been expected. On the contrary, the research activity since 1950 has provided the beginnings of insight into the underlying processes in several of our most important diseases, and there is every reason for optimism regarding the future. But it is the present that is the problem. We are, in a sense, partway along, maybe halfway along. At the same time, medicine is expected to do something for each of these illnesses, to do whatever can be done in the light of today's knowledge. Because of this obligation, we have evolved "halfway" technologies, representing the best available treatment, and the development and proliferation of these are partly responsible for the escalating costs of health care in recent years. Associated with this expansion, the diagnostic laboratories have become much more elaborate and complex in their technologies; there is no question that clinical diagnosis has become much more powerful and precise, but at a very high cost and with considerable waste resulting from overuse.

This way of looking at contemporary medicine runs against the currently general public view that the discipline has by this time come almost its full distance, that we have had a long succession of "breakthroughs" and "major advances," and that now we should go beyond our persistent concern with research on what is called "curative" medicine and give more attention to the social aspects of illness and to preventive medicine.

It does not, in fact, look much like the record of a completed job, or even of a job more than half begun, when you run through the list, one by one, of the diseases in this country which everyone will agree are the most important ones. A handy index for this sort of exercise is the annual *United States Vital Statistics Report*, in which are tabulated the ten leading causes of death, as well as the commonest non-fatal illnesses requiring attention from the health-care system.

The questions to be asked are the following: For how many of these illnesses do we now possess a decisively effective technology for cure or prevention, directed at a central disease agent or mechanism, comparable to the treatment, say, of pneumococcal lobar pneumonia with penicillin? Are we failing to employ effective measures because of deficiencies in the health-care system? To what extent do present mortality and morbidity rates simply reflect the absence of any known technology that works?

In the following section, these questions are explored. It should be emphasized here that we will not be discussing the availability of medical treatment in general. Obviously, there is a great deal that can be done for patients with the diseases considered below in the way of supportive care, the amelioration of symptoms, and sometimes the extension of life. In some conditions, this amounts to what might be called partial control of the disease, but this is not the question at hand. What we are examining here is the capacity of medicine to cure outright or to prevent completely—in situations analogous to lobar pneumonia or poliomyelitis.

Listed below are the ten leading causes of death from disease in the United States in 1974:

Cardiovascular disease (39% of total deaths in 1974): In general, cardiovascular disease lacks any decisive, conclusive technology with the power to turn off, reverse, or prevent disease. There are two possible exceptions: rheumatic heart disease is known to be preventable when the antecedent streptococcal infection can be quickly terminated by early antibiotic treatment or prevented by prophylaxis; some forms of congenital heart disease can be completely corrected by surgery. Except for these, the other therapies now available are directed at secondary results of already established disease: coronary-care units and specialized ambulances, designed primarily for coping with cardiac standstill and arrythmias, anticoagulant treatment to prevent extension and recurrence (largely given up in recent years), digitalis and diuretics for myocardial failure, drug therapy to inhibit arrythmias, and surgical replacement of already damaged coronary arteries or valves.

As to coronary disease, it is believed in some quarters that dietary lipids are an etiologic factor. It is also proposed that lack of exercise, excessive emotional stress, and various usually unstipulated environmental influences are somehow implicated in pathogenesis. The evidence for these beliefs is still inconclusive. In any event, intervention to correct them would involve grand-scale, societal reforms of living habits. Meanwhile, the actual pathologic events which cause the coronary lesions remain unknown. Until these are elucidated in some detail, a direct approach to coronary disease must await the future.

Hypertension is a separate disease state, frequently associated with cardiac disease. This will be considered below.

Cancer (19% of total deaths in 1974): Up to now, the technologies available for the treatment of cancer are all in the "halfway" category, in the sense that they deal with the already established disease and represent efforts to destroy, by one means or another (surgery, radiation, chemotherapy, immunotherapy), existing cancer cells. There are no methods for reversing the neoplastic process in cells or for preventing their emergence from normal cells. Prevention would be possible for a few types, if exposure to the known environmental carcinogens, e.g., cigarettes, asbestos, and certain industrial chemicals, could be eliminated. But prevention in the sense of eliminating the biological steps involved in the transformation of cells is not yet feasible.

Cerebrovascular diseases (11% of total deaths in 1974): Stroke results from disease of the arteries of the brain, usually associated with atherosclerosis or hypertension. Since no therapy exists for preventing or reversing atherosclerosis, this class of strokes is neither preventable nor reversible. Hypertension is considered below.

Once stroke occurs, therapy is limited to efforts at minimizing the extent of disability, largely a matter of retraining, rehabilitation, and speech therapy. No treatment exists for preventing the recurrence of stroke. Anticoagulant therapy, once attempted on a large scale, is no longer in general use.

Kidney disease (10.4% of total deaths in 1974): The major forms of kidney disease responsible for most cases of renal failure and death are chronic glomerulonephritis and pyelonephritis.

At the present time, no effective treatment exists for chronic glomerulonephritis, beyond measures aimed at compensating for the loss of renal function, e.g., electrolyte adjustment, chronic dialysis and, in a relatively few cases, kidney transplantation. Some cases are perhaps prevented by early treatment of antecedent streptococcal infection, but the initial cause in most instances is unknown. The essential lesion is a deposit of an antigen-antibody complex within the walls of glomerular capillaries, followed by injury to the vessels probably mediated by leucocytic lysosomes and complement. A direct therapeutic approach to these events cannot be conceived until more detailed scientific information becomes available.

Chronic pyelonephritis can probably be prevented in some instances by early treatment of the acute infection, but in most cases the kidney lesions develop gradually and unobtrusively, and once established they are not reversible. It is believed by some that bacterial protoplasts are involved in etiology, perhaps also with an associated immunologic injury to the tissues; even if this is so, currently available anti-microbial therapy is not effective.

Pulmonary disease (approximately 4.5% of total deaths in 1974): Included under this heading, in the *Vital Statistics Report*, are influenza and pneumonia, bronchitis, emphysema and chronic obstructive lung disease.

Almost all cases of primary bacterial and mycoplasmal pneumonia are treatable and curable by use of the appropriate antibiotic.

Influenza can be prevented in some cases by immunization, provided the antigenic strain is recognized early enough in an outbreak to prepare vaccine. Once it has occurred, there is no therapy for the influenza viral infection itself. Bacterial superinfections, when they occur, are reversible except in the occasional cases of sudden, overwhelming infection to which pregnant women and debilitated elderly people are most prone. Antibiotic treatment of uncomplicated influenza is ineffective and probably hazardous.

Bronchitis, emphysema and chronic pulmonary obstructive disease are still unsolved etiologic problems. Cigarette smoking and air pollution are suspected as causes, but the actual mechanisms underlying the injury to lung tissue remain unknown. Although technologies exist for the improvement of aeration by the damaged lungs, and thus for some prolongation of life, there are no measures available for stopping or reversing the progress of disease.

Diabetes mellitus (1.9% of total deaths in 1974): Although the discovery of insulin fifty years ago made possible the survival of most diabetics who would otherwise have died in diabetic coma, the blood-vessel disorder which is a major aspect of the disease is unaffected by insulin and remains a mystery. Hence, the disabilities and deaths of diabetics, mostly in middle-age and later, are now due to chronic kidney disease and the occlusion of arteries in one or another part of the body. Virtually nothing is known about the cause of vascular lesions, and there is no therapy to stop or reverse the process.

Cirrhosis of the liver (1.8% of total deaths in 1974): The chief cause of cirrhosis is unquestionably alcohol taken in excess and over a long period of time. If alcoholism could be prevented, cirrhosis would become a relatively rare affliction. The hepatic lesions are to some extent reversible, and the disease can sometimes be stopped and even reversed in its early stages by simple abstention.

This, however, represents about the total of today's effective therapy. The mechanism of hepatic cell injury by alcohol is not understood, nor is the process by which the liver becomes progressively atrophic and fibrosed. Nutritional deprivation, believed a few years back to play a central role, is no longer thought to be centrally involved. Once the disease is firmly established, there is no known method for turning it around. Surgical measures have been developed for reducing ascites (that is, fluid accumulation in the abdomen) and the back pressure of portal blood, with some ameliorative effort on the symptoms of cirrhosis, but the injury to the liver itself is unalterable.

Perinatal disease (1.5% of total deaths in 1974): Much of the infant mortality in the earliest days of life is associated with prematurity, and obstructive disease of the lungs accounts for much of this. At the present time, there is no effective therapy for this pulmonary disease, caused by hyaline, membranous deposits which occlude the alveolar walls. The mechanisms leading to these deposits are unknown.

Bacterial and viral infections account for a majority of other neonatal deaths. The bacterial infections are treatable with antibiotics, but often occur abruptly in overwhelming form. The viral infections are untreatable.

Hemolytic disease of the newborn, formerly a common cause of death, is now preventable by immunologic treatment during pregnancy; some cases can be cured by total blood replacement and transfusions.

Congenital malformations and deficiencies (0.7% of total deaths in 1974): Although surgical measures are available for the correction of some types of congenital malformation, such as cardiac and intestinal anomalies, most of them are untreatable. A few of the highly disabling and fatal enzyme deficiencies can be recognized during early pregnancy and thus prevented by abortion. The biochemical and genetic nature of these rare disorders is currently under investigation in many laboratories, and there is some optimism that methods for reversing the defects will eventually be found.

Peptic ulcer: Few human ailments have been subjected to as great a variety of medical and surgical treatments over the years as peptic ulcer, often with enthusiastic predictions of success, but always replaced by new and different therapies. The main problem hampering decisive progress is that the mechanism that produces peptic ulcers is not understood, and therefore there is no basis for devising a genuinely rational method of treatment or prevention. This is not to say that it is not a treatable condition, of course. There are many ways in which the symptoms and the progress of the disease can be alleviated. Nevertheless, it must be ranked as an essentially unexplained disorder.

The foregoing list accounts for approximately 80 per cent of all deaths in this country. It does not, of course, account for the major part of the work of physicians, nor the greatest element of cost for the health-care system. We are afflicted, obviously, by a great (but it must be said, finite) array of non-fatal illnesses varying in severity and duration, and it is here that the greatest demands for technology are made. For the purposes of this paper, some of the commonest of these self-limited or non-fatal diseases are listed below:

Acute respiratory infections: These and the acute gastroenteric infections and intoxications (see below) make up the great majority of transiently disabling illnesses with which people are afflicted in a year's turning.

The common cold and the array of other respiratory viral infections including influenza (sometimes called "grippe") are essentially untreatable. The measures employed for alleviating discomfort—bed rest, aspirin, a good book—are no different today from what one's grandmother would have prescribed. There is, in short, no medical technology for such illnesses. The administration of antibiotics, antihistamines, vitamin C, and various other "cold remedies" probably have no effect other than reassurance. There is a general apprehension that such illnesses may lead to other, more severe, respiratory infections, such as pneumonia, if not monitored by a physician, but there is in fact no evidence for this. By and large, people with these illnesses get better by themselves, usually within a day or two. The most frequent complications are the result of untoward reactions to unnecessary therapy, most often the antibiotics used in the hope of preventing complications.

Gastrointestinal infections: The general run of acute gastrointestinal illnesses, usually caused by a virus or salmonella infection or by staphylococcal toxin, are common, self-limited, and entirely without hazard. Intervention by medicine would be desirable, since these are unpleasant experiences for the afflicted, and there are in fact several symptomatic measures for partial relief, but the illnesses are usually so short in duration that no therapy is necessary. As in the case of acute respiratory infections, grandmother's advice is as good as any, maybe better.

Arthritis: Both rheumatoid arthritis and osteoarthritis, which account for more than 5 million illnesses each year, are unexplained, mystifying diseases for which no therapy beyond analgesic drugs is available. Rheumatoid arthritis is currently believed by a consensus of clinical investigators to be caused by an unknown infectious agent, probably with a still unidentified immunopathologic component. The partial relief provided by salicylates and related drugs, and by gold salts, are still unexplainable. In approximately 35 per cent of all cases the disease subsides spontaneously and vanishes. Prolonged, chronically disabling forms of arthritis can be partially benefited by surgical removal of inflamed synovial (joint) tissues. Prolonged hospitalization and various forms of rehabilitative care are required in some cases. In the absence of information concerning etiology, it is probable that treatment will remain at a symptomatic, empirical level not very different from the measures of fifty years ago.

Osteoarthritis remains totally unexplained. Surgical treatment is useful in some (notably hip) cases; otherwise therapy is limited to analgesic drugs.

The neuroses: It is frequently said that at least 75 per cent of the patients seeking help in doctors' offices or clinics have complaints for which there is no "organic" explanation. Some of these patients are not really ill, but simply in need of reassurance that they do not have one or another disease which they are worried about. Others are beset by family, economic, or various other social problems which seem temporarily insoluble, and for which they seek advice. Still others, an unknown number, are disabled by classical psychoneuroses.

The possible therapeutic approaches to such problems have not changed significantly in the past quarter-century. Counseling, comforting, and what is called psychotherapy are essentially the same procedures as in earlier times, without any real elements of technology, nor is there any statistical evidence for their effectiveness. An immense store of so-called "tranquilizer" drugs has been provided by pharmaceutical research in recent years, but there is little information as to the efficacy of its contents. They may provide transient symptomatic relief, but it is unlikely that they alter the underlying processes of these illnesses. In short, there is no real technology available for the treatment of "functional" illness, psychoneurosis, or the various forms of social maladaptation. It seems safe to say that nothing much has happened since 1950 to alter the situation one way or the other.

The psychoses: Schizophrenia and the manic-depressive psychoses account for the greatest part of mental illness requiring hospitalization and prolonged ambulatory care. Drug therapy evolved since 1950 has greatly improved the "manageability" of schizophrenia, but it has not much changed the disease itself. The manic-depressive psychoses are improved in some instances by pharmacologic treatment, including lithium, and also in some by electric shock. All forms of psychosis remain unexplained, however, in terms of identifiable mechanisms attributable to dysfunction in the central nervous system, and therapy directed at underlying processes has not advanced beyond what was available before 1950.

Parkinsonism: The introduction of L-Dopa as therapy for Parkinsonism in the mid-nineteen-sixties by Cotzias and his associates represents a milestone in neurological medicine. Although not all patients are uniformly benefited, and some become refractory or display untoward reactions to the drug, many do well and have their lives transformed.

Essential hypertension: In some respects, hypertension is a paradigm illustrating a central dilemma in today's health-care system. Drugs are now available with the capacity to reduce blood-pressure levels to normal. At the same time, however, the actual mechanisms of the disease remain without explanation, and it is not yet known whether the reduction of blood pressure has any effect on the underlying vascular disturbance. There is now some evidence, still incomplete, that prolonged treatment with anti-hypertensive drug decreases the incidence of stroke as a complication of hypertension. There may also be an effect on the incidence of coronary occlusion, although the evidence for this is less conclusive. There appears to be no doubt that drug treatment can prolong survival in patients with malignant hypertension.

On the basis of these observations, it has been proposed that large-scale screening programs be set up, so that all of the 10 million or more young, potentially vulnerable people with hypertension in this country can be identified and treated. This means that great numbers of patients with essential hypertension will be placed on lifelong treatment with complex pharmacologic agents, necessarily persuaded to stay under treatment because of the threat of a fatal outcome. At the same time it is a certainty that many patients with essential hypertension, if not treated, would nevertheless be able to look forward to the statistical probability of a normal life span. Indeed, there are reasons to believe that essential hypertension is a normal state of affairs for some people. The difficulty is that there is no way to predict which patients will eventually have cardiac, cerebral, or renal complications associated with hypertension; in the absence of such knowledge, all hypertensives must be treated. Meanwhile, the disease itself remains an enigma. If a mass screening and therapy program is launched it will be done in the hope that treating a symptom of disease will have long-range beneficial effects. Moreover, it will involve drug therapy, with certain predictable side effects, and perhaps still others unpredicted thus far, aimed at the protection of a minority of the patients to be treated.

The Cost of Worry in the Health-Care System

Nothing has changed so much in the health-care system over the past twenty-five years as the public's perception of its own health. The change amounts to a loss of confidence in the human form. The general belief these days seems to be that the body is fundamentally flawed, subject to disintegration at any moment, always on the verge of mortal disease, always in need of continual monitoring and support by health-care professionals. This is a new phenomenon in our society.

It can be seen most clearly in the content of television programs and, especially, television commercials, where the preponderance of material deals with the need for shoring up one's personal health. The same drift is evident in the contents of the most popular magazines and in the health columns of daily newspapers. There is a public preoccupation with disease that is assuming the dimension of a national obsession.

To some extent, the propaganda which feeds the obsession is a result of the well intentioned efforts by particular disease agencies to obtain public money for the support of research and care in their special fields. Every mail brings word of the imminent perils posed by multiple sclerosis, kidney disease, cancer, heart disease, cystic fibrosis, asthma, muscular dystrophy, and the rest.

There is, regrettably, no discernible counter-propaganda. No agencies exist for the celebration of the plain fact that most people are, in real life, abundantly healthy. No one takes public note of the truth of the matter, which is that most people in this country have a clear, unimpeded run at a longer lifetime than could have been foreseen by any earlier generation. Even the proponents of good hygiene, who argue publicly in favor of regular exercise, thinness, and abstinence from cigarettes and alcohol, base their arguments on the presumed intrinsic fallibility of human health.

Left alone, unadvised by professionals, the tendency of the human body is perceived as prone to steady failure.

Underlying this pessimistic view of health is a profound dissatisfaction with the fact of death. Dying is regarded as the ultimate failure, something that could always be avoided or averted if only the health-care system functioned more efficiently. Death has been made to seem unnatural, an outrage; when people die—at whatever age—we speak of them as having been "struck down," "felled." It is as though in a better world we would all go on forever.

It is not surprising that all this propaganda has imposed heavy, unsupportable demands on the health-care system. If people are educated to believe that they may at any moment be afflicted with one or another mortal disease and that this fate can be forestalled by access to medicine, especially "preventive" medicine, it is no wonder that clinics and doctors' offices are filled with waiting clients.

In the year 1974, 1,933,000 people died in the United States, a death rate of 9.1 per 1,000, or just under 1 per cent of the whole population, substantially lower than the birth rate for the same year. The life expectation for the whole population rose to 72 years, the highest expectancy ever attained in this country. With figures like these, it is hard to see health as a crisis, or the health-care system, apart from its huge size and high cost, as a matter needing emergency action. We really are a quite healthy society, and we should be spending more time and energy in acknowledging this, and perhaps trying to understand more clearly why it is so. We are in some danger of becoming a nation of healthy hypochondriacs.

For all its obvious defects and shortcomings, the actual technology of health care is not likely to be changed drastically in the direction of saving money—not in the short haul. Nor is it likely that changes for the better, in the sense of greater effectiveness and efficiency, can be brought about by any means other than more scientific research. The latter course, although sure, is undeniably slow and unpredictable. While it is a certainty, in my view, that rheumatoid arthritis, atherosclerosis, cancer, and senile dementia will eventually be demystified and can then become preventable disorders, there is no way of forecasting when this will happen; it could be a few years away for one or the other, or decades.

Meanwhile, we will be compelled to live with the system as we have it, changing only the parts that are in fact changeable. It is not likely that money problems can induce anyone—the professionals or the public at large, or even the third-party payers—to give up the halfway technologies that work only partially when this would mean leaving no therapeutic effort at all in place. For as long as there is a prospect of saving the lives of 50 per cent, or even only 33 per cent, of patients with cancer by today's methods for destroying cancer cells, these methods must obviously be held onto and made available to as many patients as possible. If coronary bypass surgery remains the only technical measure for relieving untractable angina in a relatively small proportion of cases, it will be continued, and very likely extended to larger numbers of cases, until something better turns up. People with incapacitating mental illness cannot simply be left to wander the streets, and we will continue to need expanding clinics and specialized hospital facilities, even though caring for the mentally ill does not mean anything like curing them. We are, in a sense, stuck with today's technology, and we will stay stuck until we have more scientific knowledge to work with.

But what we might do, if we could muster the energy and judgment for it, is to identify the areas of health care in which the spending of money represents outright waste, and then eliminate these. There are discrete examples all over the place, but what they are depends on who is responsible for citing them, and there will be bitter arguments over each one before they can be edited out of the system, one by one.

The biggest source of waste results from the general public conviction that contemporary medicine is able to accomplish a great deal more than is in fact possible. This attitude is in part the outcome of overstated claims on the part of medicine itself in recent decades, plus medicine's passive acquiescence while even more exaggerated claims were made by the media. The notion of preventive medicine as a whole new discipline in medical care is an example of this. There is an arguably solid base for the prevention of certain diseases, but it has not changed all that much since the nineteen-fifties. A few valuable measures have been added, most notably the avoidance of cigarette smoking for the prevention of lung cancer; if we had figured out a way of acting on this single bit of information, we might have achieved a spectacular triumph in the prevention of deaths from cancer, but regrettably we didn't. The same despairing thing can be said for the preventability of death from alcohol.

But there is not much more than this in the field of preventive medicine. The truth is that medicine has not become very skilled at disease prevention—not, as is sometimes claimed, because it doesn't want to or isn't interested, but because the needed information is still lacking.

Most conspicuous and costly of all are the benefits presumed to derive from "seeing the doctor." The regular complete checkup, once a year or more often, has become a cultural habit, and it is only recently that some investigators have suggested, cautiously, that it probably doesn't do much good. There are very few diseases in which early detection can lead to a significant alteration of the outcome: glaucoma, cervical cancer, and possibly breast cancer are the usually cited examples, but in any event these do not require the full, expensive array of the complete periodic checkup, EKG and all. Nevertheless, the habit has become fixed in our society, and it is a significant item in the total bill for health care.

"Seeing the doctor" also includes an overwhelming demand for reassurance. Transient upper-respiratory infections and episodes of gastroenteritis account for most of the calls on a doctor because of illness, and an even greater number of calls are made by people who have nothing at all the matter with them. It is often claimed that these are mostly unhappy individuals, suffering from psychoneuroses, in need of compassionate listening on the part of the physician, but a large number of patients who find themselves in doctors' offices or hospital clinics will acknowledge themselves to be in entirely good health; they are there because of a previous appointment in connection with an earlier illness, for a "checkup," or for a laboratory test, or simply for reassurance that they are not coming down with something serious—cancer, or heart disease, or whatever. Or they may have come to the doctor for advice about living: what should their diet be?, should they take a vacation?, what about a tranquilizer for everyone's inevitable moments of agitation and despair? I know a professor of pediatrics who has received visits from intelligent, well-educated parents who only want to know if their child should start Sunday school.

The system is being overused, swamped by expectant overdemands for services that are frequently trivial or unproductive. The public is not sufficiently informed of the facts about things that medicine can and cannot accomplish. Medicine is surely not in possession of special wisdom about how to live a life.

It needs to be said more often that human beings are fundamentally tough, resilient animals, marvelously made, most of the time capable of getting along quite well on their own. The health-care system should be designed for use when it is really needed and when it has something of genuine value to offer. If designed, or redesigned, in this way, the system would function far more effectively, and would probably cost very much less.

Conclusion

If our society wishes to be rid of the diseases, fatal and non-fatal, that plague us the most, there is really little prospect of doing so by mounting a still larger health-care system at still greater cost for delivering essentially today's kind of technology on a larger scale. We will not do so by carrying out broader programs of surveillance and screening. The truth is that we do not yet know enough. But there is also another truth of great importance: we are learning fast. The harvest of new information from the biological revolution of the past quarter-century is just now coming in, and we can probably begin now to figure out the mechanisms of major diseases which were blank mysteries a few years back as accurately and profitably as was done for the infectious diseases earlier in this century. This can be said with considerable confidence, and without risk of overpromising or raising false hopes, provided we do not set time schedules or offer dates of delivery. Sooner or later it will go this way, since clearly it can go this way. It is simply a question at this stage of events of how much we wish to invest, for the health-care system of the future, in science.

STANLEY JOEL REISER, M.D.

Therapeutic Choice and Moral Doubt
in a Technological Age

THE INSTRUMENTS AND MACHINES used by the contemporary physician are basically of two sorts: diagnostic—to perceive and evaluate the disturbances caused by illness—and therapeutic—to act to overcome these disturbances. This essay will focus on therapeutic technology, and particularly on the perplexing moral dilemmas its success has created for physicians and laymen. Certain contemporary episodes that delineate this problem and some of its roots in medical history will be examined.

In 1957, Pope Pius XII publicly discussed some questions that had been submitted to him by Dr. Bruno Haid, chief of anesthesia at the surgical clinic of the University of Innsbruck.[1] The questions concerned the morality of resuscitation, a term that was used for the techniques employed to forestall life-threatening episodes, particularly the threats posed by asphyxia, a severe lack of oxygen. Asphyxia generally causes death in several minutes unless the technology of resuscitation now available is promptly used. By the mid-nineteen-fifties the anesthesiologist no longer confined his work to the operating room, but practiced his art, more and more, during hospital emergencies that produced asphyxia, such as strangulation, open chest wounds, tetanus, poliomyelitis, poisoning by sedatives, and brain trauma.

The resuscitation of people who suffered from disorders such as these and who lapsed into a coma raised moral questions that seemed more difficult to resolve than questions of resuscitative method. In some cases the anesthesiologist, using special instruments and manual techniques to maintain respiration and provide nourishment, could support a patient long enough for spontaneous breathing to resume. But if the damage suffered by the patient was so serious that death seemed certain, the anesthesiologist was driven to doubt the value and purpose of using resuscitative techniques. For, having initiated respiratory-assisting therapies on a patient in response to an emergency, what should the anesthesiologist do if after a slight improvement the patient's condition became static, and it was clear that only the automated artificial respiratory apparatus was sustaining his life?

Dr. Haid expressed the problems which arose from the modern practice of resuscitation as three questions. First, does one have the right or obligation to use resuscitation equipment on all patients, even those whose prognosis seems hopeless to the physician? Second, does one have the right or obligation to remove the resuscitation equipment if a patient's deep unconsciousness does not begin to abate in several days, knowing that its removal will result in his death? What does the physician do if the patient's family request that the physician remove the equipment? Third, should an unconscious patient whose body functions are maintained artificially, but who does

47

not improve in several days, be considered *de facto* or *de jure* dead? Or must one wait for the heart to stop beating, the traditional criterion of death, despite the presence of the life-sustaining technology, before considering the patient dead?

Pope Pius began his answer to these questions with a statement of principle. He affirmed that natural reason and Christian morals imposed a duty on man to preserve health and life. But he maintained that in meeting this duty one was obliged to use only ordinary means (defined according to the circumstances of person, place, time, and culture) that did not impose ponderous hardships on oneself or on others. A more stringent obligation, he held, would be too burdensome for most people, and would also endanger the attainment of the higher, more important spiritual ends of life. A person might take more than the basic steps to preserve life and health, but only so long as this act did not prevent him from performing these more serious spiritual duties.

With this as a preamble, the Pope responded specifically to Dr. Haid's questions. Was one obliged to use modern respiratory technology in cases judged hopeless by the physician, and even against the wishes of the family? Since such therapy exceeded the ordinary ministrations that physicians were bound to apply, they were under no obligation to use it. Further, in the case of the unconscious patient, if resuscitation techniques imposed clear and substantial burdens on the patient's family, they could direct the physician to discontinue the use of his apparatus, and the physician could morally and lawfully comply. Should discontinuing the use of the life-sustaining apparatus cause the heart to stop beating, the act was to be considered only an indirect cause of death and not a direct assault on the life of the patient.

But if the resuscitative apparatus was left in place and a comatose patient showed no improvement after several days, when was he to be considered dead? This question perplexed the Pope. He thought that it did not truly fall within the competence of the Church to decide, but ventured a response: human life could be said to exist "as long as its vital functions—distinguished from the simple life of organs—manifest themselves spontaneously or even with the help of artificial processes."[2]

Almost a decade after the Pope delivered his statement, an ad hoc committee of Harvard faculty members, representing the disciplines of medicine, history, ethics, and law, convened to formulate new criteria of death.[3] Like the Pope, many physicians and laymen in this age of advanced resuscitative technology were troubled about the problem of determining when a person had died. This technology encouraged physicians to make greater efforts than they had in the past to sustain lives of critically injured people. But sometimes their efforts were only partially successful, and they led to situations where the heart beat continued while the brain was damaged irreversibly: the time-honored criterion of death—cessation of the heart beat—therefore seemed inadequate. The Harvard committee worked to develop criteria whose presence in such patients permitted physicians to declare that the patient had a permanently nonfunctioning brain and therefore had died. These criteria are essentially: (1) a total unawareness of externally applied stimuli; (2) the absence of spontaneous movement or breathing for at least an hour; (3) the absence of reflexes; and (4) the absence of electrical activity in the brain as detected by electroencephalograph readings during a twenty-four-hour period. If all these criteria were met, then the committee recommended that the patient be declared dead and that the artificial respirator be removed.

The issues considered by Pope Pius XII and the Harvard ad hoc committee were crystalized for the public, if not for many physicians, by the case of Karen Ann Quinlan. On the night of April 15, 1975, local police and an emergency squad were summoned to attend Karen who, for reasons yet unknown, had stopped breathing for at least two fifteen-minute periods. Friends administered mouth-to-mouth resuscitation during the first episode, and the police used a mechanical respirator during the second episode. She was taken to a local hospital in New Jersey, where attending physicians found, among other things, that the pupils of her eyes did not contract from the introduction of light and that she made no response when they administered ordinarily painful stimuli—both signs of serious brain damage probably caused by previous oxygen deprivation. She was immediately hooked up to a mechanical respirator.

When Dr. Robert Morse, a neurologist who subsequently became Karen's principal physician, examined her three days later, he found that her condition remained critical. She was still comatose and did not trigger the respirator, which meant that she was unable to breathe spontaneously or independently of it. She then was transferred to another hospital under the care of Dr. Morse. There more extensive tests were conducted, including an electroencephalogram. It was abnormal but indicated the presence of some brain activity. Dr. Morse, and several other physicians who examined her, portrayed Karen as a person whose brain had the capacity to maintain the "vegetative" aspects of neurological functioning—such as the regulation of blood pressure and swallowing—but had lost its "cognitive" capabilities—those that made possible talking, thinking, seeing, or feeling. By the yardstick of the criteria enumerated by the Harvard ad hoc committee, which had become a widely acknowledged standard in medicine, Karen was not "brain dead."

However, her physicians were unable to wean her from the respirator, and with the passage of time reached the conclusion that she could not live without it. Although attendants fed her through a tube inserted through the nose and down to the stomach, Karen became emaciated. Her posture was described as grotesque, arms and legs rigid and deformed. She was totally unaware of her surroundings and, according to her physicians, did not appear to suffer from a locked-in syndrome, a state in which a patient is conscious but totally paralyzed. Although Karen's principal physician, Dr. Morse, could not specifically foresee circumstances that would meliorate her condition, he was unwilling to declare that it was totally irreversible. Several other physicians who had examined her shared Dr. Morse's point of view and reemphasized with him that twenty-two-year-old Karen, for all her disability, did not meet the Harvard brain-death criteria.

From the outset of her illness, in the belief that she would recover, Karen's parents authorized her doctors to initiate all necessary life-preserving measures. Her parents were in constant attendance at the bedside and in close contact with Dr. Morse. But her deteriorating condition, the absence of any reasonable hope that she would get better, and Karen's own previous remarks to her parents that she never wanted to be kept alive by extraordinary measures prompted her parents to conclude, about three months after the onset of the affliction, that Karen should be removed from the respirator and nature allowed to take its course. They signed a release which freed Dr. Morse, the hospital, and the other people who attended Karen from all liability for the consequences of separating Karen from her machine. In making this decision, her parents received considerable support from their priest, who indicated that the request was permissible under the teachings of their faith, the Roman Catholic

Church, a conclusion which the priest based principally upon the 1957 statement of Pope Pius XII.

Dr. Morse refused to remove Karen from the respirator. He based his decision on his concept of the moral standards of medical practice, which he believed did not allow him to disconnect the life-sustaining equipment from a patient who was not medically dead.

The impasse between Karen's parents and her physician prompted her parents to seek the help of the courts to have the apparatus removed. The first decision on the case came from the Superior Court of New Jersey. It ruled that decisions about medical care were the responsibility of the physician. Society had given him discretion over the nature, extent, and duration of care: "What justification is there to remove it from control of the medical profession and place it in the hands of the courts?," the presiding Judge Robert Muir, Jr., asked.[4] He refused to grant the petition of Karen's father to become the sole guardian of his daughter, because of his stated intention to seek the discontinuance of what he considered the extraordinary means which kept his daughter alive. The parents appealed this decision to the Supreme Court of New Jersey. It overruled the lower court, declaring on March 31, 1976, almost a year after Karen's illness began, that no "interest of the State could compel Karen to endure the unendurable, only to vegetate a few measurable months with no realistic possibility of returning to any semblance of cognitive or sapient life."[5] The Court was convinced that Karen's parents acted as she would have acted if she had the capacity to perceive her condition. It declared that her parents could assert a right to privacy for her and request cessation of the life-sustaining technology. The Court saw an analogy between Karen's situation and one in which a competent and suffering terminally ill patient would not be kept on a respirator against his will, or resuscitated by most physicians aware of his suffering and his grave prognosis. It acknowledged the desirability, ordinarily, of resolving such dilemmas within the privacy of the physician-patient relationship. But it emphasized the benefit to society and to medicine resulting when courts introduce into the medical decision-making process the values and common moral judgments of the community at large: "The law, equity and justice must not themselves quail and be helpless in the face of modern technological marvels presenting questions hitherto unthought of."[6] The Court added that dilemmas of this kind in medicine were augmented (in this era of proliferating malpractice litigation) by the hazard of legal action faced by physicians.

The Court appointed Karen's father as guardian with the power to choose new treating physicians. It ruled that, should these new physicians conclude that no reasonable possibility existed of her emerging from coma and if a consultative body of physicians at the hospital serving as members of an ethics committee concurred, life-supporting technology could be removed without civil or criminal liability for any participant.

Karen Quinlan was removed from her respirator and did not die. She now resides in a nursing facility and is still in a coma.

The fundamental purposes of medical therapy, weighed by those who decided the issues in the Quinlan case, have been considered intermittently in medical history. One of the earliest and, for contemporary physicians, most valuable discussions of this subject took place in ancient Greece between the fifth and fourth centuries B.C., when medicine was dominated by the physician Hippocrates and his students and disciples. Their instructive thoughts have been handed down to us in a group of texts written by different hands and known collectively as the *Corpus Hippocraticum*. A problem that concerned physicians at that time, and which is explored in the *Corpus*, is the relation of the medical art to the natural processes of disease. How far can the actions of the physician influence the healing of the body? How far should the physician extend his medical techniques to fight nature? The Hippocratic writings urge restraint. For example, in one called *The Art*, the author asserts, in rejoinder to those who attributed the physician's cures to luck or to the healing power of nature, that there indeed is an art of medicine. But the treatise emphasizes that the natural forces which produce disease are powerful and that medical art has its limits: "I will define what I conceive medicine to be. In general terms, it is to do away with the sufferings of the sick, to lessen the violence of their diseases, and to refuse to treat those who are overmastered by their diseases, realizing that in such cases medicine is powerless."[7]

The author of this treatise then defends physicians against critics who censure them for sometimes refusing to treat desperately ill persons: "For if a man demand from an art a power over what does not belong to the art, or from nature a power over what does not belong to nature, his ignorance is more allied to madness than to lack of knowledge. For in cases where we may have the mastery through the means afforded by a natural constitution or by an art, there we may be craftsmen, but nowhere else. Whenever therefore a man suffers from an ill which is too strong for the means at the disposal of medicine, he surely must not even expect that it can be overcome by medicine."[8]

The Hippocratic physician was acutely aware that his therapeutic powers were limited by the forces of nature. The repetition and the austere tone of the injunction to restrain one's therapy in the face of the overwhelming power of nature and not to exceed the possibilities of the medical art elevate the counsel beyond a suggestion about technique to a moral direction; for the physician to have exceeded the possibilities of his art was to commit the sin of hubris.

Still, the reluctance of the Hippocratic physician to offend nature and to stretch the limits of his art was made easier by his knowledge that the patient had several alternatives when medicine seemed powerless and the physician could no longer help him: the patient could turn to other resources for help. He could resort to prayers and incantations. As Plutarch wrote: "Those who are ill with chronic diseases and do not succeed by the usual remedies and the customary diet turn to purifications and amulets and dreams."[9] Patients could also resort to suicide, a socially accepted escape from a life heavily burdened by disease both among those with philosophical training and among average people. Euripides wrote referring to people who patiently endured long illness: "I hate the men who would prolong their lives/ By foods and drinks and charms of magic art,/ Perverting nature's course to keep off death;/ They ought, when they no longer serve the land,/ To quit this life, and clear the way for youth."[10] Knowledge of the alternatives outside of medicine available to patients doubtless helped to relieve the physician of responsibility and to ease his conscience.

Prior to the twentieth century, physicians treated disturbances of the physiological functions of the body mainly with diet, drugs, blood-letting, and physical therapies such as bathing, massage, and exercise. The principal use of technology in medical therapy was in surgery, which was generally employed to treat wounds, injuries to bones, and lesions on the outer surface of the body such as ulcers and tumors. In the Greco-Roman period, instruments for such purposes were constructed, made of iron, steel, bronze, even gold and silver. Over the centuries surgical technologies grew in kind and number. For example, a 1674 treatise called *The Chyrurgeons Store-House* describes fifteen sorts of forceps, eleven sorts of knives, five sorts of needles; it describes lancets designed to perforate tissue and "pinchers" to extract teeth or draw out bones sticking in the throat.[11] Such an armory of instruments often frightened the patient, and surgeons were advised to consider this problem in preparing to operate. A French surgeon writing in the early eighteenth century tells us:

> 'Tis customary to send to the Patient's Chamber (some time before the Chirurgeon comes) a Servant to dispose all things in order; but frequently, by the quantity of bits of Linnen which they cut, the heaps of Lint which they make, and the spreading shew of numerous Instruments, they strike Fear and Terror into the Mind of the Patient, by giving him a cruel Idea of the Operation which they are going about. I would that the Chirurgeons would not shew themselves to their Patients, 'till the Moment appointed for the Operation; and that all things which they want, were ready prepar'd at their own Houses, or in a Chamber near the Patient, in order to spare him the sight of those Preparatives, which only inspire him with a Horror for those who make them. . . . A Chirurgeon must be naturally dextrous in Operation, and that Address must be back'd with great Experience in his Profession; whence he should learn how to place his Subject, to chuse the most proper Instruments, to invent new ones in particular Cases, and to make use of them in such a manner as shall contribute as much to the easing of the Patient, as the Satisfaction of the Spectators.[12]

In the nineteenth century, commercial firms were founded to manufacture a large number of surgical instruments. Before this time, they had usually been produced by individuals, mostly instrument makers by trade. Yet not until the end of the nineteenth century, when the problems of pain, infection, and bleeding could be handled effectively, was surgical technology widely employed to enter the interior of the body and treat a large variety of medical problems.

Machines that sustain vital physiological functions such as breathing (the mechanical respirator) or help to remove the waste products of metabolism (the artificial kidney) are essentially inventions of the twentieth century and are among the vanguard of its therapeutic technology. The manual methods of artifical respiration used in the early twentieth century were unsuited to long-term administration. And the few machines that existed to assist respiration, such as one called a pulmotor, were ineffective and sometimes injured patients. This created a need for a reliable mechanical device capable of steady work over long periods of time, which would facilitate breathing without harming the patient. The forerunners of such reliable machines, from which the respirators that sustained Karen Quinlan evolved, were the iron lungs built in the late nineteen-twenties. One of the earliest iron lungs was constructed in 1928 by the Americans Philip Drinker and Louis Shaw to alleviate the respiratory failure caused by poliomyelitis. In their first clinical test of the machine, the breathing of an eight-year-old girl afflicted with polio was maintained for 122 hours. But she succumbed to complications of her illness.[13]

A second machine that has become an important part of medical therapy is the artificial kidney, designed to cleanse the blood of waste products unexpelled when kidney function is seriously impaired. Experiments to develop an artificial kidney began in 1913. They failed for lack of a reliable drug to prevent the coagulation of the blood passed through the machine, lack of a good membrane through which the waste products could be filtered out of the blood, and the insufficient capacity of the early equipment. Willem Kolff, a Dutch physician, solved these problems and built the first clinically useful artificial kidney in Holland between 1940 and 1943. Kolff's machine could not be credited with preventing the death or producing the recovery of the first sixteen patients on which it was used. Success came only with the seventeenth patient, whose kidney function had temporarily failed as the result of an infection. After more than 11 hours on the artificial kidney, her condition improved dramatically. "The first understandable words she spoke that I remember," wrote Kolff, "were that she was going to divorce her husband, which indeed in time she did. Further recovery was uneventful."[14]

Since the nineteen-sixties, the growing availability of technological aids such as artificial respirators and artificial kidneys has engendered in both physicians and laymen a searching examination of the moral principles that should guide medical decisions. This examination, whose depth and intensity is unparalleled in medical history, has had as one of its underlying themes the notion of limits. A humility has been urged upon medicine to match the considerable technological power it has created to overcome the natural forces that produce illness. These cautionary observations are similar to those of modern ecologists, who are urging us to act with humility in dealing with the natural world. The contemporary movement in medical ethics in part asks physicians who control a powerful technological store of therapy to consider, as the ancient Greeks did, the limits imposed on therapeutic undertakings by the biological make-up of man, and the moral and therapeutic consequences of accepting these limits.

The modern patient, disquieted by recent developments, has also been prompted to consider the problem of placing limits on the use of therapeutic technology. An example is the "living will" that a number of people in the nineteen-seventies have been making up. These wills are documents in which a person can stipulate the sort of care he wishes if afflicted by an irremediable illness which might, at some stage, incapacitate and prevent him from expressing his therapeutic preferences. The wills are intended strongly to request, but not to compel, physicians to follow, if not the letter, then at least the spirit of the wishes expressed in them. To draw public attention to these documents and to enhance their legal status, some lawmakers have submitted them to state legislatures for certification. One such living will, considered but not adopted by the Massachusetts legislature in 1974, reads in part:

> The availability of medical technology does not eliminate the need for human choices regarding its use. This is especially true when a patient is irreversibly ill. The decision to cease employment of artificial means or heroic measures to prolong the life of the body belongs to the patient and/or the immediate family with the approval of the family physician. . . . In order that the rights of patients may be respected even after they are no longer able to participate actively in decisions about themselves, they may choose to indicate their wishes regarding refusal of treatment in a written statement, as follows. . . . "If there is no reasonable expectation of my recovery from physical or mental disability, as certified by two physicians, I, _____, request that I be allowed to die and not be kept alive by artificial means or heroic measures. I value life and the dignity of life, so that I am not asking that my life be directly taken, but that my dying not be unreasonably prolonged, nor the dignity of life destroyed. . . ."[15]

The availability of therapeutic technology has also prompted concern by society that touches limits of another kind—financial. For example, in the mid-nineteen-sixties, when the demand grew for artificial-kidney machines among people with chronic and potentially fatal kidney disease, a patient treated twice weekly with the machine at the Veterans Hospital in Los Angeles could run up a bill of twenty-eight thousand dollars a year.[16] Because of the high cost, and the inadequate supply of artificial kidneys in relation to the demand for them, sometimes certain patients were given preferences over other patients in allocating the scarce therapeutic resource. The distributive decisions made by an advisory committee at the Seattle Artificial Kidney Center, composed of physicians and laymen who were supposed to represent the public interest, received wide publicity because the committee's decisions represented one of the first modern peace-time efforts to allocate important but scarce medical resources among specific individuals. The Center developed a set of admission criteria which it followed closely. They were essentially: a slow deterioration of renal function; an absence of longstanding hypertension and its permanent complications; the patient's emotional maturity and responsibility; his demonstrated willingness to cooperate; a "physiological" age of between 17 and 50; six months' residence in the five-state area around Seattle; the amount of his financial resources; his value to the community; potential for rehabilitation; and psychological and psychiatric status. In addition to this advisory committee on which laymen sat, all candidates for kidney machines were reviewed by a medical committee and the Center's medical director. A physician at the Center discussed some of the patients who were rejected in this selection process:

> There was the beatnik—in his mid-twenties, doing poorly in college (in spite of considerable effort on the part of the faculty sponsor), poor job record, and apparently without funds or plans for the future. He just did not seem to fulfill the criteria of value to the community and rehabilitation potential. There was the lady of ill repute (a veritable Camille) and altho she had plenty of financial support, it was not felt that she could be considered a responsible citizen and her potential (interest) for rehabilitation seemed limited. A final example is the logger who seemed to qualify in every way, except that our staff and his employer simply were unable to put together any semblance of a financial package for his continued care. He expired the same day a letter of rejection and explanation went to his wife. . . . Rejection invariably has called forth lengthy soul-searching by the various deliberative bodies. In a sense rejection has made some of the staff feel they have failed the candidate. We have been accused of "playing God" by this process of selection, but with limited facilities and limited financial backing and nowhere else to turn for help, we experienced (many of us for the first time) the choice of taking patients on a first come, first served basis or by means of a super-triage system. We elected the latter course. Altho it may smack of smugness, we have been fairly well satisfied with our procedure. . . .[17]

The decision process used at the Seattle Center evoked a variety of reactions. Many questioned the standards used to make these life and death determinations. The Center's emphasis on social and economic considerations in making their choices drew particular criticism. An article published in the *UCLA Law Review* in 1968 by a physician and an attorney characterized the selection process as a "disturbing picture of the bourgeoisie sparing the bourgeoisie."[18] A number of the decisions made by the Seattle Center seemed to penalize non-conformity, and the authors commented that "the Pacific Northwest is no place for a Henry David Thoreau with bad kidneys."[19]

One ethicist strongly argued, in 1970, that when determinations which involve the sacrificing of life must be made, procedures which require human choices should yield to procedures which produce random choices, such as a lottery or a first-come, first-served method. If the value of human life transcends all other values, then it should not be subjected to a bartering strategy in which one person's worth is weighed against another's. Random selection seemed preferable, "because we have no way of knowing how really and truly to estimate a man's societal worth or his worth to others or to himself. . . . When tragically not all can be saved the rule of practice must be the equality of one life with every other life. . . ."[20] Popular literature discussed the Center's deliberations in articles often having provocative titles such as "They Decide Who Lives, Who Dies"[21] and "The Rest Are Simply Left to Die."[22]

Because many people were deeply disturbed by such allocative problems and some of the decisions they generated, the United States Congress, in 1972, passed legislation which required the federal government to assume financial responsibility for almost all patients who needed treatment with the artificial kidney, or who required a kidney transplantation.[23] By 1975, over 20,000 patients were receiving kidney dialysis. But its annual price, in excess of $300 million, surpassed original estimates by approximately 50 per cent.[24] The cost overruns of the artificial kidney program, as well as of government programs, such as Medicare and Medicaid, that subsidize general health needs, have created a quandary for our society as we decide how to match almost limitless health-care needs with limited medical resources, and all in the context of a strongly held belief in the United States that health care is a social right. Interpretation of the meaning of this right is controversial. However, one can think of it not as a right to all the medical assistance that it is possible to receive (health care like all other things of value is limited), but rather a right of equal access to any national program of health benefits enacted, whatever its limits may be.[25]

Although technology has enabled the modern physician to advance beyond the therapeutic boundaries of his predecessors, he faces perplexing questions about the goals of its use. Moreover complicated and expensive apparatus and finding or training the experts needed to run it have created a problem of scarcity in relation to demand, and dilemmas of allocation and selection have become increasingly common features of medical care. These problems have helped to reveal that scientific and technological advances alone cannot produce optimum medical care. It is paradoxical, perhaps, that to apply the creations of our newest scientific disciplines, physicians must reexamine the moral principles by which they act, and turn to ethics, one of our oldest humanistic disciplines.

REFERENCES

[1]Pope Pius XII, "The Prolongation of Life," *The Pope Speaks*, 4 (1958), pp. 393-98.

[2]*Ibid.*, p. 398.

[3]"A Definition of Irreversible Coma: Report of the Ad Hoc Committee of the Harvard Medical School to Examine the Definition of Brain Death," *Journal of the American Medical Association*, 205 (1968), pp. 337-40.

[4]*In the Matter of Karen Quinlan, An Alleged Incompetent*, 348 A. 2d 801 at 818 (1976).

[5]*In the Matter of Karen Quinlan, An Alleged Incompetent*, 355 A. 2d 647 at 663 (1976).

[6]*Ibid.*, 355 A. 2d at 665 (1976).

[7]W. H. S. Jones, *Hippocrates*, 2 (Cambridge, Mass., 1923), p. 193.

[8]*Ibid.*, pp. 203, 205.

[9]Ludwig Edelstein, "Greek Medicine in Its Relation to Religion and Magic," in Owsei Temkin and C. Lilian Temkin, eds., *Ancient Medicine: Selected Papers of Ludwig Edelstein* (Baltimore, 1967), p. 245. A valuable discussion of Greek medicine is also found in P. Lain Entralgo, *Doctor and Patient* (New York, 1969).

[10]Ludwig Edelstein, "The Distinctive Hellenism of Greek Medicine," in Temkin and Temkin, *Ancient Medicine*, p. 382.

[11]Johannes Scultetus, *The Chyrurgeons Store-House* (London, 1674).

[12]Pierre Dionis, *A Course of Chirurgical Operations, Demonstrated in the Royal Garden At Paris* (London, 1710), pp. 8-9.

[13]Philip Drinker and Charles F. McKhann, "The Use of a New Apparatus for the Prolonged Administration of Artificial Respiration," *Journal of the American Medical Association*, 92 (1929), pp. 1658-60.

[14]Willem J. Kolff, "First Clinical Experience with the Artificial Kidney," *Annals of Internal Medicine*, 62 (1963), p. 617.

[15]John S. Ames, III, "An Act Relating to Certain Medical Treatment," Legislative Proposal to Commonwealth of Massachusetts, 1974. Further discussion of the living will and a proposed new document is found in Sissela Bok. "Patient Directions for Care at the End of Life," *New England Journal of Medicine*, 295 (1976), pp. 367-69.

[16]David Sanders and Jesse Dukeminier, Jr., "Medical Advance and Legal Lag: Hemodialysis and Kidney Transplantation," *UCLA Law Review*, 15 (1968), p. 362.

[17]James W. Haviland, "Experiences in Establishing a Community Artificial Kidney Center," *Transactions of the American Clinical and Climatological Association*, 77 (1966), pp. 133-34.

[18]Sanders and Dukeminier, "Medical Advance and Legal Lag," p. 378.

[19]*Ibid.*

[20]Paul Ramsey, *The Patient as Person* (New Haven, 1970), pp. 256, 259.

[21]Shana Alexander, "They Decide Who Lives, Who Dies," *Life*, November 9, 1962, p. 102.

[22]Jhan Robbins and June Robbins, "The Rest Are Simply Left to Die," *Redbook*, November, 1967, p. 81.

[23]U.S. Congress, *Social Security Amendments*, Public Law 92-603, Sec. 299I, 92nd Cong., 1st Sess., 1972.

[24]*New York Times*, September 25, 1975, p. 24.

[25]See, for an excellent analysis of this issue, David Mechanic, "Rationing Health Care: Public Policy and the Medical Market Place," *Hastings Center Report*, 6:1 (February, 1976), pp. 34-37; Charles Fried, "Equality and Rights in Medical Care," *ibid.*, pp. 29-34; and Eugene Outka, "Social Justice and Equal Access to Health Care," *Journal of Religious Ethics*, 2:1 (1974), pp. 11-32.

JOHN H. KNOWLES, M.D.

The Responsibility of the Individual

THE HEALTH OF HUMAN BEINGS IS DETERMINED by their behavior, their food, and the nature of their environment. The first agricultural revolution occurred 10,000 years ago with the domestication of plants and animals. Nomadic hunter-gatherers settled around their flocks and fields. Nutrition improved, with a resultant fall in mortality and rise in birth rates. The population expanded, but its growth was checked periodically by crop failures and famine, tribal war over scarce resources, infectious disease now easily transmitted by air, water, and food among settled people, and the common practice of infanticide. The population was under 10 million people.

By 1750, the number of people in the world had grown to 750 million, by 1830 to one billion, by 1930 to two billion, by 1960 to three billion, and then to four billion today. This massive growth of population resulted from the fall in mortality rates attendant upon steadily increasing food supplies. Improved nutrition again increased birth rates and resistance to infectious disease. The greater availability of food also reduced the practice of infanticide.

The second agricultural revolution had begun in the eighteenth century; it included increased land use, extensive manuring to restore soil fertility, crop rotation, winter feeding, and the widespread cultivation of potatoes and maize. A massive increase in available food was extended still further by the Industrial Revolution of the nineteenth and twentieth centuries through mechanization, extensive irrigation, chemical fertilizers, and pesticides. The "Green Revolution" of the past thirty years further increased food production, and was based on genetic manipulations which produced hardier and more productive varieties of crops, responsive to the more intensive use of water and fertilizer.

More than half the reduction in mortality rates over the past three centuries occurred before 1900 and was due in nearly equal measure to improved nutrition and reduced exposure to air-and water-borne infection. The provision of safe water and milk supplies, the improvement in both personal and food hygiene, and the efficient disposal of sewage all helped to reduce the incidence of infectious disease. Vaccination further reduced mortality rates from smallpox in the nineteenth century and from diphtheria, pertussis, tetanus, poliomyelitis, measles, and tuberculosis in the twentieth century, although the contribution of vaccinations to the overall reduction in mortality rates over the past hundred years is small (perhaps as small as 10 per cent) as contrasted with that due to improved nutrition and reduction in the transmission of infectious disease.[1] An even smaller contribution has been made by

the introduction of medical and surgical therapy, namely antibiotics and the excision
of tumors, in the twentieth century.

Over the past 100 years, infanticide has declined in the developed countries as
changes in reproductive practice, such as the use of contraceptives, have been
introduced to contain family size and reduce national growth rates of population, thus
sustaining the improvement in health and standards of living. The population of
England and Wales trebled between 1700 and 1850 without any significant importation of food. If the birth rate had been maintained, the population by now would be
some 140 million instead of the 46 million it actually is. Changes in reproductive
behavior maintained a rough balance between food production and population growth
and allowed standards of living to rise. A similarly remarkable change in reproductive
behavior occurred in Ireland following the potato famines of the eighteen-forties, and
birth rates have been sustained voluntarily at a low level to this day in that largely
Catholic country.

Improvement in health resulted from changes in personal behavior (hygiene,
reproductive practices) and in environmental conditions (food supplies, provision of
safe milk and water, and sewage disposal). Cartesian rationalism, Baconian empiricism, and the results of the Industrial Revolution led the medical profession into
scientific and technical approaches to disease. The engineering approach to the
human machine was strengthened by the germ theory of disease which followed the
work of Pasteur and Koch in the late nineteenth century. The idea was simple,
unitary, and compelling: one germ—one disease—one therapy. Population factors,
personal behavior, and environmental conditions were neglected in such a pure model
or paradigm of approach and were picked up by elements less powerful and perceived
increasingly as marginal to health, i.e., politicians, state departments, and schools of
public health. The medical profession hitched its wagon to the rising stars of science
and technology. The results have been spectacular for some individuals in terms of
cure, containment of disease, and alleviation of suffering; as spectacular in terms of
the horrendous costs compounding now at a rate of 15 per cent annually; and even
more spectacular to some because allocation of more and more men and women,
money, and machines has affected mortality and morbidity rates only marginally.
The problem of diminishing returns, if current trends continue, will loom as large
and pregnant to the American people in the future as the mushrooming atomic cloud
does today.

I will not berate the medical profession, its practitioners and its professors—they
reflect our culture, its values, beliefs, rites, and symbols. Central to the culture is faith
in progress through science, technology, and industrial growth; increasingly peripheral to it is the idea, vis-à-vis health, that over 99 per cent of us are born healthy and
made sick as a result of personal misbehavior and environmental conditions. The
solution to the problems of ill health in modern American society involves individual
responsibility, in the first instance, and social responsibility through public legislative
and private voluntary efforts, in the second instance. Alas, the medical profession
isn't interested, because the intellectual, emotional, and financial rewards of the
present system are too great and because there is no incentive and very little demand
to change. But the problems of rising costs; the allocation of scarce national resources
among competing claims for improving life; diminishing returns on health from the
system of acute, curative, high-cost, hospital-based medicine; and increasing evidence
that personal behavior, food, and the nature of the environment around us are the

prime determinants of health and disease will present us with critical choices and will inevitably force change.

Most individuals do not worry about their health until they lose it. Uncertain attempts at healthy living may be thwarted by the temptations of a culture whose economy depends on high production and high consumption. Asceticism is reserved for hair-shirted clerics and constipated cranks, and everytime one of them dies in the age of 50, the hedonist smiles, inhales deeply, and takes another drink. Everyone is a gambler and knows someone who has lived it up and hit 90 years, so bad nurture doesn't necessarily spell doom. For others, a genetic fatalism takes hold: Nature—your parents' genes—will decide your fate no matter what you do. For those who remain undecided, there is always the reassuring story—and we all know it—of someone with living parents who has led a temperate, viceless life and died of a heart attack at the age of 45. As for stress, how about Winston Churchill at the age of 90! And he drank brandy, smoked cigars, never exercised, and was grossly overweight! Facing the insufferable insult of extinction with the years, and knowing how we might improve our health, we still don't do much about it. The reasons for this peculiar behavior may include: (1) a denial of death and disease coupled with the demand for instant gratification and the orientation of most people in most cultures to living day by day; (2) the feeling that nature, including death and disease, can be conquered through scientific and technologic advance or overcome by personal will; (3) the dispiriting conditions of old people leads to a decision by some that they don't want infirmities and unhappiness and would just as soon die early; (4) chronic depression in some individuals to the extent that they wish consciously or unconsciously for death and have no desire to take care of themselves; and (5) the disinterest of the one person to whom we ascribe the ultimate wisdom about health—the physician.

Prevention of disease means forsaking the bad habits which many people enjoy—overeating, too much drinking, taking pills, staying up at night, engaging in promiscuous sex, driving too fast, and smoking cigarettes—or, put another way, it means doing things which require special effort—exercising regularly, going to the dentist, practicing contraception, ensuring harmonious family life, submitting to screening examinations. The idea of individual responsibility flies in the face of American history which has seen a people steadfastly sanctifying individual freedom while progressively narrowing it through the development of the beneficent state. On the one hand, Social Darwinism maintains its hold on the American mind despite the best intentions of the neo-liberals. Those who aren't supine before the Federal Leviathan proclaim the survival of the fittest. On the other, the idea of individual responsibility has been submerged to individual rights—rights, or demands, to be guaranteed by government and delivered by public and private institutions. The cost of sloth, gluttony, alcoholic intemperance, reckless driving, sexual frenzy, and smoking is now a national, and not an individual, responsibility. This is justified as individual freedom—but one man's freedom in health is another man's shackle in taxes and insurance premiums. I believe the idea of a "right" to health should be replaced by the idea of an individual moral obligation to preserve one's own health—a public duty if you will. The individual then has the "right" to expect help with information, accessible services of good quality, and minimal financial barriers. Meanwhile, the people have been led to believe that national health insurance, more doctors, and greater use of high-cost, hospital-based technologies will improve health. Unfortunately none of them will.

More and more the artificer of the possible is "society"—not the individual; he thereby becomes more dependent on things external and less on his own inner resources. The paranoid style of consumer groups demands a fight against something, usually a Big Bureaucracy. In the case of health, it is the hospitals, the doctors, the medical schools, the Medicaid-Medicare combine, the government. Nader's Raiders have yet to allow that the next major advances in the health of the American people will come from the assumption of individual responsibility for one's own health and a necessary change in habits for the majority of Americans. We do spend over $30 billion annually for cigarettes and whiskey.

The behavior of Americans might be changed if there were adequate programs of health education in primary and secondary schools and even colleges—but there aren't. School health programs are abysmal at best, confining themselves to preemptory sick calls and posters on brushing teeth and eating three meals a day; there are no examinations to determine if anything's been learned. Awareness of danger to body and mind isn't acquired until the mid-twenties in our culture, and by then patterns of behavior are set which are hard to change. Children tire of "scrub your teeth," "don't eat that junk," "leave your dingy alone," "go to bed," and "get some exercise." By the time they are sixteen, society says they shall have cars, drink beer, smoke, eat junk at drive-ins, and have a go at fornication. If they demur, they are sissies or queer or both. The pressure of the peer group to do wrong is hardly balanced by the limp protestations of permissive parents, nervously keeping up with the Joneses in suburban ranch houses crammed with snacks and mobile bars.

The barriers to the assumption of individual responsibility for one's own health are lack of knowledge (implicating the inadequacies of formal education, the all-too-powerful force of advertising, and of the informal systems of continuing education), lack of sufficient interest in, and knowledge about, what is preventable and the "cost-to-benefit" ratios of nationwide health programs (thereby implicating all the powerful interests in the health establishment, which couldn't be less interested, and calling for a much larger investment in fundamental and applied research), and a culture which has progressively eroded the idea of individual responsibility while stressing individual rights, the responsibility of society-at-large, and the steady growth of production and consumption ("We have met the enemy and it is us!"). Changing human behavior involves sustaining and repeating an intelligible message, reinforcing it through peer pressure and approval, and establishing clearly perceived rewards which materialize in as short a time as possible. Advertising agencies know this, but it is easier to sell deodorants, pantyhose, and automobiles than it is health.

What is the problem? During the nineteenth and early twentieth centuries, communicable disease was the major health problem in the United States. In 1900, the average life expectancy at birth was 49.2 years. By 1966, it had increased to 70.1 years, due mainly to marked reduction in infant and child mortality (between birth and age 15). By mid-century, accidents were by far the leading cause of death in youngsters, and the majority of accidents were related to excessive use of alcohol by their parents, by adults generally, and even occasionally by themselves. While 21 years were added to life expectancy at birth, only 2.7 years were added to it at age 65—the remaining life expectancy at age 65 being 11.9 years in 1900 and 14.6 in 1966. The marked increase in life expectancy at birth was due to the control and eradication of infectious disease, directly through improved nutrition and personal hygiene, and environmental changes, namely, the provision for safe water and milk supplies and for sewage disposal.

Today, the major health problems in the United States are the chronic diseases of middle and later age, mainly heart disease, cancer, and strokes. Death and disability in middle age is premature and potentially preventable. For those under 44 years, the leading causes of death are accidents, heart disease, cancer, homicide, and suicide. For those under 25 years, accidents are by far the most common cause of death, with homicide and suicide the next leading causes. Of the roughly 2 million deaths in the United States in 1969, 50 per cent were due to heart disease (40%) and strokes (10%); 16 per cent to cancer; and 8 per cent to accidents (6%), homicide (1%), and suicide (1%). But death statistics tell only a small part of the story. For every successful suicide, an estimated ten others, or 200,000 people, have made the attempt. For every death due to accidents, hundreds of others are injured, and many of those are permanently disabled. Over 17 per cent, or 36 million people, have serious disabilities limiting their activities.

Premature death and disability are far too common. For the 178,000 people between the ages of 45 and 64 years who died of heart disease in 1969, 1.2 million (or 3 per cent of the 40.5 million people in this age group) were chronically disabled because of heart disease.[2] For the over 30,000 people who died of cirrhosis of the liver in 1969—a disease related directly to excessive ingestion of alcohol together with poor nutrition—as many as 10 million people suffer from alcoholism and varying degrees of malnutrition. Twenty-six million Americans, 11 million of whom receive no federal food assistance, live below the federally defined poverty level, a level which does not support an adequate diet.

The control of communicable disease depended as much (or even more) on broad changes in the environment attendant upon economic development (improved housing and nutrition, sanitary engineering for safe water supplies, and sewage disposal) as it did on the individual's knowledge and behavior (need for immunization, personal hygiene, and cooperation with case finding). However, control of the present major health problems in the United States depends directly on modification of the individual's behavior and habits of living. The need for improved nutrition remains unchanged. The knowledge required to persuade the individual to change his habits is far more complex, far less dramatic in its results, far more difficult to organize and convey—in short, far less appealing and compelling than the need for immunization, getting rid of sewage, and drinking safe water. Even the problems of immunizing the population in contemporary America are difficult, however—witness the failure to eradicate measles ten years after the technical means became available.

Studies by Breslow and Belloc[3] of nearly 7,000 adults followed for five and one-half years showed that life expectancy and health are significantly related to the following basic health habits:

1) three meals a day at regular times and no snacking;
2) breakfast every day;
3) moderate exercise two or three times a week;
4) adequate sleep (7 or 8 hours a night);
5) no smoking;
6) moderate weight;
7) no alcohol or only in moderation.

A 45-year-old man who practices 0-3 of these habits has a remaining life expectancy of 21.6 years (to age 67), while one with 6-7 of these habits has a life expectancy of 33.1 years (to age 78). In other words, 11 years could be added to life expectancy by relatively simple changes in habits of living, recalling that only 2.7 years were added to the life expectancy at age 65 between 1900 and 1966. Breslow also found that the health status of those who practiced all seven habits was similar to those 30 years younger who observed none.

A large percentage of deaths (estimates up to 80 per cent) due to cardiovascular disease and cancer are "premature," that is, occur in relatively young individuals and are related to the individual's bad habits. Heart disease and strokes are related to dietary factors, cigarette smoking, potentially treatable but undetected hypertension, and lack of exercise. Cancer is related to smoking (oral, buccal, lung, and bladder cancer) and probably to diets rich in fat and refined foodstuffs and low in residue (gastrointestinal and perhaps breast and prostatic cancer) and to the ingestion of food additives and certain drugs, or the inhalation of a wide variety of noxious agents. Certain occupational exposures and personal hygienic factors account for a small but important fraction of the total deaths due to cancer. Theoretically, all deaths due to accidents, homicide, and suicide are preventable.

Stress appears to play a critical role in disease. The stress of adjusting to change may generate a wide variety of diseases, and change is the hallmark of modern society. It is known that the death rate for widows and widowers is 10 times higher in the first year of bereavement than it is for others of comparable age; in the year following divorce the divorced persons have 12 times the incidence of disease that married persons have. People living in primitive societies insulated from change have low blood pressures and blood cholesterol levels which do not vary from youth to old age. Blood pressure and cholesterol tend to rise with age in our culture and are thought to be a prime cause of heart attacks and strokes. Studies indicate that up to 80 per cent of serious physical illnesses seem to develop at a time when the individual feels helpless or hopeless. Studies on cancer patients have revealed lives marked by chronic anxiety, depression, or hostility and a lack of close emotional ties with parents—significantly greater than in a control group.

Despite the well-known hazards of smoking, per-capita consumption of cigarettes is expected to increase in 1975-76 after having been relatively stable between 1963—when the Surgeon General sounded the warning against smoking—and 1973, at 211 packs annually per person over 18 years. Some 15 per cent of boys and girls under 18 years smoke cigarettes. Cigarette production is increasing at about 3.5 per cent per year due to population growth and to a marked increase in smoking in teenage girls, which has risen from 8 to 15 per cent in the past several years. If cigarette smoking were to be eliminated entirely, a 20 per cent reduction in deaths due to cancer would result (based on the assumption that 85 per cent of lung cancer is causally related to cigarette smoking). If all contributing environmental factors and personal bad health habits were eliminated, it is possible that cancer could be virtually eliminated as a cause of death. This would increase the average life expectancy at birth by 6 to 7 years, and at age 65 by 1.4 years for men and 2.1 years for women. The use of averages gives an erroneous impression, however, for one out of six people die of cancer. The elimination of cancer would mean that one out of six people would live 10.8 years longer.

Bad nutritional status (of the too-much-fat-intake-resulting-in-obesity type) can predispose the individual to heart attacks, strokes, cancer of the gastrointestinal tract, diabetes, liver and gall-bladder disease, degenerative arthritis of the hips, knees, and ankles, and injuries. It is estimated that 16 per cent of Americans under the age of 30 years are obese, while 40 per cent of the total population, or 80 million Americans, are 20 or more pounds above the ideal weight for their height, sex, and age. Over 30 per cent of all men between 50 and 59 years are 20 per cent overweight and 60 per cent are at least 10 per cent overweight.

Excessive use of alcohol is directly related to accidents and to liver disease (cirrhosis) as well as to a wide variety of other disorders, including vitamin deficiencies, inflammation of the pancreas, esophagus, and stomach, and muscular and neurologic diseases. Alcohol is a strong "risk factor" in cancer of the mouth, pharynx, larynx, and esophagus. More than 50 per cent and probably nearer to 75 per cent of all deaths and injuries due to automobile accidents are associated with the excessive use of alcohol. Alcoholism in one or both parents is significantly associated with home injuries to children (more than 50 per cent in some studies). The prevalence of "heavy-escape" drinkers in the United States has been estimated at 6.5 million people (5.4 per cent of total adult population), and the figures for those who use alcohol chronically and excessively range up to 10 million adults. Teenage drinking is now nearly universal. A study of high school students revealed that 36 per cent reported getting drunk at least four times a year (remember, 15 per cent smoke!). An increased frequency of cancer of the mouth, pharynx, larynx, and esophagus is seen in those who both smoke and drink and is less frequent, but still significantly higher than normal, in those who only smoke or only drink.

Dietary factors play a major role in cardiovascular disease and cancer. The major variable, as deduced from studies of migrant populations, seems to be fat content. For example, cancer of the large bowel as well as that of the breast and prostate is much more common in the United States than in Japan, and seems to be related to the difference in fat intake. The American derives 40 to 45 per cent of his calories from fat, whereas the Japanese obtains only 15 to 20 per cent of his calories from that source. Japanese descendants living in the United States have an incidence of bowel cancer similar to that seen in native Americans. Although the mechanism has not been established, it would appear that high fat intake (usually with resultant obesity) predisposes the American to both cancer and cardiovascular disease. Data from a long-term study of cardiovascular disease in Framingham, Massachusetts, indicate that each 10 per cent reduction in weight in men 35-55 years old would result in a 20 per cent decrease in the incidence of coronary disease. A 10 per cent increase in weight would result in a 30 per cent increase in coronary disease.[4]

The incidence of cancer of the colon and rectum in Americans both white and black is 10 times the incidence estimated for rural Africans. The removal of dietary fiber and a high intake of refined carbohydrates typical of diets in developed countries such as the United States result in a slowed transit time of food through the intestines. This is thought to facilitate the development of cancer, along with such diseases as diverticulitis, appendicitis, and even hemorrhoids. Prudence would dictate a reduction in fat and refined carbohydrates (and therefore increased fiber content) in the American diet. High-carbohydrate diets typical in the American culture also lead to dental caries, and may, over time, increase the risk of acquiring diabetes.

Knowledge of cancer and evidence for its multiple causes have increased to the point where the statement can be made with confidence that over 80 per cent of human neoplasms depend either directly or indirectly on environmental factors. The term "environmental factors" includes cancer-provoking substances or carcinogens in the food and the drugs we ingest, the air we breathe, the water we drink, the occupations we pursue, and the habits we indulge. There are three major groups at high risk of cancer: (1) those with known host factors such as genetic and other congenital defects and immunologic-deficiency diseases; (2) those with exposure to environmental contaminants known to produce cancer; and (3) those with certain demographic characteristics which reflect as yet unknown carcinogenic factors such as place of residence or migration.[5]

The familial occurrence of cancer is a well-known phenomenon. A significant two to four times excess occurrence in relatives of patients has been noted in cancer of the stomach, breast, large intestine, uterus, and lung. Increased familial incidence has also been noted in leukemia, brain tumors in children, and sarcomas. Individuals with hereditary deficiencies of the immune system of the body develop malignant diseases of the blood vessels and lymphatic system. Acquired immunodeficiency also leads to the development of cancer. When patients with kidney transplants are given drugs over a long time to suppress the immune system in order to prevent rejection of the grafted kidney, cancer of the lymphatic system (lymphoma of the reticulum-cell-sarcoma type), frequently confined to the brain, and cancer of the skin develop in a significant proportion of the patients. Women who have had genital herpes (herpes simplex virus 2) have an increased incidence of cancer of the cervix of the uterus and constitute a high-risk population. People with pernicious anemia with associated gastritis develop cancer of the stomach at five times the rate of the normal population. Cirrhosis is associated with an increased incidence of cancer of the liver. Patients with diabetes have two times the incidence of cancer of the pancreas as normal individuals. The presence of gallstones and kidney stones increases the risk of developing cancer in the respective organs. Single episodes of trauma have been implicated in cancer of the bone, breast, and testicles. Chronic irritation of a skin mole may lead to cancerous degeneration, called malignant melanoma.

Environmental factors include tobacco, alcohol, radiation, occupation, drugs, air pollutants, diet, viruses, and other organisms, and sexual factors. The evidence on cigarette smoking is incontrovertible. It greatly increases the risk of lung cancer as well as cancer of the mouth, pharynx, larynx, esophagus, and urinary bladder. The incidence of cancer in cigarette smokers is higher in urban than rural dwellers, suggesting that air pollutants are additional major causative factors. Occupational exposure to asbestos fibers results in lung cancer, but here again the incidence is higher in those who smoke. Alcohol as a carcinogenic agent in malignancy of the mouth, larynx, esophagus, and liver (in association with cirrhosis) has been noted. A major long-term effect of radiation is cancer. Radiologists are ten times more likely to die of leukemia than are physicians not exposed to x-rays.

The list of drugs known or thought to be carcinogenic also continues to expand. Studies have shown that post-menopausal women given estrogens (so-called "replace-ment therapy" to diminish menopausal complaints and advertised to "keep women feminine") are five to fourteen times more likely to develop cancer of the uterus (endometrial cancer) than post-menopausal women not given the drug. (Other factors known to be associated with uterine cancer such as obesity, high blood pressure, never having borne a child, and age were not significant variables in these studies.) The risk increased with dosage size and duration of estrogen therapy. Other studies have shown beyond a doubt that the daughters of women given diethylstilbestrol (DES) during pregnancy are at higher risk of developing a rare form of cancer of the vagina. Despite this knowledge, DES is still being given to pregnant women to prevent spontaneous abortion. Most astounding has been the discovery of over 100 cases of liver tumors in women taking oral contraceptive pills. Most of the tumors were benign, but some showed cancerous degeneration and others ruptured with hemorrhage into the abdomen. Many carcinogenic agents incite the disease only many years after the initial exposure (e.g., atomic-bomb radiation) or after prolonged use, so it is not known whether an epidemic of liver tumors will ultimately develop in oral-contraceptive users. (The "pill" also causes a small but significant risk for heart attacks in users.) Long-term epidemiologic research is needed to establish knowledge necessary for control programs, but there is sufficient knowledge now to suggest that we should sharply restrict the use of many drugs.

Sexual factors (both hormonal and behavioral) play a role in the causation of cancer of the breast and uterus (cervix and body of the uterus), penis, prostate, and testis. Cancer of the cervix occurs much more frequently in women who have had many sexual partners beginning at an early age, who come from a lower socioeconomic status, and who have had infection with Herpes simplex virus type 2, which is transmitted venereally. Celibate women are at very low risk, although they are at high risk for cancer of the breast. Cancer of the penis occurs in those who have poor penile hygiene and are uncircumcised in infancy (circumcision after the age of two years does not protect against the disease).

Attempts to prevent disease and improve and maintain health involve multifaceted strategies and expertise from many disciplines. Fundamental to any and all such attempts is sufficient empirical knowledge, i.e., knowledge gained through observation and trial-and-error experimentation that allows the advocate to convey his information with sufficient conviction to change the behavior of his audience. Although a great deal of information is available, the whole field of preventive medicine and health education needs far more fundamental research and long-term field experimentation. The biological and epidemiological effects of a wide variety of pollutants, the cost-benefit ratios of many available screening services, the influence of financial sanctions on changing health behavior, the use of the mass media and their effect on cognition and behavior, the long-term effects of various therapeutic regimens on the morbidity and mortality of individuals with asymptomatic high blood pressure, the long-term effects of marked reduction of fat in the diet on the incidence of cancer and heart disease, the influence of personal income on the development of cancer and coronary disease (the death rate from both lung cancer and coronary disease is significantly lower for the affluent than for the poor) are all examples of problems that need study. These problems demand for their solution the participation and integration of the disciplines of the biological sciences, the behavioral and social sciences (social, psychology, economics, cultural anthropology, political science), and public health (epidemiology and biostatistics).

It is a sad fact that of a total annual national expenditure on health of $120 billion, only 2 to 2.5 per cent is spent on disease prevention and control measures, and only 0.5 per cent each for health education and for improving the organization and delivery of health services. The national (federal) outlay for environmental-health research is around 0.25 per cent of total health expenditures. These relatively meagre expenditures speak for the lack of interest in fields that rationally demand a much heavier commitment. The support of fundamental biomedical research has also flagged alarmingly in the past several years. The basic biological mechanisms of most of the common diseases are still not well enough known to give clear direction to preventive measures.

Strategies for improving health must include the incorporation of preventive measures into personal health services and into the environment, and individual and mass educational efforts.[6] For example, in dealing with the health problem of heart attacks, preventive measures would include screening for high-risk factors (high blood pressure, elevated blood cholesterol and fat levels, overweight, cigarette smoking, stress, and family history) and making available emergency services and measures for rapid transit to hospital-based coronary-care units; environmental measures would include altering food supply to reduce the intake of fat (i.e., those substances that raise blood cholesterol) and encouraging experiments in reducing work-related stress; and individual and mass educational efforts would include encouraging the use of screening examinations, the cessation of smoking, the maintenance of optimal weight with a balanced, low-fat diet, and obtaining regular exercise. Carrying out such a strategy involves many variables—convincing the doctor to play his pivotal role (and most medical educators and physicians are singularly uninterested in prevention), altering financing mechanisms to provide incentives to use preventive services (and most health insurance is, in fact, "disease insurance" which does not cover health education and preventive measures), and stimulating public as well as private efforts to exercise restraint on advertising and to exert positive sanctions for dissemination of health information through the mass media.

The health catastrophe related to automobile accidents presents a different type of problem. Here, personal-health services include availability of rapid transportation and first aid, emergency medical services, and definitive acute-care services in regional general hospitals; environmental measures would relate to road and highway construction (including lighting, warning signs, speed limits, safety rails), and the design and construction of automobiles for safety; and educational measures would include driver training, relicensing with eye examination, avoidance of alcohol and other drugs before driving, and reduction of speed. Which of these efforts will produce the most benefit at least cost? An interesting answer was provided during the oil-embargo energy crisis which necessitated reductions in speed limits and in the use of vehicles. The result in California was a 40 per cent reduction in death rates from automobile accidents during the month of February, 1974, as contrasted with the previous February. Accidents on the New Jersey Turnpike dropped by one-fifth from 1973 to 1974, and fatalities were down by almost one-half, the lowest figure since 1966. Meanwhile, many people won't change their habits and wear seat belts, stop drinking, or reduce speed—and are annoyed with the restrictions on their freedom when someone tries to make them.

Dental health involves the personal services of the dentist and dental hygienist, the environmental measures of fluoridation of water supplies and the dietary restriction of refined carbohydrates, and the educational measures of prudent dietary habits, brushing the teeth, and visiting the dentist regularly. Where is the greatest benefit-cost ratio to be found? There is unequivocal evidence that fluoridation of water supplies will reduce dental caries by as much as 60 per cent. It is safe and inexpensive, costing only 20 cents a year per person to prevent dental decay in children. Fluoridation of water supplies began about 1950. By 1967 over 3,000 communities with some 60 million people had adopted fluoridation. But the pace of change has slowed considerably, and the majority of people still lack fluoridated water due to fears of poisoning and resistance to what is perceived as an encroachment on their freedom. This highest benefit-cost dental-health program is still unavailable to the majority of Americans. Personal dental services are unavailable to large segments of our population and qualify as a luxury item

Conceptually, it is useful to subdivide preventive medicine into three classes: primary prevention and the measures employed to prevent disease, such as vaccination against measles; secondary prevention, that is, the early detection of disease so that active therapeutic intervention can be employed to cure or arrest the progress of the disease—examples are the detection of high blood pressure or the use of mammography to detect cancer of the breast; and tertiary prevention, which comprises those measures that will slow the progress or avoid the complications of established (chronic) disease—an example is the education of the patient with diabetes in the nature of the disease and its treatment: insulin administration, diet control, exercise, urine testing, and care of the feet. Well-conceived programs of patient education can reduce the rate of hospital readmission due to decompensation or complications of the disease by as much as 50 per cent. The statement is frequently made that if one wants to lead a long and healthy life, develop a chronic disease and take good care of it! This has to be tempered by the knowledge obtained at the McMaster University Medical Center at Hamilton, Ontario: ambulatory patients are unlikely to take more than 50 per cent of the medications prescribed for them. Nor does the degree of compliance have anything to do with how much the patient knows about his disease.

All three forms of prevention require the organization of personal health services, reinforced by environmental measures and mass education. The most good can be obtained, relative to the cost, where large populations can be reached over time, e.g., school, hospital clinic, place of work, or the doctor's office. The providers of personal health services are attuned largely to acute, curative medicine in a "complaint-responsive" system geared to the individual, and they have not assumed responsibility for health maintenance in population groups. Health (i.e., disease) insurance has solidified the behavior of both producers and consumers in such a way that neither is interested in, or rewarded for, health-maintenance efforts. A successful long-term strategy for improving and maintaining health must place equal responsibility on individual producers and individual consumers—and substantial change in the behavior of both will be required before health is improved measurably in the United States. At the moment the producers are flagellated to a fare-thee-well and studiously avoid the subject, while the consumers recognize only rights, not responsibilities.

Preventive medicine can concentrate on special disease problems (heart disease, cancer) or on special population groups largely based on age (pregnant women, school children, industrial workers). Special disease problems present a good point of departure. Their discussion exemplifies some of the complexities of developing adequate programs, both from the standpoint of needed knowledge and that of changing behavior:

Immunization against infectious disease: Vaccines are available against smallpox, mumps, rubella (German measles), measles, diphtheria, pertussis (whooping cough), tetanus, and poliomyelitis. The benefit-cost ratio favors vaccination for measles, rubella, poliomyelitis, diphtheria, pertussis, and mumps. Mumps is a minor public health problem but the ease of combining mumps vaccine with those against measles and rubella into one "shot" adds a small advantage at insignificant cost. Despite the high benefit-cost advantage of measles-rubella and poliomyelitis vaccination, the percentage of the population protected against these diseases waxes and wanes. We have not eradicated measles ten years after the technical means were made available. There was a resurgence of measles between 1969 and 1971, and, in 1974, 40 per cent of children in the critical age between 1 and 4 were not immunized against measles, and 44 per cent were unprotected against rubella. Recent declines in levels of immunization against poliomyelitis are also cause for alarm and for renewed efforts. Inadequacies in the delivery system and in the behavior of the population at large— based on everything from lack of information to superstition—are obvious, and it is not easy to improve the delivery system or change the behavior of people. Here again, more intensive research is needed on the factors that influence compliance with public health programs.

Smallpox vaccination presents an interesting and valuable lesson. By 1968, the "costs" of vaccination outweighed the benefits and included 8,024 complications, of which 152 were major, including 9 deaths (1 per million vaccinations); the last cases of smallpox in the United States were reported in 1949. Because risk of acquiring the disease is now so small and the costs of vaccination so large relative to the benefits, the United States Public Health Service and the Academy of Pediatrics recommended that routine smallpox immunization be terminated. Perhaps revaccination for hospital employees is worthwhile, but even here the risk of exposure to the disease imported from another country is minimal. Worldwide obliteration of the disease is, in fact, at hand. Recommending against smallpox vaccination is a fine example of terminating a once vital program when the costs exceed the benefits.

Venereal disease: Sexual activity seems to have increased in the United States. A marked rise in the incidence of gonorrhea and syphilis began in 1957, and the trend has continued to the present. Nearly 900,000 cases of gonorrhea and 25,000 cases of syphilis were reported in 1974. Officially reported cases represent the absolute minimum numbers affected. The Public Health Service estimated 2,700,000 new cases of gonorrhea and 80,000 new cases of syphilis in 1974. More recently, herpes virus has been added to the roster of venereal diseases, and there is evidence that hepatitis virus can be transmitted among homosexuals (the virus is present in saliva and semen). Recent surveys have indicated that asymptomatic infection with gonor-rhea exists in 1 to 5 per cent of various groups of young women, thereby maintaining a substantial reservoir of infection with which to sustain the disease at epidemic levels. Control of such epidemics is extremely difficult and includes: (1) sex education in high school (effectively prevented by horrified parents in many school districts); (2) screening of sexually active women for gonorrhea and syphilis, with treatment of the individual and active case-finding for the contacts of the individual (far too few doctors and hospital clinics and emergency wards are organized or even interested in this—and contacts don't like to be investigated!); and (3) massive public education. When the "V.D. Blues" was shown over WNET-New York several years ago, thousands thronged the clinics with the belief they had the disease. Several weeks later, attendance figures were down again. If the message is not sustained, a change in behavior will not be sustained. The issue is not just the public health problem. In 1974, there were 600,000 births to teenagers, the majority of which were illegitimate, a doubling of the figure from 1965; nearly all were unplanned and unwanted.

Increased efforts are required to control venereal disease (which would also decrease the number of illegitimate births), and a number of programs have been successful. The long-range benefits justify the costs, but the most effective ways and the most favorable benefit-cost ratios are known only theoretically. If the President of the United States declared a National V.D. Eradication Week each year, giving detailed instructions to providers and consumers, could we eliminate the disease? Or would the President be thought daft or offensive and voted out of office? Should failure to be screened annually for venereal disease be punishable by imprisonment? How many policemen and prisons would then be necessary, and would the benefits justify the costs? If the President is to use his precious time for health matters, why not give detailed instructions on heart disease, cancer, stroke, and accidents which are far more costly to our society? But then, the American people are tired of restraints on their freedom and they want a treat, not a treatment. Turn the President off! The dilemma remains: How do we maintain individual freedom and still achieve desirable social ends? How do we change behavior and reinforce individual responsibility?

High blood pressure: It is estimated that some 24 million Americans have hypertension. Nationwide surveys in 1971 showed that nearly half of those afflicted didn't know it, and only one-sixth (4 million people) were receiving adequate therapy (rest and judicious exercise, diet to reduce weight and restrict salt, reduction or avoidance of stress, and drug therapy)—this in the face of the fact that high blood pressure is the primary cause of 60,000 deaths a year and is a significant causative factor in the more than 1,500,000 heart attacks and strokes suffered annually by Americans. Screening surveys allow us to estimate that 30 per cent of the roughly one million blacks in New York City have hypertension—a disease more prevalent among blacks than whites and associated with a particularly malignant course. Approximately 1,250,000 excess deaths occur in hypertensives (blood pressure greater than 160 mm Hg systolic, 95 mm Hg diastolic) between the ages of 35 and 64 years over a 10-year period as contrasted with a comparable group with normal blood pressure. Within this age group are another 11 million persons with borderline hypertension (between 160/95 and 140/95) among whom an estimated 500,000 excess deaths occur over the 10-year period.

It is obvious that hypertension is a massive public health problem with tremendous costs, emotional and financial, to the American people. It is easy to measure the blood pressure, so why not just do it and treat the cases found? First of all, we lack sufficient knowledge to carry out the program with conviction. We should be unwilling to bear the considerable costs of detecting and then treating perhaps 10 to 15 million people (recognizing that as many as 50 per cent of them won't follow instructions anyway) to justify unknown, or at best uncertain, benefits. For example, it is known that detection and treatment of those with diastolic pressure above 115 mm Hg reduce morbidity and mortality. It is not known whether those with milder degrees of hypertension (diastolic pressure 95 to 110 mm Hg) will benefit from treatment. In the absence of this information (and long-range studies are currently being conducted by the Veterans Administration), the costs cannot be justified, and the mass screening of millions of people is simply not worth the effort. Assuming that it was worth the effort, we would then face the knotty problems of public education and compliance with therapeutic regimens, to say nothing of the need for new facilities and manpower-training programs. The balance of costs and benefits must be known, and this requires further research.

In the meantime, maintaining the ideal weight, restricting the use of salt and alcohol, ceasing to smoke, and exercising regularly will do much to maintain vascular tone and reduce the morbidity and mortality from heart attacks and probably also hypertension. But how many of us are willing to do these things? There is good news. In 1972, government and private agencies began a coordinated program to educate the public about the disease. Over the next three years the number who didn't know they had the disease decreased from 49 per cent to 29 per cent and the numbers receiving adequate therapy doubled, from 4·to 8 million people. There are still, however, 5 million others who know they have the disease and won't do anything about it.

Breast cancer: Cancer of the breast is the leading cause in women of death from cancer. There were 33,000 deaths and 90,000 new cases in 1974. This incidence is increasing rapidly in black women, although it remains more frequent—and it is also still increasing—in white women. Clinical examination and mammography (an x-ray technique enabling one to "see" into the breast tissue) in selected age groups have not given sufficiently clear-cut results in terms of early detection and reduction in mortality to warrant a massive national expansion of screening procedures. Further research into costs and benefits in various age groups using a variety of techniques of detection is needed, and some is already being done. One study of women aged 40 to 64 showed that mammography and clinical examination reduced the short-term mortality by one-third. Just as important, 35 per cent of those offered the examination declined to participate in the program. And bear in mind that mammography carries with it the hazard of radiation damage to the individual if done too frequently.

Cancer of the cervix of the uterus: This cancer can be detected in the pre-invasive stage of the disease and cured by surgery and/or radiation. The widespread use of cervical smears is probably justified. I say "probably," because it still isn't known how many cases of pre-invasive cancer (also called cancer-in-situ) will become "invasive," meaning malignant and life threatening. Therefore rigorous benefit-cost analysis is not available as yet. Present evidence suggests that screening of adult women at two-year intervals is worth the effort (an example of secondary prevention). A major problem is that those most susceptible, i.e., black women, who suffer the disease at twice the incidence of white women, are least likely to use the available screening services. Here, lack of education, financial barriers, inaccessibility of services, early onset of sexual activity in teenage girls, and multiple births all play a role and have to be contended with if a campaign of prevention is to be effective. Jewish women are most apt to use available services, but least apt to develop the disease. This is thought to be due to their better education and personal hygiene, later onset of sexual activity, and fewer births. In addition, circumcision in Jewish males is thought to prevent the accumulation of a carcinogen under the foreskin that would otherwise be transmitted to the female through intercourse.

Multiphasic screening: The above are examples of diseases where specific interventions and the questions surrounding them offer a variety of strategies for improving health, while calling for a far larger national commitment to research. In principle, the use of an automated series of tests on the blood, urine, and stool, combined with examination of sputum and cervical secretions and various other procedures (x-rays, blood-pressure measurement, proctoscopy, electrocardiogram) should be effective primary and secondary preventive measures. Economies of scale and convenience would seem to offer the best way to improve and maintain health. Here again, not enough is known of the costs and benefits to launch a national program with any degree of conviction—the conviction needed to enhance participation and sustain a long-term effort. Effectiveness must be established before one worries about efficiency and availability, which have nothing to do with whether the procedure is harmful or helpful (both psychologically and physically) to the patient.

Even when all is known, compliance or participation of the target population is still difficult to obtain in our "free" society. In one study conducted by the Kaiser-Permanente Medical Foundation, 65 per cent of a study group agreed to participate in multiphasic screening in each of seven years—which means that 35 per cent did not (and remember, 50 per cent of patients will not take medications as prescribed). After 7 years, there was an insignificant overall effect on the health of those who participated. A control group which did not undergo screening suffered 400 deaths during the 7-year period, of which only 60 (15 per cent) were judged to be "potentially postponable" through specific preventive-medicine measures. Much more research is needed to identify those age-specific measures of detection and prevention that have acceptable costs for the benefits obtained.

Screening tests can detect serious and correctable defects in school children, and here there are very favorable benefit-cost ratios. Once detected, however, an inadequate system of health services may prevent necessary action. We should not launch mass surveys if we are unwilling or unable to take care of what we find. This is particularly true of those most vulnerable and in need, namely, children in impoverished, inner-city areas. An OEO Youth Health Program in Boston reported in 1968 that 354, or 31 per cent, of 1,191 youths examined had "one or more medical conditions requiring more definitive diagnostic and/or treatment services." Ninety per cent needed some form of dental care. In Washington, D.C., more than one-quarter of a largely black population of children ages 6 months through 3 years were anemic; in another group, ages 4 through 11 years, one-quarter failed a comprehensive vision screening examination. Twenty per cent of all the children had evidence of middle-ear disease, and 7 per cent of those between 4 and 11 years had hearing loss in the speech frequencies—enough to interfere with learning. In both the Boston and the Washington studies, the detection of such gross health problems led neither to adequate follow-up and treatment, nor to the implementation of large-scale programs of detection and prevention. If such programs had been launched, the system of health services would have been swamped. Nonetheless, the highest long-range benefits will accrue in programs geared to the needs of impoverished, inner-city children.

Specific programs can be structured according to age groups or to the geographic location of "captive populations" (doctor's office, hospital clinics, work location, public health departments, school systems). Both approaches are important, and they frequently overlap. Such programs are constrained by the availability of manpower, technical facilities, financing mechanisms, and the participation and compliance of the producer, as well as of the recipient population. Those most in need are frequently those least educated and most inaccessible in terms of distance or ability to communicate (remember, between 20 and 40 per cent of our population is functionally illiterate). There is a lack of conviction on the part of both purveyors and recipients about the long-range value of such services when compared with their costs. The latter are more accurately perceived in terms of time, convenience, and money.

An example of the range of preventive procedures that might be utilized in middle-aged adults (36 to 64 years old) is presented in Table I. Clearly if every adult in

TABLE I

PREVENTIVE MEDICINE PROCEDURES: MIDDLE-AGE ADULT

Procedure	*Detection-Prevention-Treatment-Implications*
History	Symptoms, environmental exposures, habits, mental status
Height and weight	Obesity, malnutrition, metabolic disease
Blood pressure	Hypertension
Electrocardiogram	Heart disease; baseline for future
Vision (including pressure measurement-tonometry)	Myopia of aging; glaucoma
Spirometry	Breathing disorders: bronchitis, emphysema
Physical examination including dental	Span of physical abnormalities
Breast examination	Cancer (also occurs rarely in males)
Rectal examination	Cancer of rectum and prostate
Sigmoidoscopy	Cancer of rectum and colon
Pelvic examination	Cancer of vagina, cervix, uterus, and ovary
Laboratory Examinations:	
Multiphasic Screening	
Blood cholesterol & triglycerides	Heart disease
Sugar	Diabetes
Uric acid	Gout, heart disease, kidney disease
SGOT	Liver disease
Hemoglobin-hematocrit	Anemia (nutrition, cancer, iron deficiency)
Urea nitrogen	Kidney disease
Creatinine	Kidney disease
Urine examination	Bladder and kidney infection or disease; cancer
VDRL	Syphilis
Tuberculin test	Tuberculosis
Gonococcal culture (usually females)	Gonorrhea
Pap smear (females)	Cancer of cervix of uterus
Stool guiac	Occult blood in stool: bowel cancer
Mammography (females)	Cancer of breast
Chest x-ray	Cancer, emphysema, tuberculosis of lung, heart disease
Tetanus and diphtheria boosters	Infectious disease
Counseling: Health Education	
Nutrition	Heart disease, cancer, liver disease
Smoking	Cancer, heart and lung disease
Alcohol and drugs	Liver disease, accidents
Contraception	Family planning, mongolism
Exercise	Heart disease, vascular disease
Sleep	General health, accidents
Accidents	Alcohol, orthopedic problems
Mental status	Male and female menopause, work, stress
Abortion	Genetic disease; maternal health

the United States between the ages of 36 and 64 years (66 million people) were to have the complete "works" listed in Table I, the costs would far exceed the benefits and the health-delivery system would collapse. Furthermore, there is no assurance that a clean bill of health won't get dirty the day after you've seen the doctor. The number of people who have dropped dead or developed incurable cancer within weeks or months of being told that "all systems are go" attests to this. It must also be noted that technology, automated and computerized, can never be substituted for the judgment, the support, or the reassurance of the compassionate and wise physician.

So what do I do at the age of 50 years? I see my physician once a year for a general history and physical examination (including blood pressure, rectal-prostate exam), chest x-ray, hematocrit, stool test for blood, blood sugar and cholesterol tests, height and weight, immunizations when needed. My wife does the same, plus breast and pelvic examination. We both get regular moderate exercise, sleep eight hours a night, keep trim, and enjoy the odd cocktail. I will continue to have difficulty wrestling with seat belts and to be incensed with the pollution of my ears when the damned buzzer won't go off until I plug the belt in.

Mental illness and mental retardation: These present special problems for preventive-medicine efforts. Here social, cultural, and genetic factors all play decisive roles and lead to the difficulties of structuring rational programs. Schizophrenia is an extremely serious public health problem. Nearly one million episodes of patient care were estimated to have taken place in 1971 in outpatient and inpatient facilities. The incidence of the disease is estimated to be somewhere between 50 and 250 cases per 100,000 population. Further estimates tell us that somewhere between 28 and 140 cases will occur during the lifetime of each thousand newly born individuals. With over 3 million new births in the United States in 1973, that means that something like 84,000 to 320,000 new cases of schizophrenia will appear during the lifetime of that group. The cause of the disease remains unknown, but strong evidence has turned up for genetic predisposition. There is a 10 per cent chance of schizophrenia developing in offspring if one parent has the disease; this jumps to 40 per cent if both parents are affected. The risk is sufficiently high to justify genetic counseling as a primary preventive measure. Beyond this, early detection and treatment of the psychotic individual can reverse the disease and restore the individual to a productive life, although the relapse rate is high at 20 to 30 per cent in the first year, and 50 to 70 per cent in five years. Without early treatment the disease can become chronic and much more difficult to reverse.

The affective disorders of mania and depression constitute another major public health problem. In 1971, over 600,000 patients with these disorders were under care in facilities reporting to the National Institutes of Mental Health. For every one reported, there may be another not diagnosed or being cared for. There is growing evidence for genetic transmission in depressive psychoses that calls for greater efforts in making genetic-counseling services available as a form of primary prevention. Secondary prevention makes use of antidepressant drugs, which facilitate the successful treatment of 70 to 80 per cent of depressive episodes. The use of lithium and phenothiazines in the treatment of manic states has markedly altered the previously dismal prognosis for these diseases. Relapses and chronicity, suicide and injury can now be avoided with early secondary-prevention measures.

Finally, included within the problems of mental illness are the large number of people who are sufficiently troubled psychologically to handicap them seriously in work, love, and play. Some surveys have shown that as many as 25 per cent of a community's population are in need of psychological testing and services. The roots of this malaise are multiple; they include the effects on the offspring of inadequate spacing of pregnancies, too early pregnancies among teenagers, inadequate maternal nutrition, inadequate infant nutrition, inadequate maternal and paternal caring, inadequate cognitive environment—in short, social impoverishment of the worst form. Leon Eisenberg has referred to this complex of maladjusted individuals as suffering from developmental attrition—"a sequential and cumulative failure to attain levels of cognitive and affective development sufficient for personal and social competence."[7] The infant who represents the unwanted birth may be abused or neglected and cannot attain personal and social competence; poor nutrition in the last trimester of pregnancy and the first two years of life can stunt both intellectual and physical growth; inadequate affective and cognitive stimulation for the developing infant and child results in inadequate personality and intellectual development.

What form should preventive medicine take so that coming generations will not suffer from developmental attrition? Primary prevention must include family-planning services and therapeutic abortions, maternal- and child-health services with emphasis on good nutrition for everyone—and *food* for the poor, family counseling to help preserve its integrity, the full support of foster care and progressive adoption policies, the development of day-care centers for pre-school children of working mothers, and adult education emphasizing cognitive and affective development in infant and child care. Alleviation of poverty and a much higher national priority on the developmental needs of infants and children and their families are necessary, if this tremendous loss of human energy and potential is to be corrected.

Quite aside from the mental retardation due to developmental attrition or brain damage at birth, there are other diseases causing retardation which are inherited or are present from conception, namely Tay-Sachs disease, Down's syndrome, and phenylketonuria (PKU). In each of these, preventive measures can be utilized to avoid the abnormality, i.e., either through genetic counseling and avoidance of conception, in-utero diagnosis of the condition by amniocentesis and abortion, if desired, or screening at birth with dietary treatment to avoid retardation in the case of PKU.

Down's syndrome or mongolism occurs approximately once in every 600 births. The older the mother, the greater the risk. The average mother faces a 1-in-900 risk of producing a mongoloid infant, while the mother over 40 years of age faces a 1-in-50 risk. Amniocentesis (withdrawal of fluid from the fetal sac in the pregnant uterus and examination of the cells in the fluid) can detect from about the fifteenth week of pregnancy the chromosomal abnormality that signals the condition. Selective abortions can then be offered the prospective parents. Without the test of amniocentesis and selective abortion, roughly 57,000 to 83,000 mongoloid children (depending on birth rates) would be born in the United States between 1970 and 1980. The estimated cost today of caring for mongoloids is $1.7 billion. The financial and emotional costs to parents and society-at-large are still more staggering. Prevention consists of primary efforts to counsel against childbearing in older women and secondary efforts of amniocentesis and selective abortion in those populations at high risk, e.g., pregnant women over forty years of age.

In summary, it is estimated that 30 per cent of severe forms of mental retardation could be avoided in the United States if all currently available scientific information were utilized, namely, identification of parents carrying recessive genes, birth control, amniocentesis and induced abortion, screening and treatment at birth, and intensified efforts to enhance cognitive and affective development of infants and children.

But what is the responsibility of the individual in matters pertaining to health? The United States now spends more on health in absolute terms and as a percentage of the gross national product than any other nation in the world—from $39 billion or 5.9 per cent of the GNP in 1965 to $120 billion or 8.3 per cent of the GNP in 1975 (over $550 per person per year). No one—but no one—can deny the fact that billions of dollars could be saved directly—and billions more indirectly (in terms of family suffering, time lost, and the erosion of human capital)—if our present knowledge of health and disease could be utilized in programs of primary, secondary, and tertiary prevention. The greatest portion of our national expenditure goes for the caring of the major causes of premature, and therefore preventable, death and/or disability in the United States, i.e., heart disease, cancer, strokes, accidents, bronchitis and emphysema, cirrhosis of the liver, mental illness and retardation, dental caries, suicide and homicide, venereal disease, and other infections. If no one smoked cigarettes or consumed alcohol and everyone exercised regularly, maintained optimal weight on a low fat, low refined-carbohydrate, high fiber-content diet, reduced stress by simplifying their lives, obtained adequate rest and recreation, understood the needs of infants and children for the proper nutrition and nurturing of their intellectual and affective development, had available to them, and would use, genetic counseling and selective abortion, drank fluoridated water, followed the doctor's orders for medications and self-care once disease was detected, used available health services at the appropriate time for screening examinations and health education-preventive medicine programs, the savings to the country would be mammoth in terms of billions of dollars, a vast reduction in human misery, and an attendant marked improvement in the quality of life. Our country would be strengthened immeasurably, and we could divert our energies—human and financial—to other pressing issues of national and international concern.

But so much conspires against this rational ideal: our historic emphasis on rugged individualism, social Darwinism, and unrestricted freedom together with our recent emphasis on individual rights as contrasted with responsibilities; a neo-liberal ideology which has stressed societal responsibility and the obligations of the beneficent state, resulting in an erosion of individual responsibility and initiative; a credit-minded culture which does it now and pays for it later, whether in drinking and eating or in buying cars and houses; an economy which depends on profligate production and consumption regardless of the results to individual health, or to the public health in terms of a wide variety of environmental pollutants; ignorance (and therefore a lack of conviction and commitment) on the part of both producers and consumers as to exact costs and benefits of many preventive and health-education measures, a reflection of the sparse national commitment to research in these areas; the failure, conceptually, to view health holistically, i.e., its interdependence with educational attainment, poverty, the availability of work, housing and the density of populations, degree of environmental pollution (air, water, noise, mass-media offerings), and levels of stress in work, play, and love; and finally, the values and habits of the health establishment itself. One cannot hope to develop a rational health system if the parts of the whole that bear on health are moving in irrational ways.

Within the health system, medical educators and the teaching hospitals display only acute curative, after-the-fact medicine. The rewards—intellectually, financially, and emotionally—for specialist care far outweight those for the low-status generalist (primary-care physician) or public health worker. The specialty organizations (surgeons, internists, radiologists, for example), the American Medical Association, the Association of American Medical Colleges, the American Hospital Association, the "disease-insurance" companies, as well as governmental insurance programs (Medicare-Medicaid), pay lip service or no service to reordering priorities and sanctions to the needs of the people for prevention and health education. Present plans for national health insurance do not contend with the issues of preventive medicine and health education. Over 65 per cent of the 4.5 million workers in the health system are employed in hospitals, and their interests demand more expenditures and an even higher priority for acute, curative, after-the-fact medicine and the care of those with chronic disease. There is one health educator for every 17,000 people, while there is one physician for every 650 and one nurse for every 280 people.

Research priorities stress biological and not epidemiological, social, and environmental research. Even here, we should be willing to take decisive action when inferential evidence, e.g., the production of cancer in animals by drugs, is available, unacceptable as this may be to scientists. I cannot believe that man was meant to ingest drugs and artificial-food substances, breathe polluted air, or have his ears banged mercilessly by the uproar of industrial society. Those who do work in the field of prevention and health education have too often stressed social control (some have called them "health fascists") rather than social change and have become curiously indifferent to the needs and aspirations of families, communities, and particularly minority groups. Those places where benefit-cost ratios are potentially most favorable for programs of health education and prevention—and where long-range research could be conducted—have been neglected: the schools and universities, places of work, hospitals and clinics, and, obviously, doctors' offices. Very little is known about how television functions as a cognitive medium; little sophistication is shown by interested experts in developing sanctions, i.e., financial or other incentives, to modify bad habits of living. Those in the health professions play a minimal role in supporting the needs of minority groups for better housing and jobs, higher income, and improved transportation—not realizing that the fulfillment of these needs will reduce stress and anxiety and therefore improve health by reducing susceptibility to disease or to the disease-provoking habits of smoking and drinking.

If the health establishment isn't interested and the consumers don't want or demand health education and preventive medicine, what is to be done? First of all we should look at a few concrete changes in behavior which, through a variety of mechanisms, have improved health:

1) When the Surgeon General issued his report on the hazards of smoking in 1964, 52 per cent of the male population smoked cigarettes. Through massive public educational programs and restrictions on advertising, the percentage was reduced over a 10-year period to roughly 42 per cent. (This desirable change has been accompanied, however, by an equally undesirable increase in teen-age smoking, particularly among females, and no change in the 41 per cent of 17-to-25-year-olds who smoke.)

2) During World War I, the United Kingdom increased taxes on alcohol, reduced

the amount of alcohol available for consumption, and restricted the hours of sale. Consumption of alcohol fell and, with it, deaths from cirrhosis of the liver—from 10.3 per 100,000 people in 1914 to 4.5 in 1920. Following the war, the regulations governing the amount of alcohol allowed for consumption and the hours of its sale were relaxed, but taxes on alcoholic beverages were continually increased. By 1936, the death rate due to cirrhosis was down to 3.1 per 100,000, and it has remained at this level in that country. In the United States, wartime prohibition also reduced the cirrhosis death rate, from 11.8 per 100,000 in 1916 to 7.1 per 100,000 in 1920; it was still 7.2 in 1932, the year before prohibition was ended. But following the repeal of prohibition, the death rate from cirrhosis climbed steadily to an all-time high of 16.0 deaths per 100,000 in 1973, five times the rate in Great Britain. These results suggest a national strategy for the United States of (a) steadily increasing taxes on alcoholic beverages, (b) a massive public education program on the hazards of alcohol plus restrictions on all advertising, (c) aid to farmers and companies to help them shift to other crops and products. Increased tax income should temporarily help to defray the costs of public health education. The same strategy should be applied to cigarettes.

3) The marked reduction in auto fatalities and injuries during the oil crisis suggests that a permanent reduction of speed limits combined with sanctions to limit the use of automobiles would more than justify the cost of enforcing such a program.

4) A program to improve the self-care of patients with diabetes (tertiary prevention) at the University of Southern California resulted in a 50 per cent reduction in emergency-ward visits, a decrease in the number of patients with diabetic coma from 300 to 100 over a two-year period, and the avoidance of 2,300 visits for medications. The theme was, "You must take responsibility for your own health." Savings were estimated at $1.7 million. In other studies involving the care and education of diabetics, hemophiliacs, and others, hospital readmissions decreased by over 50 per cent. These efforts resulted in tremendous savings of time and money and reflected vastly improved self-care in cases of chronic disease.

5) A heart-disease-prevention program run by Stanford University similarly demonstrated that an intensive program of health education and preventive medicine—utilizing personal instructions, television spots, and printed material—resulted in a markedly higher level of information about the disease by the community and a marked improvement in dietary habits and in the reduction of smoking among those at high risk.

There are many other examples. Some encouragement can also be obtained from the results of occupational health programs, an occasional school health program, the efforts of the Kaiser Foundation Medical Program with its stress on prevention, the new attention being paid the subject in medical schools, largely through a renewed emphasis on the production of family or primary physicians, and the increasing numbers of legislative proposals which stress expansion of health education and preventive-medicine programs. A steadily growing number of newspapers and journals have health columns, and television and radio seem to be paying more attention to the subject. Industrial-medicine programs and socially responsible advertising and pamphleteering by insurance companies have done a great deal of good. The public's appetite for books on dieting and for Dr. Spock's *Infant and Child Care* speaks for a definite interest despite continuing bad habits.

Following extensive hearings before the Senate Subcommittee on Health of the Committee on Labor and Public Welfare during 1975,[8] a new National Health

Information and Health Promotion Act (Public Law 94-317) was signed into law in 1976. It is designed to encourage healthier living habits and to enhance the federal role in disease prevention and control. It signals a new public interest and, depending on the level of implementation of its consumer health education and information programs to be run from an office within HEW, it could represent a shift in the direction of the nation's health effort.

The individual must realize that a perpetuation of the present system of high cost, after-the-fact medicine will only result in higher costs and greater frustration. The next major advances in the health of the American people will be determined by what the individual is willing to do for himself and for society-at-large. If he is willing to follow Breslow's seven rules for healthy living, he can extend his life and enhance his own and the nation's productivity. If he is willing to reassert his authority with his children, he can provide for their optimal mental and physical development. If he participates fully in private and public efforts to reduce the hazards of the environment, he can reduce the causes of premature death and disability. If he is unwilling to do these things, he should stop complaining about the steadily rising costs of medical care and the disproportionate share of the GNP that is consumed by health care. This is his primary critical choice: to change his personal bad habits or stop complaining. He can either remain the problem or become the solution to it; Beneficent Government cannot—indeed, should not—do it for him or to him.

In terms of public policy and the social responsibility of the individual, I believe he should consider the following:

1) Support vastly increased funding to develop the best possible integration of health education into the school system, stressing measures that the individual can take to preserve his own health and knowledge about environmental hazards. There are over 45 million children enrolled in grades kindergarten through 12 in nearly 17,000 school districts comprising 115,000 schools and 2.1 million teachers. These children are at the most impressionable stage of development, and, for the long range, this population—its attitudes, knowledge, and habits—will determine the health of the nation. In the majority of schools, health education is assigned low or no priority. Curricular material needs to be developed, school health educators recruited and trained, and courses on health education given the same central importance (with examinations) as reading, writing, arithmetic, and athletics!

2) Support a far greater national commitment for research in health education and preventive medicine with emphasis on epidemiologic studies, benefit-cost analysis, and the most effective and least offensive ways of changing human behavior. Arbitrarily, the less than 0.5 per cent for health education and 2.5 per cent for preventive medicine (services and research) of the total national health expenditure now spent should be increased to at least 5 and preferably 10 per cent of that total. Ten billion dollars could be saved and made available for such programs, if by some miracle all unnecessary surgery were abolished, or all cigarette smoking stopped, or all alcohol consumption ceased in the United States. More realistically, a 20 per cent increase in taxes on the $30 billion annual expenditure on cigarettes and whisky would produce the $6 billion needed annually for this program. Beyond this, there remains the need for increased support for fundamental biological research on the mechanism of disease-producing environmental contaminants.

3) With respect to cigarettes and whisky, the individual should support greatly

increased taxes on the consumption of both, massive public education programs on the hazards of their use, and severe restrictions on advertising. New tax money generated could be used to defray the costs of public education. Consumption should fall and health improve with the above measures. A more extreme additional measure would be to limit amounts available for consumption and to provide subsidies to help producers change to other products.

4) Support the development of genetic-counseling services, family planning services, and selective abortion.

5) Support the development of age-specific preventive measures, which would include selective screening and counseling services. Preventive services must be tied into a comprehensive system of personal-health services to provide for continuous follow-up. Programs to expand the numbers of qualified individuals in the disciplines of health education and preventive-medicine services and research must be supported.

6) "Disease insurance" should be converted to health insurance. Coverage for preventive medicine and health education would change the behavior of both consumers and producers by introducing economic sanctions. We have barely scratched the surface in our search for those that would be most effective.

7) More attention should be devoted to the family as the basic social unit of the nation. The responsibilities of parents—for using genetic counseling and family planning, for pursuing the proper intellectual, affective, and physical development of their children both at home and in school, and for setting the example of individual responsibility and prudence in their own life styles—are paramount. A nation is only as strong as its children and as good as its parents.

8) The shadows of disease and unhealthy habits follow poverty and ignorance. The greatest costs are incurred, but the greatest benefits can be obtained, through preventive medicine and health-education measures aimed specifically at impoverished minority groups in inner city as well as rural areas. Quite beyond these direct measures, one must understand that total health depends on the eradication of poverty and ignorance, the availability of jobs, adequate transportation, recreation and housing, the level of public safety, and an aesthetically pleasing and physically benevolent environment. Improve health—improve those elements equally which are central to the quality of life.

Ironically, we can be grateful for some of our failures in health education, for at least, as Guy Steuart has said, "we have been spared the realization of the dreadful specter of an Orwellian society in which our daily behavior would be motivated primarily by health considerations, in which hangovers would yield to hang-ups, Shakespeare to plays about unsaturated fats, and Beethoven to the ecstatic crunch of raw broccoli."[9] I agree, but Madison Avenue and television almost have us there now by an alternative route. Instead of fats and broccoli, we have cigarettes and belly-wash, and an abysmally low level of national support for the arts and humanities—those areas of human endeavor which give joy to life, enhance human understanding, and glorify the human condition.

I began by saying that the health of human beings is determined by their behavior, their food, and the nature of their environment. Over 99 per cent of us are born healthy and suffer premature death and disability only as a result of personal misbehavior and environmental conditions. The sociocultural effects of urban industrial life are profound in terms of stress, an unnatural sedentary existence, bad habits, and unhealthy environmental influences.[10] The individual has the power—indeed, the moral responsibility—to maintain his own health by the observance of simple, prudent rules of behavior relating to sleep, exercise, diet and weight, alcohol, and smoking. In addition, he should avoid where possible the long-term use of drugs. He should be aware of the dangers of stress and the need for precautionary measures during periods of sudden change, such as bereavement, divorce, or new employment. He should submit to selective medical examination and screening procedures.

These simple rules can be understood and observed by the majority of Americans, namely the white, well-educated, and affluent middle class. But how do individuals in minority groups follow these rules, when their members include disproportionately large numbers of the impoverished and the illiterate, among whom fear, ignorance, desperation, and superstition conspire against even the desire to remain healthy? Here we must rely on social policies *first*, in order to improve education, employment, civil rights, and economic levels, along with efforts to develop accessible health services.

Beyond these measures, the individual is powerless to control disease-provoking environmental contaminants, be they drugs, air and water pollutants, or food additives, except as he becomes knowledgeable enough to participate in public debate and in support of governmental controls. Here, we must depend on the wisdom of experts, the results of research, and the national will to legislate controls for our protection, as damaging as they may be, in the short run, to our national economy.

When all is said and done, let us not forget that he who hates sin, hates humanity. Life is meant to be enjoyed, and each one of us in the end is still able in our own country to steer his vessel to his own port of desire. But the costs of individual irresponsibility in health have now become prohibitive. The choice is individual responsibility or social failure. Responsibility and duty must gain some degree of parity with right and freedom.

REFERENCES

[1]T. McKeown, *The Modern Rise of Population* (London, 1976), pp. 152-63.

[2]M. Susser, ed., *Prevention and Health Maintenance Revisited* (*Bulletin of the New York Academy of Medicine*, 51 [January, 1975], pp. 5-243), p. 96.

[3]N. B. Belloc and L. Breslow, "The Relation of Physical Health Status and Health Practices," *Preventive Medicine*, 1 (August, 1972), pp. 409-21; see also "Relationship of Health Practices and Mortality," *Preventive Medicine*, 2 (1973), pp. 67-81.

[4]F. W. Ashley, Jr., and W. B. Kannel, "Relation of Weight Change to Changes in Atherogenic Traits: The Framingham Study," *Journal of Chronic Diseases*, 27 (March, 1974), pp. 103-14.

[5]J. F. Fraumeni, ed., *Persons at High Risk of Cancer: An Approach to Cancer Etiology and Control* (New York, 1975), p. 526.

[6]L. Breslow, "Research in a Strategy for Health Improvement," *International Journal of Health Services*, 3 (1973), pp. 7-16.

[7]Susser (cited above, note 3), p. 124.

[8]*Disease Control and Health Education and Promotion, 1975. Hearings before the Subcommittee on Health of the Committee on Labor and Public Welfare, U.S. Senate, 94th Congress* (U.S. Government Printing Office, 1975), p. 1306.

[9]Susser (cited above, note 3), p. 179.

[10]J. H. Knowles, *Health in America. Health Service Prospects: An International Survey* (London, 1973), pp. 307-34.

DAVID E. ROGERS, M.D.

The Challenge of Primary Care

IN RECENT YEARS AMERICANS HAVE COME TO BELIEVE that the United States is not supplying general medical care with suitable dispatch, dignity, and equity to all its citizens. The problem is not new. Inequities in the delivery of medical services have always been, and probably always will be, with us. Until recently, expressions of concern came primarily from and about groups that are underprivileged because of race, poverty, or geographic location. Because these groups have less of everything— status, money, and political power—the complaints went largely unheeded except by those who worked with them and by those examining broader problems of medical-care delivery. Americans generally continued to be proud of the successes of biomedical science and of the high quality of the care in American hospitals.

However, as the costs of medical care, and particularly of hospital care, escalated, public attention focused on medical services. From all socioeconomic levels and widely divergent political persuasions, complaints increased regarding the difficulty of finding a personal physician and in developing a satisfactory professional rapport with him. The absence of readily accessible general practitioners and the difficulties people encountered in finding medical care outside a hospital during the evening, on Wednesday afternoons, and on weekends came to be regarded as serious problems, and demands that ambulatory medical care be improved have since continued to increase.

Pressures for changes in the training and distribution of medical manpower and the implementation of new knowledge in biomedical science and medical care are very much with us. The medical profession has been quite successful in treating certain kinds of acute and complex life-threatening problems, and in this regard it continues to have the trust and confidence of most Americans. But how American medicine can be adapted to meet the more general medical needs—real or perceived—of a broader public at reasonable cost now represents the major challenge.

Before examining primary care, I should first attempt to define it and to determine how the current dichotomy between what is regarded as desirable and what is actually supplied has come to pass. I will also consider whether it is reasonable even to try to develop a better primary-care system when there are so many other pressing social problems competing for resources, and, if it is, what broader changes in society it will have to contend with in the quarter-century ahead. Finally, I shall outline the options that must be weighed, if strengthening general medical-care services continues as an important national objective.

The term "primary care" is usually used to describe the range of care traditionally rendered by physicians in community practice. It is the point of first contact for an individual with a physician, but it also has several other important dimensions. First, it is care of a continuing kind; implicit in the notion is responsibility for a particular patient over many years. The responsibility may at times be delegated or relinquished, but it is not terminated so long as both patient and physician remain satisfied with the relationship. But primary care is more than the medical care of individuals; primary-care practitioners also have responsibilities for groups of people, usually in a defined geographic area. Finally, its interests are comprehensive: primary care, regardless of how it is rendered or by whom, is concerned with the psychological and social as well as the physical aspects of illness. This kind of general medical care might be provided by family practitioners, by groups of internists and pediatricians or obstetrician-gynecologists, or by some other combination of physicians and other health professionals. But, however constituted, it is the point of entry into the health system and of continuing contact with it. Its patients are usually ambulatory and able to function at home, although it utilizes, and probably will continue to utilize, some hospital services.

A satisfactory national system for delivering primary or general medical care must have certain basic capabilities: (1) ready access to a physician or some other health professional who can effectively cope with ordinary medical problems; (2) the ability to identify, from innocent-appearing situations, those few that are potentially serious and provide properly for them; (3) science-based humanistic support for those that it serves; (4) care on a continuing basis; (5) distribution of care with reasonable equity; (6) the delivery system must be stable and self-renewing: those who work in it must find it sufficiently rewarding to want to stay in, and others must wish to enter, the field; (7) it must be compatible with the life, culture, and needs of the people it serves and adapt to the wide differences that exist in various areas of the country; (8) it must be able to compete effectively for resources with other social needs. Using these criteria, our primary health-care system is generally regarded as inadequate, and the supply of physicians specifically trained for, and willing to offer, primary health care as a significant part of their practice has been steadily declining for the last forty years.

One of the questions often asked of American health care is why this apparently vital service has been so neglected in the progress of medicine—why has the medical profession, traditionally so responsive to human needs, strayed so far from its generalist heritage, where the major focus has always been care of the individual patient by the individual physician?

The trend away from the general, all-purpose physician and toward the more narrowly oriented, highly trained specialist was, at the outset, a logical response to advancing knowledge about the causes of disease and increasing understanding of the biologic workings of the human body. The recognition of the microbial etiology of many of the serious infectious plagues of mankind in the late nineteenth century led to rapid advances in public health. Improvements in environmental sanitation, the development of clean water supplies, indoor plumbing, clean food, control of insect vectors, and immunizations eliminated or contributed to a profound decline in the incidence of many common diseases of high morbidity and mortality, thus improving health in large segments of the population. The advent of anesthesia, which allowed complicated surgical procedures to be undertaken, led rapidly to the belief that surgery should be done only by those with extensive training in it. Although specialties were already well developed in Europe, in America it was the availability of anesthetic agents which separated surgery from general medicine and led to the establishment of the American College of Surgeons early in the twentieth century. World War I furthered the trend toward specialization as it revealed that many physicians were simply not equipped or trained to handle new surgical technologies, and demands to require further training for those electing to treat particular diseases intensified.

In the early nineteen-twenties, science-based medicine also began to place more and more powerful tools in the hands of the personal physician who did not practice surgery. Starting with the discovery of insulin and proceeding through the development of the sulfonamides, antibiotics, and other potent drugs for the management of hypertension, cardiac failure, malignancies, and other maladies, many new and highly successful techniques were found for modifying or curing disease. To use these tools precisely and appropriately required new knowledge and skills. No longer could the all-purpose physician command sufficient competence to deal with all the ills of all his patients. The need for specialists was obvious and incontrovertible.

Pressures toward specialization, however, were also coming from the patients. As the public became more and more aware of the complexities of science-based medicine, consumers of medical care, particularly upper- and middle-class people in metropolitan areas, began to insist on consultation and care by physicians with "specialist" labels, and respect for the generalist correspondingly fell. Maintaining the availability of the services of the all-purpose physician was not at first viewed as a problem: specialists came from the ranks of all-purpose physicians, who made up the bulk of the profession, specialization required unusual effort, and those who chose to become specialists fully understood the need for generalists, for they had "been there."

In time, however, a number of factors and events converged to accelerate the change from general to specialty careers at rates and to degrees which were not anticipated. Under the impact of the Flexner Report of 1910, medical schools underwent a profound change—beginning with the Johns Hopkins medical school, founded on the European model in 1893. A strong research base was introduced in academic medical centers. Full-time salaried physicians who brought special scientific and technical skills increasingly replaced the largely non-specific generalist on medical-school faculties. Consequently, those who practiced general medicine had less and less contact with those who were in the process of becoming doctors. The generalist became in the main a dropout of postdoctoral training, and internists, surgeons, pediatricians, obstetrician-gynecologists, psychiatrists, and a rising number of medical and surgical subspecialists became the models for aspiring physicians. World War II accentuated the race toward specialization by rewarding medical specialists with higher rank and pay in the armed forces than were given general physicians.

Thus by the late nineteen-forties medical students in training in the academic medical centers had little, if any, contact with those practicing general medicine. Further, academic training of medical students took place more and more within the hospitals, effectively removing them and their teachers from contact with most of the illnesses that confront people in their daily lives. The classic report of Kerr White and his colleagues in the early sixties—pointing out that in an adult population of 1,000 people, 750 have some illness monthly, 250 of those see a physician, and only one is referred for care to a medical-training center—was largely ignored.[1] To the detriment of medical education and medicine and society in general, virtually all the experience of students involved only that tiny subset of sick people who gain entry to the academic medical center.

Part of this emphasis on the hospitalized patient is logical and defensible. To recognize and know how to manage serious or life-threatening disease are the skills basic to medicine. These skills are generally viewed as more important than those of managing self-limiting or nuisance illnesses for which medicine has no solutions. Further, medical educators have always had great difficulty in designing effective training in the care of ambulatory patients within the limits of the student years, and this has pushed medical schools in other directions.

The problem of the disproportion between the kinds of doctors needed and those produced has been further compounded by the large number of academic medical-training centers. In this country, there are 114 of them, each, for the most part, free to pursue its own objectives. Moreover, medicine has remained a laissez-faire enterprise in the United States: there are no overall national plans or objectives for the training, the numbers, or the distribution of the generalists and medical and surgical specialists that are admitted into the profession. Thus, while individual academic medical centers work responsibly and energetically to achieve excellence in the physicians they train, they do not plan their particular output of physicians to reflect national needs for specific types of medical manpower. Consequently, most schools place emphasis on the training of specialists, hoping that other schools will fill the gap in the requirements for general physicians. This has resulted in a collective lack of responsibility for the needs of the profession at large, albeit for understandable reasons.

As a result we are left with a problem now perceived as serious. This is the apparent inability of American medicine to deal with the simple, day-to-day medical needs of our population. First is the worrisome lack of correlation between the kinds of physicians most agree should be available to handle the common medical problems of American society and the kinds of physicians actually trained and available. While approximately 60 per cent of patient visits to physicians are for basic, general, or primary medical care, only 1 per cent of the hospital residencies available in 1970 offered specific training in general or family practice. This is now changing rapidly, however, and the numbers of primary-care residencies and of family-practice programs are growing steadily.

As noted in Figures 1 and 2, the distribution of physicians by specialty status shows that the number of those practicing general medicine was in a steady decline through 1973. Indeed, on the basis of those trends, Fahs and Peterson predicted in 1968 that general practice as we now know it would completely disappear by the year 2000.[2] Obviously these general needs were not entirely abandoned; they were assumed by physicians with specialist labels, primarily internists, pediatricians, and, to a lesser extent, obstetrician-gynecologists, but the extent of the "generalist"-care function served by these groups is not known. It is largely a "hidden" system for primary care, and this has made the structuring of national health-manpower training programs frustrating and difficult.

There are also wide geographic variations in the distribution of physicians. Rural areas, particularly in the South, and city ghetto areas have far fewer health

FIGURE 1

THE DECLINE IN GENERAL PRACTITIONERS
IN THE UNITED STATES BETWEEN 1949-1973

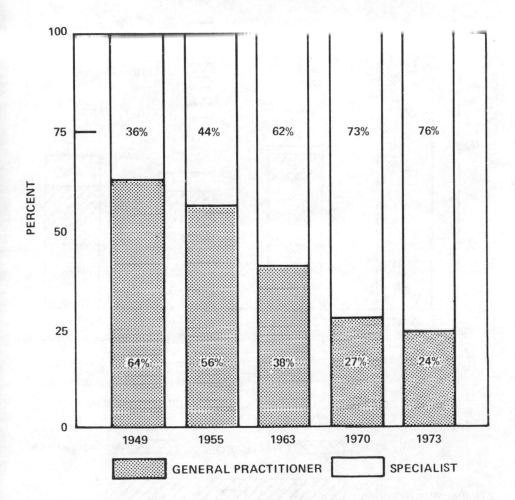

professionals than do affluent suburbs. While the Boston area can claim 239 physicians per 100,000 population, certain rural areas have less than 45. Although New York state has 228 physicians per 100,000 residents, the state of Mississippi has only 82 and certain sections of The Bronx have less than 50. Unfortunately, these inequities have grown over the years. Similarly the differences in the availability of physicians to those who are well-to-do versus those who are poor show wide disparities. As noted in Figure 3, non-poverty areas have twice as many physicians as poverty areas, and specialists are in short supply in poorer sections and communities.

The difficulties in using these kinds of data to determine the adequacy of care provided are obvious and well known: the ratios of physicians to populations have no necessary relation to either quality or extent of services. For example, health indices are similar for New York and Nebraska despite gross differences in the numbers of available physicians. The statistics do, however, give some yardsticks for comparison

FIGURE 2

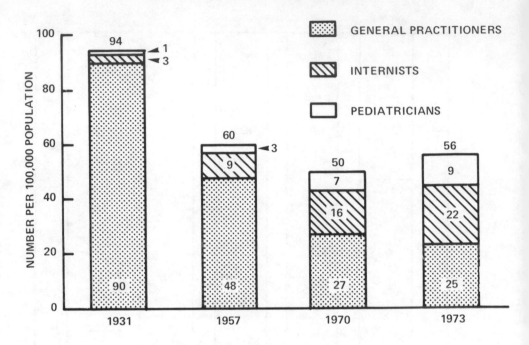

PHYSICIANS IN PRIMARY - CARE PRACTICE
PER 100,000 POPULATION 1931, 1957, 1970, 1973

FIGURE 3

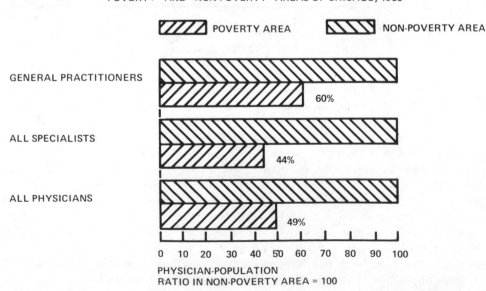

THE RELATIVE SUPPLY OF PHYSICIANS BY SPECIALTY STATUS IN
"POVERTY" AND "NON-POVERTY" AREAS OF CHICAGO, 1966

of the potential availability of physician services. Certainly, 500 per cent variations suggest that America is not functioning optimally in the organization of these services in either well-supplied or sparsely-doctored sectors.

At the present time, the United States is undergoing a period of self-analysis. The sharp downturn in our economic-growth rate and the realization that the period of the "great society" of the sixties did not eliminate many serious social problems despite the expenditure of large amounts of money to do so have led to greater caution about expecting too much from social reform. Some are consequently asking if it is sensible or fiscally reasonable to develop a better system for delivery of primary-care services in this country. In our inequitable world, we will never have a fully equitable distribution of our resources. Further, many other needs which add to the betterment of life, such as adequate income, nutritious foods, decent housing, better educational opportunities, and the like, must inevitably compete for limited resources. There is, in fact, much to suggest that improvement in any of these areas has a clear potential for improving health. Indeed, many would argue that improvements in them would have a considerably greater positive impact on health than universally accessible primary medical care.

It seems clear that during the last decade we have oversold health—or, more accurately, what the availability of adequate medical care can do to improve or maintain health. Some thoughtful students suggest that we should spend more on basic research and the development of genuinely decisive medical technologies, analogous to those of modern immunization against diphtheria, tetanus, or measles, or surgery for osteoarthritic joints, or the contemporary use of antibiotics, rather than spending vast sums on "supportive" therapy and the very expensive "half-way" treatments which we now use to modify or delay the incapacitating effects of certain diseases about which we know little. Many adult illnesses, especially major ones, are accidents of nature, and we have little knowledge and only tentative ideas about how to avoid them. In most instances, we are relatively ineffective in preventing disease or preserving health by medical intervention. We are unlikely to become more effective unless we learn a great deal more about the mechanisms of disease. Several decades of heavy investment in training mental-health workers and developing mental-health centers have not made schizophrenia go away. Nor has it been shown that readily available primary care can maintain the general good health of a community. Our present use of phrases such as "health maintenance" are conjuring up hopes that are not likely to be fulfilled, and we must clearly realize that more medical care will not in itself result in better health.

It is also worth pointing out that the development of a primary-care system in which the physician and other health professionals offer continuing care to a defined population group contains a serious and troublesome contradiction which worries thoughtful physicians. To maintain modern scientific and technologic skills requires that the physician have frequent contact with patients suffering from complex disease processes which demand the repeated use of his skills. However, commitment to providing continuous personal care limits the number of patients for an individual physician to such a small sample of the population (2,500 to 4,000 people) that challenges to his technical skills and specialized knowledge are comparatively infrequent. Thus he faces the hazard of having his expertise atrophy from disuse. This dilemma must be dealt with in the design of any sensible system for primary care. Large organized systems, such as the Kaiser-Permanente plan and other comprehensive group practices, are designed in part to cope with this problem, but the answers to this dilemma are not as simple as some would suggest.

Given these constraints—the expense of developing a more equitable system, the lack of correlation between the availability of front-line medical care and health, and the limits which responsibilities for a defined group place on the continuous updating and refinement of the physicians' skills—we should perhaps now ask the question: Should this nation spend more of its precious and limited resources for social welfare on attempts to upgrade and distribute more equitably our system of general medical care? Obviously, this is a question which American society at large and, through it, its social planners must answer. It is a question of values.

There are, however, some data to support the belief that development of more adequate and more comprehensive primary-care service can, under certain circumstances, reduce mortality and the needs for hospitalization and prevent certain kinds of serious, crippling disease. The following are examples that merit attention:

1) The introduction of maternal and infant-care-treatment centers into low-income areas in the nineteen-sixties resulted in an overall reduction of neonatal death rates from 20.0 to 15.4 per 1,000 live births, or a 23 per cent decline in infant mortality in the predominantly black and high-risk populations served in this program.[3] In slum areas of specific cities across the nation, the results are compelling: in Denver in the 25 census tracts served, a fall in infant mortality from 34.2 per 1,000 live births in 1964 to 21.5 per 1,000 in 1969, and in Birmingham, Alabama, a decrease from 24.5 in 1965 to 14.3 in 1969. Most dramatic, the maternal- and infant-care project in Omaha, Nebraska, resulted in a reduction in infant deaths from 33.4 per 1,000 live births in 1964 to 13.4 in 1969, a 60 per cent decline in infant wastage.[4] These remarkable achievements have received little publicity and therefore have gone largely unnoticed.

2) Available statistics suggest that medical-care programs in children and youth clinics reduced the incidence of serious illness and hospitalization and lowered the long-term costs of providing medical care. The number of days of hospitalization per 1,000 children-and-youth-clinic registrants dropped from 101 days to 42 days between the inception of the program in 1968 and 1972. Further, the annual cost per registrant fell from $201 to $131 during this same period.[5] These are impressive gains.

3) A striking indication that costly and serious chronic illness can be prevented was provided by a careful study of the impact of a comprehensive-care program on the incidence of rheumatic fever in Baltimore children during the late nineteen-sixties. The results showed a 60 per cent reduction in new cases of the disease in children within the comprehensive-care tracts, the attack rate falling from 27 cases per 100,000 to less than 11. During this same period the incidence of rheumatic fever remained unchanged in the non-eligible children in the same city.[6]

There is an additional, pragmatic reason for working toward a better system for delivering out-of-hospital medical care. The major cause of the rapidly rising cost of medical care is hospitalization (see Figure 4). While we can probably make hospitals more efficient, the continuing technological advances of medicine dictate that the costs of a day in a hospital bed will continue to rise. But there is good evidence to show that a well-organized ambulatory-care system for certain groups can significantly reduce the amount of hospital care needed per person. A program that would cut hospitalization for each patient now admitted to a hospital in the United States each

FIGURE 4

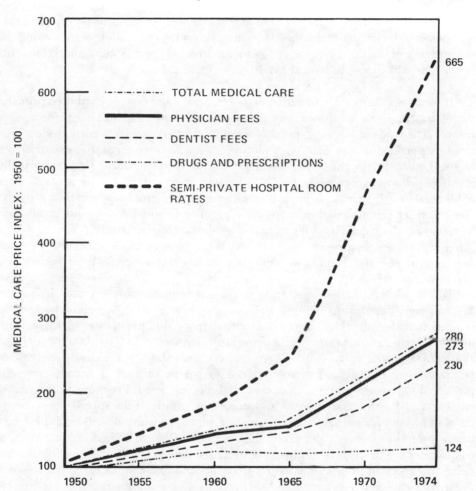

THE INCREASING COSTS OF MEDICAL CARE
U.S.A., 1950 1974

year by just one day would save two billion dollars. Obviously, logic suggests that we strive toward a system in which less hospitalization is required, if we are to contain the costs of medical care within tolerable limits.

I also believe that having access to a more effective primary-care system constitutes a profound human need. Our contemporary society is witnessing the fragmentation of families and a decline in the importance of the church as a social organization, while at the same time it is increasingly troubled by the stresses of modern life; the combination tends to make medicine and the services it renders an important human coping system as well as a medical one. The professional management of simple, straightforward illnesses, including those that resolve themselves, and of chronic illness, despite medicine's inability to eliminate it, are viewed by society as important, whatever their cost. Relief from anxiety—the child does not have meningitis, the lump is not cancerous—and allowing the individual to function with crippling rheumatoid arthritis or serious heart disease are important to our way of life. It will be difficult to show the cost-effectiveness of an efficient, well-distributed system for primary care, but I believe there is little doubt that we will put one in place. While human interactions and interventions that add to the quality of life are often difficult to evaluate or to measure in quantitative cost-effective terms, primary medical care that places more emphasis than it has in the past on the prevention of illness and the maintenance of health will be viewed as an important support system, and I think that Americans will choose to have it available.

If we do decide to move toward a more responsive and better distributed primary-care network, with what things must the system be prepared to deal in the foreseeable future? The kinds of physical, psychological, and social problems currently encountered by a generalist or primary-care physician have been shown in studies carried out in the United States and other countries of the Western world to have virtually identical patterns everywhere. Tables 1–5, taken from a study by the Royal College of General Practitioners in Britain, illustrate the sorts of problems seen by a primary-care physician serving a defined population group in the nineteen-seventies; they will be found on the pages that follow, and they deserve careful study.[7] The problems listed in them are, in general, not complex. What changes might we expect between now and the year 2000, and how might they modify this picture? My projections are as follows:

1) We will have a modest increase in the size of our population from its present 219 million to approximately 260 million by the year 2000.[8] Current projections suggest that the supply of physicians will outpace this population increase, with doctor-to-population ratios rising from approximately 135/100,000 in 1975 to 183/100,000 in the year 2000.[9] There is every indication that a steady increase in other kinds of health professionals trained to handle many of the problems now presented to primary-care practitioners can also be expected. Programs to train nurse clinicians and nurse practitioners are increasing rapidly. Educational programs to develop physician's assistants have flourished, and approximately 2,000 of these new health professionals now enter the United States work force annually. New kinds of community health workers, health associates, and emergency medical technicians are being incorporated in experiments to deliver general first-contact care, and this will eventually change the character and perhaps the scope of primary-care practice.

2) We will, as a nation, have more and more old people in our society. With the fall in birth rate and the increasing longevity of Americans, the numbers of persons 65 and over will rise by 9 million between 1970 and 2000, approximately 45 per cent.[10] This will alter the character of families and communities. It will add to the number of individuals with chronic disease, and it will add to the problems of how we plan for the support of those no longer able to care for themselves.

3) The fragmentation of the extended families of yesteryear will continue. According to the United States Census Bureau, there are now 4.2 million "single-parent" families in the nation.[11] In certain sections of New York City, over one-third of the families are one-adult families. The slow but consistent decline in church attendance will also continue: for example, Roman Catholic church attendance has

TABLE 1

Persons consulting for minor illnesses in a year in a hypothetical average practice of 2,500

Conditions	Consultations per 2,500 patients
General	
Upper respiratory infections	500
Emotional disorders	300
Gastro - intestinal disorders	250
Skin disorders	225
Specific	
Acute tonsillitis	100
Middle ear infection	75
Ear wax	50
Acute urinary infections	50
Acute back syndrome	50
Migraine headache	30
Hay Fever	25

declined by 16 per cent in the past decade, and the trend is still evident.[12] Thus the kinds of people who depended in the past on the extended life-support system supplied by families and by the church systems which aided in the management of many transient and chronic problems of illness will increasingly seek help from other social institutions.

4) The proportion of working women with young children will continue to grow. In 1950, 28 per cent of women with children 6 to 17 years of age worked outside the home. By 1975, over 50 per cent of women with children were members of the work force.[13] These data combined with the numbers of single-parent families suggest that families will become more dependent upon institutions for services formerly supplied by parents in the home.

5) Problems associated with the incidence of mental illness will increase. The number of cases involving aberrations regarded as "mental illness" have been on the rise in recent years. Whether this increase in mental illness is real or simply represents

TABLE 2

Persons consulting for acute major (life threatening) illnesses in a hypothetical average practice of 2,500

Condition	Consultations per 2,500 patients
Acute bronchitis and pneumonia	50
Severe depression	12
Acute myocardial infarction	7
Acute appendicitis	5
Acute strokes	5
All new cancers	5
Cancer of lung	1-2 per year
Cancer of breast	1 per year
Cancer of large bowel	2 every 3 years
Cancer of stomach	1 every 2 years
Cancer of bladder	1 every 3 years
Cancer of cervix	1 every 3 years
Cancer of ovary	1 every 5 years
Cancer of esophagus	1 every 7 years
Cancer of brain	1 every 10 years
Cancer of the uterus	1 every 12 years
Lymphoma	1 every 15 years
Cancer of thyroid	1 every 20 years
Suicidal attempts	3
Deaths in road traffic accidents	1 every 3 years
Suicide	1 every 4 years

TABLE 3

Persons consulting for chronic illness in a year in a hypothetical average practice of 2,500

Conditions	Consultations per 2,500 patients
Chronic arthritis	100
Chronic mental illness	55
Chronic bronchitis	50
Anemia: iron deficiency	40
Anemia: pernicious anemia	3
Chronic heart failure	30
High blood pressure	25
Asthma	25
Peptic ulcer	25
Coronary artery disease	20
Cerebrovascular disease	15
Epilepsy	10
Diabetes	10
Parkinsonism	3
Multiple sclerosis	2
Chronic pyelonephritis	Less than 1
Tuberculosis	Less than 1

changing definitions of emotional well-being is not really known, but society may nevertheless be heading for a crisis in the volume of problems of stress or psychological illness which it carries. A recent study of 200,000 residents of New York City showed some type of "neurosis" (an ill-defined term) in 43 per cent of individuals from higher socioeconomic groups, and in 25 per cent of the poor. The prevalence of overt psychosis was 4 per cent and 13 percent respectively.[14] Whether a primary-care

TABLE 4

Social pathology in a population of 2,500

Conditions	Persons
Aged over 65	350
Poverty	150
Aged over 75	100
Severe physical handicaps	70
Broken homes: one parent families with children under 15	60
Male homosexuals	50
Chronic alcoholics (Edwards, 1968)	5 (known)
	25 (unknown)
Deaf (requiring hearing aids)	25
Severe mental handicaps	10
Blind	7
Problem families	5-10
Juvenile delinquents	5-7
Divorce	3-4
Illegitimate births	3
Adults in prison	1

system and health workers generally should be the ones to cope with these behavioral variances remains to be seen, but at the moment it is clear that physicians and the medical-care system will at least be heavily involved.

These projections are based on data reflecting trends of the last several decades and can thus be made with some degree of confidence. Predictions of changes in technology and biomedical science which may also alter the patterns of practice for those dealing with ambulatory patients are necessarily more tentative, but they must

TABLE 5

Vital statistics in a population of 2,500

Annual vital statistics in a population of 2,500	Numbers
Marriages	17
Divorces	3-4
Pregnancies	40
Deaths	26
Cardiovascular	10
Cancer	5
Strokes	4
Accidents	1
Children under 15	600
Aged over 65	350

be included if we are to try to visualize what medical care might be in the next quarter-century.

6) People will have swifter access to health facilities geographically distant from their places of residence. New roads and more efficient methods of transportation will offer new options and changes in the requirements for placement of health facilities.

7) New communications technologies may also increase the ways in which medical care can be made available. Two-way television via satellite or cable is already being tested in health systems in certain locales. A number of communications and information-handling technologies may result in increased productivity of the individual physician and the effectiveness of those who work with him.

8) New biomedical technologies may permit medicine to deal considerably more effectively with—perhaps even eradicate—certain diseases ranging from the common cold to cancer. The evidence is mounting that some forms of cancer are caused by viruses. It seems possible that during the next quarter-century, tumor prophylaxis by vaccine and antiviral chemotherapy for certain kinds of cancers may become realities. Immunologic advances also raise the possibility that biological and chemical agents will be employed to induce immunity against, or block the action of agents responsible for, some cancers. Specific serologic tests for the detection of certain malignancies at earlier, more treatable stages seems a reasonable prospect.

Many of the "nuisance" viral diseases which now cause the illnesses that result in most of the loss in days of work and interference with feelings of good health may also be brought under control. The prevention of diseases of the vascular system looks less promising, but management may at least become less costly or less time consuming. More effective health education of the young and the elimination of certain environmental health hazards could alter this picture.

These changes in society and in technology and biomedical science will affect the role of the primary-care physician and his colleagues and will have to be taken into account in planning any future programs designed to make general medical care more broadly available.

Over the past ten years, many attempts to identify ways of improving and strengthening the delivery of general medical-care services in this country have been made. Given the culture, the times, and what is already in place, the options appear relatively straightforward. Broadly speaking, one set of options rests on the hypothesis that the number of primary-medical-care practitioners has declined because the right kinds of students for medicine are not being selected. Those who would find such careers attractive have not been admitted to medical school, or have not received medical educations that show the appeal of a general medical-care career.

Another set of options is based on the hypothesis that the large-scale avoidance of general primary-care careers by American physicians is a permanent phenomenon in this country—the scientific and technologic requirements for a career in modern medicine are so demanding as to be irreconcilable with the generalist role. If this is true, it follows that any strategy for improving ambulatory care must include new institutional forms and new professional support systems which would fulfill the function of general care.

Obviously neither of these hypotheses is mutually exclusive; indeed they are in many ways interdependent. One can, by combining them, set forth a number of options which might fit within the limits of social choice for the United States.[15]

Option 1. Recast the criteria for admission to medical school to select more men and women interested in general medicine careers; change the emphasis in the medical-school curriculum to strengthen the interest and preparation of such students for this role: Evidence, notably that of Funkenstein[16] and of Gough and his associates,[17] indicates that students with certain specific characteristics are apt to be inclined toward primary- or general-care roles in medicine, suggesting that it may be possible to identify early on prospective medical students who might follow such careers. Combining this with a recasting of the curriculum so that these students would have a broader exposure than they now have to the problems of out-patient care might help reverse the trend toward specialty careers.

This approach is being tried in some academic medical centers. However, as previously mentioned, medical educators have had only limited success through the years in teaching the medicine of sophisticated ambulatory care. There are difficulties in providing practical experience in ambulatory care for medical students because of the constraints of the relatively short time involved in medical education. A medical student caring for a patient in a hospital bed is doing what he will be doing all his professional life when called upon to care for a hospitalized patient. The biologic events in the hospitalized patient often show rapid changes. Because both the patient and the student are continuously present, the student can see and react to these changing events at any time of the day or night. Thus it is relatively easy to fit an intense educational experience into the confines of a limited time. By contrast, changes in the character of illness, particularly chronic illness, in ambulatory patients often occur gradually over months or years, a period long beyond that which can readily be fitted into any medical-school curriculum without drastic revision in philosophy or format. The "hit and run" kinds of ambulatory programs now generally offered are usually not sufficiently rigorous or challenging; they often simply convince the student that general medicine is not a very attractive career.

This approach has yet another hazard. Because of the need for biomedical scientists and specialists who require a very different kind of education, in all probability a two-track system would emerge, and the hazard that these two tracks would be of unequal standing is great. The difficulty of teaching ambulatory care, however, should not prevent us from trying, but the pitfalls should be recognized.

Option 2. Train two kinds of physicians: If the needs and requirements for specialists and generalists are different, educating and training two kinds of physicians—one a rapidly trained practitioner, the other a graduate similar to that of today—deserves consideration. Historically, the development of any two-track system which might lead to "first-class" and "second-class" physicians has been vigorously resisted in this country. It would probably be feasible only if there was a marked shortening of the premedical and medical education for the practitioner whose primary interest was ambulatory care. It would perhaps be more acceptable if it were regarded as a responsibility to be assumed at a given stage in every physician's development: those who wished to become specialists or superspecialists would be permitted to return for further training only after a period of fulfilling this role. Such a system is similar to that which obtained in this country in the nineteen-twenties, before specialization became an early postgraduate option, and that which still obtains in many other countries today.

Option 3. Restructure the postgraduate training of physicians materially to increase the number of primary-care and family-practice physicians; couple this with restriction of entry into the specialties: Because the ambulatory aspects of general medical care cannot be readily taught within the time constraints of medical-school training, the most logical time to begin them might be the postgraduate period, during which the various forms of training are genuinely differentiated. Well-designed residency programs should allow involvement in ambulatory care for sufficiently long periods for the student to gain competence. The program should be conducted by skilled clinicians in well-organized programs geared to care of patients in families or patients in groups.

A number of opportunities for experience in family residencies which immerse young physicians in the realities of family practice are already available, and the number is growing rapidly—from 62 approved programs in 1970 to 219 in 1974—all supported by federal funds. Primary-care tracks designed to give internists or pediatricians the tools necessary to be effective in general-medical-care settings are also now available in some of our academic medical centers.

Probably the major deficiency in this strategy is that postgraduate programs come late in the educational experience of young physicians. Unless there are profound changes in the attitude of undergraduate teachers toward general-care programs, they will not be effective in persuading significant numbers of young people to enter the field. The choice of career within medicine is generally made well before graduation. It often reflects to a significant degree the orientation of the specialist resident staff who do much of the clinical training. Hence a vigorous and attractive residency program which demonstrates what physicians can gain from, and give to, general medicine might well influence career selection toward general care.

A potent but coercive method for encouraging this choice would be simultaneously to limit entry into the specialties. There are numerous ways in which this could be accomplished, some probably more socially acceptable than others. The number of residency positions in any specialty could be determined by a central authorizing body. The geographic mobility of specialists could be limited, i.e., their practices confined to hospital settings. Such regulation would run counter to some deeply held American values: the right to free choice of career and of the place where one lives is fundamental. But we must realize that virtually any design for encouraging the development of general-practice careers will require voluntary or involuntary curtailment of unrestricted entry into specialty training if present trends are to be modified significantly.

Option 4. Economic incentives to encourage entry into primary or general medical careers: Establishing special facilities that could be offered to individuals entering general medical practices which would permit them to avoid the initial costs of establishing themselves in practice is well within the capacity of many communities. Tax rebates for doctors willing to practice in underserved areas is another possibility. Educational-loan programs with "forgiveness clauses" for those who elect a period of service in primary care are also being seriously considered, and, indeed, one such program may soon become law.

It should be borne in mind, however, that many experiments have already been tried with these options and that none has proved very effective. On the other hand, the interest of some young individuals today in escaping from large-city environments and the high cost of education combine to suggest that a loan-forgiveness program might prove more effective in the future than it has been in the past.

The first four options are based on the assumption that more young people would enter general medical careers if the right individuals were chosen, properly educated, and properly motivated. The next six options focus on modifying the setting or system in which medical care is delivered rather than on changing the kind of individual who enters medicine as a career.

Option 5. Consider general medical practice as a stage in a physician's development or career: The time required for a medical education has been shortened in many institutions, and many educators feel that the recent graduate is still reasonably well prepared for general medical service. Thus, serious consideration might be given to the development of a system in which all graduates of medical schools enter general medical-care training immediately after graduation for a defined period of time. General medical care would be regarded simply as a stage in a physician's career and not necessarily as an end in itself. It would, in many respects, return us to the situation that prevailed when specialties first emerged and when most, if not all, young physicians were first generalists, returning to specialty training only after a period in general medical care. This system would probably be effective in fulfilling many of the functions of general medical care. It would mean the entry of 14,000 to 15,000 young men and women into the field each year. However, those most conversant with the subtleties and complexities of primary-care practice maintain that it would fall far short of the ideal.

But this alone would not solve the primary-care problem. While it seems likely that some would elect to stay in general practice, it would not satisfy one of the basic requirements for primary care, namely, its continuity. It would resemble, rather, medical care given to our armed services by young men serving two-year tours of duty before going on to other pursuits. This is clearly satisfactory care, but it lacks the continuing interaction with one's physician regarded by many as being so desirable. It also fails to recognize the "specialty" nature of primary care; less education is not regarded as satisfactory preparation by those in the field.

Option 6. Use non-physicians to deliver most primary medical care: All evidence suggests that individuals other than physicians can be trained to deliver a major portion of primary or general care, using the physician as backup. It is clear that a good deal of care for commonplace ills and some aspects of psychologic support could be provided by such individuals. But one requirement outlined earlier, namely, that the system should have "the ability to identify, from innocent-appearing situations, those few that are potentially serious and provide properly for them," might not be so well handled. Such a system would probably be, at least initially, most acceptable to the two areas that currently have the most serious problems in general medical care— rural areas of low-patient density and heavily congested, inner-city areas now deprived of physicians. It is less certain that it would be accepted in higher income areas, and thus eventually it would also be stoutly resisted by the first two groups because of its obvious inequities. Again, it runs the hazard of perpetuating a "two-class" system, unless nurse practitioners, physician assistants, and the like, are part of a system of care which intimately involves physicians.

Option 7. Use foreign medical graduates for the bulk of general medical care: The physician-manpower pool in this country is currently replenished from two sources, the graduates of American medical schools and the graduates of foreign institutions. Foreign medical graduates now represent almost 50 per cent of the new American medical-manpower pool each year. Because of this, we have been able to avoid thinking about some of the problems of the shortage of medical manpower.

The strategy of using foreign medical graduates, however, disregards their present career patterns. While it is true that they often take residency training in hospitals not affiliated with academic centers and fill posts that American graduates find undesirable, foreign medical graduates have in fact generally chosen specialty careers in a way indistinguishable from that of their American counterparts, and they clearly therefore will not solve the problem of primary health care in the long run. Further, the psychological and social aspects of primary care would not be well served by this strategy. Even if language barriers are ignored, the culture of physicians from other countries and their approach to subtle human problems are often different, if understandably so, from the needs and habits of the people to be served. Even if they were willing to accept primary-care roles permanently, there is little evidence that we could develop an equitable system based on a group viewed as often poorly trained and as less familiar with the culture in which it will work. Such a system would inevitably come to be viewed as "two-class" and therefore unacceptable.

Option 8. Rely on the "hidden" system of general medical care, and create special subsystems and facilities to take care of the remainder of the population: It is perfectly clear that the largely specialist-oriented private sector of medicine now handles the primary-care needs of most of the population. This system has two very real problems: it is hidden, and it requires a special ticket for entry (e.g., a surgeon may handle the primary-care needs of a patient who originally came to him for surgery, but not as a first-contact physician for a patient with undifferentiated problems). A large study is now underway to determine just how much primary care is given by those in various subspecialty areas. Some figures have been published suggesting that certain "specialists," notably pediatricians, internists, and obstetricians, do much more general practice than they are generally willing to admit.[18] Eighty per cent of the disease processes most frequently managed by pediatricians and internists are the same as those handled by general practitioners. Further, if a "specialist" can be defined as one who sees patients on referral from other physicians, referred patients are not a major part of these specialty practices. Only 8 per cent of the pediatrician's patients, 26 per cent of the internist's, and 19 per cent of the obstetrician's fall into this category. These data strongly suggest that the hidden system of primary or general medical care is heavily subserved by physicians entering those fields. Thus redesigning their training to prepare them for what they in fact will be doing anyway might decrease the criticism of specialty-oriented programs, while improving the availability and quality of general care.

Option 9. Develop multi-specialty groups: This strategy would not actually place more individual physicians in primary or general care, but it could be designed collectively to handle primary-care needs. It has the further advantages that continuous interchange of information among members of the group would help to keep each physician's skills current and that it builds on a system already in operation in our society. It is an approach that is already being explored in some parts of the country.

Option 10. Organize a mixed public/private system of ambulatory care in which individuals or families become the responsibility of a medical-care facility, principally a hospital-based or hospital-linked unit: This is really a variant of Option 9. It is one of the modes of organizing group practice to serve defined populations. It has been used in the development of comprehensive programs such as Kaiser-Permanente, Group Health Cooperative of Puget Sound, the Group Health Association of Washington, D.C., and the Health Insurance Plan of New York City. Legislation encouraging the development of health-maintenance organizations has incorporated some of the knowledge gained from these experiments, and many similar groups are now in various stages of development. Such programs have demonstrated that the clientele can be satisfied, that the amounts of hospitalization required by the population served can be reduced, and that promising mechanisms for the maintenance of professional expertise and for the monitoring of the quality of medical care can be developed.

On the negative side, group health programs have been very expensive in their initial stages and have often been slow to reach a size sufficient for economic viability. They are also dimly viewed by many physicians because of the restrictions which the organizational structure imposes upon them.

Any comprehensive system of primary care should make use of the network of 7,000 hospitals now in existence in this country. Encouraging the organization of a system which permits groups, individual doctors, and clinic staffs the use of a hospital base with a system of common records, sharing of expensive equipment, and collective experience with complex problems would seem promising. Again, it builds on a system already in place. It could, perhaps, be subdivided into smaller units to facilitate the continuous and personal-caring elements of medicine while assuming complete responsibility for defined population groups. It might also develop the flexibility needed to adapt readily to new changes in technology.

I have earlier stated my conviction that the nation will opt for the development of a more responsive system for the equitable distribution and delivery of primary medical care, but one more obvious and potent force compelling us to do this has not yet been mentioned. This is the advent of universal entitlement to medical care—or at least to some form of national health insurance. Although we have proceeded by fits and starts, all evidence suggests that we will have some national mechanism for financing medical care in the foreseeable future. Changes in methods of paying for medical care, even if only partially removing the fee-for-service barrier, will place profound stress on medical-care practitioners and on the facilities in which they work. A careful study of the effects of shifting the payment mechanism from individuals to some collective agency, public or private, suggests more, not less, difficulty in finding a personal physician, longer waits for care, more impersonal treatment, and potentially a lowering of the quality of care rendered, if more effective ways to deliver ambulatory care are not developed. [19] This has not gone unnoticed by those designing fiscal plans for medical care, and the pressures for redressing the situation will inevitably intensify as we move toward some form of national health insurance.

While there may be ways to strengthen primary-care services other than those summarized here, we have not yet been able to identify them. Which option will we elect? In our pluralistic and individualistic society, it seems safest to answer: Some or all of them.

There are, however, a few general observations which might be made. First, I believe that we will try incentives to encourage the growth of primary-care services and will shy away form negative sanctions to promote change. The carrot, rather than the stick, has been the general approach favored by our political process, at least initially. Second, while it seems clear that medicine will become an increasingly regulated profession, I believe we will continue to place more emphasis on local, state, or regional initiatives than on centrally directed services. While mechanisms of payment for medical services, the location of health facilities, and the services they offer will be under increasing regulation, I think it most unlikely that physicians will become employees of a centralized system such as they are in Britain or Sweden.

Americans continue to feel that decentralization of authority and placement of responsibilities in the hands of many individuals are preferable to imposition of control from above, despite the sluggishness and greater costs such a system often displays. Consequently, I do not believe that there will be any basic shift in this attitude during the next quarter-century; indeed, there are many indications that individualism is on the upsurge.

In viewing the options available, I believe the first move will be toward filling the gaps in the current "hidden" system of primary care. The training of family practitioners will be expanded, and the training of internists, pediatricians, and obstetrician-gynecologists will be modified to prepare them more adequately for generalist roles and for the medical care of defined groups of people. New arrangements and new groupings of physicians, joined with an enlarged corps of new health professionals, will be encouraged in order to increase the numbers of patients who can be managed by each individual physician. In this way, the physician will be able to keep his skills up to date while continuing to serve in his capacity as personal physician. Our network of community hospitals will increasingly become an important base for these primary-care practices, and more rational regionalization of costly and less frequently utilized services will result.

Strengthening the "hidden" system also offers the greatest opportunity for the private professional sector to remain autonomous, which is viewed as desirable by most Americans. It would, however, require a drastic reorientation of the role of professional and specialty organizations. If these groups decide to accept responsibilities for the delivery of their services, it might be possible for physicians practicing a given specialty in a particular region to organize themselves and the facilities they use in a more rational fashion than exists today.

Comprehensive prepaid programs will continue to increase in number, though at rates slower than their proponents might wish. Clearly the way in which medical care is paid for is a potent force for reordering the priorities in medicine. Changes in the way we finance medical care could cause shifts in the kinds of health professionals produced, the nature and distribution of their services, and the allocation of funds to medicine and health care. Those in government responsible for the large federal share of medical-care costs will push strongly in this direction. Many in the profession of medicine will resist it.

In the process of developing a more visible primary-care system, I believe we will see internal changes in location, content, and attitude in a number of medical specialties. Many, such as the surgeon and the surgical and medical subspecialists and the pediatric neonatologists, will become more hospital-based and function more exclusively on a referral basis as consultants; thus continuity of care will again be the function of the generalist, whether internist, pediatrician, or family practitioner.

With the focus of primary care on the health and care of groups, we will begin to see further development in the scientific content, so necessary for academic disciplines to flourish, of primary-care programs. New skills in epidemiology, demography, the behavioral sciences, and other disciplines now rarely employed by physicians in their practices, may prove to be potent tools for bettering medical care. Consequently, the practice of general medicine may become intellectually richer, more exciting, and more challenging for aspiring physicians. And this, in turn, may begin to alter the status of specialty training and shift its emphasis in medical education, altering career choices among those who enter medical school.

We will, in the final analysis, continue to have inequities in the availability and in the quality of medical care and gaps between what people want and expect from medical services and what medicine can deliver. We can, however, reduce them to more acceptable dimensions without a total dismemberment of the medical establishment. We can build on structures already in place, if Americans in sufficient numbers decide it is worth the effort. Every indication suggests that we will move in this direction during the next several decades.

REFERENCES
    Note: The sources for Figures 1, 2, 4 are the Medical Care Chartbook (5th ed., Ann Arbor, Michigan, 1972), and the American Medical Association Statistical Department; the source for Figure 3 is the Chicago Board of Health Medical Report for 1966.

[1]K. L. White, T. F. Williams, and B. G. Greenberg, "The Ecology of Medical Care," *New England Journal of Medicine*, 265 (1961), p. 885.

[2]I. J. Fahs and O. L. Peterson, "The Decline in General Practice," *Public Health Reports*, 83 (1968), p. 267.

[3]*Infant Mortality Rates, Socioeconomic Factors*, Series 22, No. 14, U.S. Department of Health, Education, and Welfare, National Center for Health Statistics, Publication No. (HSM) 72-1045 (1972).

[4]D. S. Kessner, *Infant Death: An Analysis of Maternal Risk and Health Care* (Institute of Medicine, National Academy of Sciences, 1973).

[5]*Children and Youth Projects Report Series 18 and 20, Quarterly Summary Reports*, Minnesota Systems Research, April-June, 1972; October-December, 1972

[6]L. Gordis, "Effectiveness of Comprehensive Care Programs in Preventing Rheumatic Fever," *New England Journal of Medicine*, 289 (1973), p. 331

[7]*Present State and Future Needs of General Practice*, Royal College of General Practitioners (3rd ed., London, 1973).

[8]*Population of the United States: Trends and Prospects 1950-1990*, U.S. Department of Commerce (1974).

[9]*The Supply of Health Manpower: Profiles and Projections*, U.S. Department of Health, Education, and Welfare, No. 75-28 (1974).

[10]C. F. Westoft and R. Parker, "Demographic and Social Aspects of Population Growth," *Growth of the Population of the United States in the Twentieth Century* (U.S. Government Printing Office, Washington, D.C., 1972).

[11]Georgia Dullea, "The Increasing Single Parent Families," *New York Times*, December 3, 1974, p. 46.

[12]Gallup Poll on Religion in America (Princeton, 1975).

[13]*Statistical Abstract of the United States, 1973* (U.S. Government Printing Office, Washington, D. C., 1973).

[14]P. Selby, *Health in 1980-1990: A Predictive Study Based on an International Inquiry* (Basel, 1974).

[15]W. McDermott, "General Medical Care: Identification and Analysis of Alternative Approaches," *Johns Hopkins Medical Journal*, 135 (1974), p. 292.

[16]D. H. Funkenstein, "The Changing Pool of Medical School Applicants," *Harvard Medical Alumni Bulletin*, 41 (1967), p. 18.

[17]H. B. Gough and W. B. Hull, "A Prospective Study of Personality Changes in Students in Medicine, Dentistry, and Nursing," *Research in Higher Education*, 162 (1973), p. 127.

[18]K. M. Endicott, *The Distribution of Physicians Geographically and by Specialty* (Institute of Medicine, Washington, D.C., 1974).

[19]J. P. Newhouse, C. E. Phelps, and W. B. Schwartz, "Policy Options and the Impact of National Health Insurance," *New England Journal of Medicine*, 290 (1974), p. 1345.

AARON WILDAVSKY

Doing Better and Feeling Worse:
The Political Pathology of Health Policy

ACCORDING TO THE GREAT EQUATION, Medical Care equals Health. But the Great Equation is wrong. More available medical care does not equal better health. The best estimates are that the medical system (doctors, drugs, hospitals) affects about 10 per cent of the usual indices for measuring health: whether you live at all (infant mortality), how well you live (days lost due to sickness), how long you live (adult mortality). The remaining 90 per cent are determined by factors over which doctors have little or no control, from individual life style (smoking, exercise, worry), to social conditions (income, eating habits, physiological inheritance), to the physical environment (air and water quality). Most of the bad things that happen to people are at present beyond the reach of medicine.

Everyone knows that doctors do help. They can mend broken bones, stop infections with drugs, operate successfully on swollen appendices. Innoculations, internal infections, and external repairs are other good reasons for keeping doctors, drugs, and hospitals around. More of the same, however, is counterproductive. Nobody needs unnecessary operations; and excessive use of drugs can create dependence or allergic reactions or merely enrich the nation's urine.

More money alone, then, cannot cure old complaints. In the absence of medical knowledge gained through new research, or of administrative knowledge to convert common practice into best practice, current medicine has gone as far as it can. It will not burn brighter if more money is poured on it. No one is saying that medicine is good for nothing, only that it is not good for everything. Thus the marginal value of one—or one billion—dollars spent on medical care will be close to zero in improving health. And, for purposes of public policy, it is not the bulk of present medical expenditures, which do have value, but the proposed future spending, which is of dubious value, that should be our main concern.

When people are polled, they are liable, depending on what they are asked, to say that they are getting good care but that there is a crisis in the medical-care system. Three-quarters to four-fifths of the population, depending on the survey, are satisfied with their doctors and the care they give; but one-third to two-thirds think the system that produces these results is in bad shape. Opinions about the family doctor, of course, are formed from personal experience. "The system," on the other hand, is an abstract entity—and here people may well imitate the attitudes of those interested and vocal elites who insist the system is in crisis. People do, however, have specific complaints related to their class position. The rich don't like waiting, the poor don't like high prices, and those in the middle don't like both. Everyone would like easier

105

access to a private physician in time of need. As we shall see, the widespread belief that doctors are good but the system is bad has a plausible explanation. That's the trouble: everyone behaves reasonably; it is only the systemic effects of all this reasonable behavior that are unreasonable.

If most people are healthier today than people like themselves have ever been, and if access to medical care now is more evenly distributed among rich and poor, why is there said to be a crisis in medical care that requires massive change? If the bulk of the population is satisfied with the care it is getting, why is there so much pressure in government for change? Why, in brief, are we doing better but feeling worse? Let us try to create a theory of the political pathology of health policy.

Paradoxes, Principles, Axioms, Identities, and Laws

The fallacy of the Great Equation is based on the Paradox of Time: past successes lead to future failures. As life expectancy increases and as formerly disabling diseases are conquered, medicine is faced with an older population whose disabilities are more difficult to defeat. The cost of cure is higher, both because the easier ills have already been dealt with and because the patients to be treated are older. Each increment of knowledge is harder won; each improvement in health is more expensive. Thus time converts one decade's achievements into the next decade's dilemmas. Yesterday's victims of tuberculosis are today's geriatric cases. The Paradox of Time is that success lies in the past and (possibly) the future, but never the present.

The Great Equation is rescued by the Principle of Goal Displacement, which states that any objective that cannot be attained will be replaced by one that can be approximated. Every program needs an opportunity to be successful; if it cannot succeed in terms of its ostensible goals, its sponsors may shift to goals whose achievement they can control. The process subtly becomes the purpose. And that is exactly what has happened as "health" has become equivalent to "equal access to" medicine.

When government goes into public housing, it actually provides apartments; when it goes into health, all it can provide is medicine. But medicine is far from health. So what the government can do then is try to equalize access to medicine, whether or not that access is related to improved health. If the question is, "Does health increase with government expenditure on medicine?," the answer is likely to be "No." Just alter the question—"Has access to medicine been improved by government programs?"—and the answer is most certainly, with a little qualification, "Yes."

By "access," of course, we mean quantity, not quality, of care. Access, moreover, can be measured, and progress toward an equal number of visits to doctors can be reported. But better access is not the same as better health. Something has to be done about the distressing stickiness of health rates, which fail to keep up with access. After all, if medical care does not equal health, access to medical care is irrelevant to health— unless, of course, health is not the real goal but merely a cover for something more fundamental, which might be called "mental health" (reverently), or "shamanism" (irreverently), or "caring" (most accurately).

Any doctor will tell you, say sophisticates, that most patients are not sick, at least physically, and that the best medicine for them is reassurance. Tranquilizers, painkillers, and aspirin would seem to be the functional equivalents, for these are the drugs most often prescribed. Wait a minute, says the medical sociologist (the student not merely of medicine's manifest, but also of its latent, functions), pain is just as real when it's mental as when it's physical. If people want to know somebody loves them, if today they prefer doctors of medicine to doctors of theology, they are entitled to get what they want.

Once "caring" has been substituted for (or made equivalent to) "doctoring," access immediately becomes a better measure of attainment. The number of times a person sees a doctor is probably a better measure of the number of times he has been reassured than of his well-being or a decline in his disease. So what looks like a single goal substitution (access to medicine in place of better health) is actually a double displacement: caring instead of health, and access instead of caring.

This double displacement is fraught with consequences. Determining how much medical care is sufficient is difficult enough; determining how much "caring" is, is virtually impossible. The treatment of physical ills is partially subjective; the treatment of mental ills is almost entirely subjective. If a person is in pain, he alone can judge how much it hurts. How much caring he needs depends upon how much he wants. In the old days he took his tension chiefly to the private sector, and there he got as much attention as he could pay for. But now with government subsidy of medicine looming so large, the question of how much caring he should get inevitably becomes public.

By what standard should this public question be decided? One objective criterion—equality of access—inevitably stands out among the rest. For if we don't quite know what caring is or how much of it there should be, we can always say that at least it should be equally distributed. Medicaid has just about equalized the number of doctor visits per year between the poor and the rich. In fact, the upper class is showing a decrease in visits, and the life expectancy of richer males is going down somewhat. Presumably, no one is suggesting remedial action in favor of rich men. Equality, not health, is the issue.

Equality

One can always assert that even if the results of medical treatment are illusory, the poor are entitled to their share. This looks like a powerful argument, but it neglects the Axiom of Inequality. That axiom states that every move to increase equality in one dimension necessarily decreases it in another. Consider space. The United States has unequal rates of development. Different geographic areas vary considerably in such matters as income, custom, and expectation. Establishing a uniform national policy disregards these differences; allowing local variation means that some areas are more unequal than others. Think of time. People not only have unequal incomes, they also differ in the amount of time they are prepared to devote to medical care. In equalizing the effects of money on medical care—by removing money as a consideration—care is likely to be allocated by the distribution of available time. To the extent that the pursuit of money takes time, people with a monetary advantage will have a temporal disadvantage. You can't have it both ways, as the Axiom of Allocation makes abundantly clear.

"No system of care in the world," says David Mechanic, summing up the Axiom of Allocation, "is willing to provide as much care as people will use, and all such systems develop mechanisms that ration . . . services." Just as there is no free lunch, so there is no free medicine. Rationing can be done by time (waiting lists, lines), by distance (people farther from facilities use them less than those who are closer), by complexity (forms, repeated visits, communications difficulties), by space (limiting the number of hospital beds and available doctors), or by any or all of these methods in combination. But why do people want more medical service than any system is willing to provide? The answer has to do with uncertainty.

If medicine is only partially and imperfectly related to health, it follows that doctor and patient both will often be uncertain as to what is wrong or what to do about it. Otherwise—if medicine were perfectly related to health—either there would be no health problem or it would be a very different one. Health rates would be on one side and health resources on the other; costs and benefits could be neatly compared. But they can't, because we often don't know how to produce the desired benefits. Uncertainty exists because medicine is a quasi-science—more science than, say, political science; less science than physics. How the participants in the medical system resolve their uncertainties matters a great deal.

The Medical Uncertainty Principle states that there is always one more thing that might be done—another consultation, a new drug, a different treatment. Uncertainty is resolved by doing more: the patient asks for more, the doctor orders more. The patient's simple rule for resolving uncertainty is to seek care up to the level of his insurance. If everyone uses all the care he can, total costs will rise; but the individual has so little control over the total that he does not appreciate the connection between his individual choice and the collective result. A corresponding phenomenon occurs among doctors. They can resolve uncertainty by prescribing up to the level of the patient's insurance, a rule reinforced by the high cost of malpractice. Patients bringing suit do not consider the relationship between their own success and higher medical costs for everyone. The patient is anxious, the doctor insecure; this combination is unbeatable until the irresistible force meets the immovable object—the Medical Identity.

The Medical Identity states that use is limited by availability. Only so much can be gotten out of so much. Thus, if medical uncertainty suggests that existing services will be used, Identity reminds us to add the words "up to the available supply." That supply is primarily doctors, who advise on the kind of care to provide and the number of hospital beds to maintain. But patients, considering only their own desires in time of need, want to maximize supply, a phenomenon that follows inexorably from the Principle of Perspective.

That principle states that social conditions and individual feelings are not the same thing. A happy social statistic may obscure a sad personal situation. A statistical equilibrium may hide a family crisis. Morbidity and mortality, in tabulating aggregate rates of disease and death, describe you and me but do not touch us. We do not think of ourselves as "rates." Our chances may be better or worse than the aggregate. To say that doctors are not wholly (or even largely) successful in alleviating certain symptoms is not to say that they don't help some people and that one of those people won't be me. Taking the chance that it will be me often seems to make sense, even if there is reason to believe that most people can't be helped and that some may actually be harmed. Most people, told that the same funds spent on other purposes may increase social benefits, will put their personal needs first. This is why expenditures on medical care are always larger than any estimate of the social benefit received. Now we can understand, by combining into one law the previous principles and Medical Identity, why costs rise so far and so fast.

The Law of Medical Money states that medical costs rise to equal the sum of all private insurance and government subsidy. This occurs because no one knows how much medical care ought to cost. The patient is not sure he is getting all he should, and the doctor does not want to be faulted for doing less than he might. Consider the triangular relationship between doctor, patient, and hospital. With private insurance, the doctor can use the hospital resources that are covered by the insurance while holding down his patient's own expenditures. With public subsidies, the doctor may charge his highest usual fee, abandon charitable work, and ignore the financial benefits of eliminating defaults on payments. His income rises. His patient doesn't have to pay, and his hospital expands. The patient, if he is covered by a government program or private insurance (as about 90 per cent are) finds that his out-of-pocket expenses have remained the same. His insurance costs more, but either it comes out of his paycheck, looking like a fixed expense, or it is taken off his income tax as a deduction. Hospitals work on a cost-plus basis. They offer the latest and the best, thus pleasing both doctor and patient. They pay their help better; or, rather, they get others to pay their help. It's on the house—or at least on the insurance.

Perhaps our triangle ought to be a square: maybe we should include insurance companies. Why are they left out of almost all discussions of this sort? Why don't they play a cost-cutting role in medical care as they do in other industries? After all, the less the outlay, the more income for the company. Here the simplest explanation seems the best: insurance companies make no difference because they are no different from the rest of the health-care industry. The largest, Blue Cross and Blue Shield, are run by the hospital establishment on behalf of doctors. After all, hospitals do not so much have patients as they have doctors who have patients. Doctors run hospitals, not the other way around. Insurance companies not willing to play this game have left the field.

What process ultimately limits medical costs? If the Law of Medical Money predicts that costs will increase to the level of available funds, then that level must be limited to keep costs down. Insurance may stop increasing when out-of-pocket payments exceed the growth in the standard of living; at that point individuals may not be willing to buy more. Subsidy may hold steady when government wants to spend more on other things or when it wants to keep its total tax take down. Costs will be limited when either individuals or governments reduce the amount they put into medicine.

No doubt the Law of Medical Money is crude, even rude. No doubt it ignores individual instances of self-sacrifice. But it has the virtue of being a powerful and parsimonious predictor. Costs have risen (and are continuing to rise) to the level of insurance and subsidy.

Why There Is a Crisis

If more than three-quarters of the population are satisfied with their medical care, why is there a crisis? Surveys on this subject are inadequate, but invariably they reveal two things: (1) the vast majority are satisfied, but (2) they wish medical care didn't cost so much and they would like to be assured of contact with their own doctor. So far as the people are concerned, then, the basic problems are cost and access. Why, to begin at the end, aren't doctors where patients want them to be?

To talk about physicians being maldistributed is to turn the truth upside down: it is the potential patients who are maldistributed. For doctors to be in the wrong place, they would have to be where people aren't, and yet they are accused of sticking to the main population centers. If distant places with little crowding and less pollution, far away from the curses of civilization, attracted the same people who advocate their virtues, doctors would live there, too. Obviously, they prefer the amenities of metropolitan areas. Are they wrong to live where they want to live? Or are the rural and remote wrong to demand that others come where they are?

Doctors can be offered a government subsidy—more money, better facilities— on the grounds that it is a national policy for medical care to be available wherever citizens choose to live. Virtually all students in medical schools are heavily subsidized, so it would not be entirely unjust to demand that they serve several years in places not of their own choosing. The reason such policies do not work well— from Russia to the "Ruritanias" of this world—is that people who are forced to live in places they don't like make endless efforts to escape.

Because the distribution of physicians is determined by rational choice—doctors locate where their psychic as well as economic income is highest—there is no need for special laws to explain what happens. But the political pathology of health policy—the more the government spends on medicine, the less credit it gets— does require explanation.

The syndrome of "the more, the less" has to be looked at as it developed over time. First we passed Medicare for the elderly and Medicaid for the poor. The idea was to get more people into the mainstream of good medical care. Following the Law of Medical Money, however, the immediate effect was to increase costs, not merely for the poor and elderly but for all the groups in between. You can't simply add the costs of the new coverage to the costs of the old; you have to multiply them both by higher figures up to the limits of the joint coverage. This is where the Axiom of Inequality takes over. The wealthier aged, who can afford to pay, receive not merely the same benefits as the aged poor, but even more, because they are better able to negotiate the system. Class tells. Inequalities are immediately created within the same category. Worse still is the "notch effect" under Medicaid, through which those just above the eligibles in income may be worse off than those below. Whatever the cutoff point, there must always be a "near poor" who are made more unequal. And so is everybody else who pays twice, first in taxes to support care for others and again in increased costs for themselves. Moreover, with increased utilization of medicine, the system becomes crowded; medical care is not only more costly but harder to get. So there we have the Paradox of Time—as things get better, they get worse.

The politics of medical care becomes a minus-sum game in which every institutional player leaves the table poorer than when he sat down. In the beginning, the number of new patients grows arithmetically while costs rise geometrically. The immediate crisis is cost. Medicaid throws state and federal budgets out of whack. The talk is all about chiselers, profiteers, and reductions. Forms and obstacles multiply. The Medical Identity is put in place. Uncle Sam becomes Uncle Scrooge. One would hardly gather that billions more are actually being spent on medicine for the poor. But the federal government is not the only participant who is doing better and feeling worse.

Unequal levels of development within states pit one location against another. A level of benefits adequate for New York City would result in coverage of half or more of the population in upstate areas as well as nearly all of Alaska's Eskimos and Arizona's Indians. The rich pay more; the poor get hassled. Patients are urged to take more of their medicine only to discover they are targets of restrictive practices. They are expected to pay deductibles before seeing a doctor and to contribute a co-payment (part of the cost) afterward. Black doctors are criticized if their practice consists predominantly of white patients, but they are held up to scorn if they increase their income by treating large numbers of the poor and aged in the ghettos. Doctors are urged to provide more patients with better medicine, and then they are criticized for making more money. The Principle of Perspective leads each patient to want the best for himself, disregarding the social cost; and, at the same time, doctors are criticized for giving high-cost care to people who want it. The same holds true for hospitals: keeping wages down is exploitation of workers; raising them is taking advantage of insurance. Vast financial incentives are offered to encourage the establishment of nursing homes to serve the aged, and the operators are then condemned for taking advantage of the opportunity.

Does anyone win? Just try to abolish Medicare and Medicaid. Crimes against the poor and aged would be the least of the accusations. Few argue that the country would be better off without these programs than with them. Yet, as the programs operate, the smoke they generate is so dense that their supporters are hard to find.

By now it should be clear how growing proportions of people in need of medicine can be getting it in the midst of what is universally decried as a crisis in health care. Governments face phenomenal increases in cost. Administrators alternately fear charges of incompetence for failing to restrain real financial abuse and charges of niggardliness toward the needy. Patients are worried about higher costs, especially as serious or prolonged illnesses threaten them with financial catastrophe. That proportionally few people suffer this way does not decrease the concern, because it *can* happen to anyone. Doctors fear federal control, because efforts to lower costs lead to more stringent regulations. The proliferation of forms makes them feel like bureaucrats; the profusion of review committees threatens to keep them permanently on trial. New complaints increase faster than old ones can be remedied. Specialists in public health sing their ancient songs—you are what you eat, as old as you feel, as good as the air you breathe—with more conviction and less effect. True but trite: what can be done isn't worth doing; what is worth doing can't be done. The watchwords are malaise, stasis, crisis.

If money is a barrier to medicine, the system is discriminatory. If money is no barrier, the system gets overcrowded. If everyone is insured, costs rise to the level of the insurance. If many remain underinsured, their income drops to the level of whatever medical disaster befalls them. Inability to break out of this bind has made the politics of health policy pathological.

Political Pathology

Health policy began with a laudable effort to help people by resolving the polarized conflict between supporters of universal, national health insurance ("socialized" medicine) and the proponents of private medicine. Neither side believed a word uttered by the other. The issue was sidestepped by successfully implementing medical care for the aged under Social Security. Agreement that the aged needed help was easier to achieve than consensus on any overall medical system. The obvious defect was that the poor, who needed financial help the most, were left out unless they were also old and covered by Social Security. The next move, therefore, was Medicaid for the poor, at least for those reached by state programs.

Even if one still believed that medicine equaled health, it became impossible to ignore the evidence that availability of medical services was not the same as their delivery and use. Seeing a doctor was not the same as actually doing what he prescribed. It is hard to alleviate stress in the doctor's office when the patient goes back to the same stress at home and on the street.

"Health delivery" became the catchword. At times it almost seemed as if the welcome wagon was supposed to roll up to the door and deliver health, wrapped in a neat package. One approach brought services to the poor through neighborhood health centers. The idea was that local control would increase sensitivity to the patients' needs. But experience showed that this "sensitivity" had its price. Local "needs" encompassed a wider range of services, including employment. The costs per patient-visit for seeing a doctor or social worker were three to four times those for seeing a private practitioner. Achieving local control meant control by inside laymen rather than outside professionals, a condition doctors were loath to accept. Innovation both in medical practice and in power relationships proved a greater burden than distant federal sponsors could bear, so they tried to co-opt the medical powers by getting them to sponsor health centers. The price was paid in higher costs and lower local control. Amid universal complaints, programs were maintained where feasible, phased out where necessary, and forgotten where possible.

By now the elite participants have exceeded their thresholds of pain: government can't make good on its promises to deliver services; administrators are blamed for everything from malpractice by doctors to overcharges by hospitals; doctors find their professional prerogatives invaded by local activists from below and by state and federal bureaucrats from above. From the left come charges that the system is biased against the poor because local residents are unable to obtain, or maintain, control of medical facilities, and because the rates by which health is measured are worse for them than for the better off. Loss of health is tied to lack of power. From the right come charges that the system penalizes the professional and the productive: excessive governmental intervention leads to lower medical standards and higher costs of bureaucracy, so that costs go up while health does not.

As neighborhood health centers (NHCs) phased out, the new favorites, the health-maintenance organizations (HMOs), phased in. If the idea behind the NHCs was to bring services to the people, the idea behind the HMOs is to bring the people to the services. If a rationale for NHCs was to exert lay control over doctors, the rationale for HMOs is to exert medical control over costs. The concept is ancient. Doctors gather together in a group facility. Individuals or groups, such as unions and universities, join the HMO at a fixed rate for specified services. Through efficiencies in the division of labor and through features such as bonuses to doctors for less utilization, downward control is exerted on costs.

Since the basic method of cutting costs is to reduce the supply of hospital beds and physician services (the Medical Identity), HMOs work by making people wait. Since physicians are on salary, they must be given a quota of patients or a cost objective against which to judge their efforts. Both incentives may have adverse effects on patients. HMO patients complain about the difficulty of building up a personal relationship with a doctor who can be seen quickly when the need arises. Establishing such a relationship requires communication skills most likely to be found among the middle class. The patient's ability to shop around for different opinions is minimized, unless he is willing to pay extra by going outside the system. Doctors are motivated to engage in preventive practices, though evidence on the efficacy of these practices is hard to come by. They are also motivated to engage in bureaucratic routines to minimize the patients' demands on their time; and they may divert patients to various specialties or ask them to return, so as to fit them into each physician's assigned quota. In a word, HMOs are a mixed bag, with no one quite sure yet what the trade-off is between efficiency and effectiveness. Turning the Great Equation into an Identity—where Health = Health Maintenance Organization—does, however, solve a lot of problems by definition.

HMOs may be hailed by some as an answer to the problem of medical information. How is the patient-consumer to know whether he is getting proper care at reasonable cost? If it were possible to rate HMOs, and if they were in competition, people might find it easier to choose among them than among myriads of private doctors. Instead of being required to know whether all those tests and special consultations were necessary, or how much an operation should cost, the patients (or better still, their sponsoring organizations) might compare records of each HMO's ability to judge. Our measures of medical quality and cost, however, are still primitive. Treatment standards are notoriously subjective. Health rates are so tenuously connected to medicine that they are bound to be similar among similar populations so long as everyone has even limited access to care.

If health is only minimally related to care, less expertise may be about as good as more professional training. If by "care" many or most people mean simply a sympathetic listener as much as, or more than, they mean a highly trained, cold diagnostician, cheaper help may be as good as, or even better than, expensive assistance. Enter the nurse-practitioner or the medical corpsman or the old Russian *feldsher*—medical assistants trained to deal with emergencies, make simple diagnoses, and refer more complicated problems to medical doctors. They cost less, and they actually make home visits. The main disadvantage is their apparent challenge to the prestige of doctors, but it could work the other way around: doctors might be elevated because they deal with more complicated matters. But the success of the medical assistant might nonetheless raise questions about the mystique of medical doctors. In response the doctors might deny that anyone else can really know what is going on and what needs to be done, and they might then use assistants as additions to (but not substitutes for) their services. That would mean another input into the medical system and therefore an additional cost. The politics of medicine is just as much about the power of doctors as it is about the authority of politicians.

Now we see again, but from a different angle, why the medical system seems in crisis although most people are satisfied with the care they are receiving. At any one time, most people are reasonably healthy. When they do need help, they can get it. The quality of care is generally impressive; or whatever ails them goes away of its own accord. But these comments apply only to the mass of patients. The elite participants—doctors, administrators, politicians—are all frustrated. Anything they turn to rebounds against them. Damned if they do and cursed if they don't, it is not surprising that they feel that any future position is bound to be less uncomfortable than the one they hold today. Things can always get worse, of course, but it is not easy for them to see that.

Governmental Legitimacy: Curing the Sickness of Health

Why should government pay billions for health and get back not even token tribute? If government is going to be accused of abusing the poor, neglecting the middle classes, and milking the rich; if it is to be condemned for bureaucratizing the patient and coercing the doctor, it can manage all that without spending billions. Slanders and calumnies are easier to bear when they are cost-free. Spending more for worse treatment is as bad a policy for government as it would be for any of us. The only defendant without counsel is the government. What should it do?

The Axiom of Inequality cannot be changed; it is built into the nature of things. What government can do is to choose the kinds of inequalities with which it is prepared to live. Increasing the waiting time of the rich, for instance—that is, having them wait as long as everybody else—may not seem outrageous. Decreasing subsidies in New York City and increasing them in Jacksonville may seem a reasonable price to pay for national uniformity. From the standpoint of government, however, the political problem is not to achieve equal treatment but to get support, at least from those it intends to benefit. Government needs gratitude, not ingrates.

The Principle of Goal Displacement, through the double-displacement effect, succeeds only in substituting access to care for health; it by no means guarantees that people will value the access they get. Equal access to care will not necessarily be equated with the best care available or with all that patients believe they require. Government's task is to resolve the Paradox of Time so that, as things get better, people will see themselves as better off.

Proposals for governmental support of medical care have ranged from modest subsidies to private insurance (the AMA's Medicredit) to public control of the medical industry on the British model. The latter has never had much support in this country, because of widespread opposition to socializing doctors by turning them into de facto government employees. The former has lost whatever support it once had as respect for the AMA has declined, its internal unity has diminished, and its congressional supporters have nearly vanished. Private insurance seems as much the problem as the solution.

The two most prominent proposals would resolve the political problems of medical care in contrasting ways, but substantively they are similar. Both the Comprehensive Health Insurance Plan (CHIP), introduced in the last days of the Nixon administration, and the Kennedy-Mills proposal would involve billions of dollars in additional expenditures. Estimates put each of them at $42 billion to start, less substantial existing expenditures—but then no estimates in this field have ever come remotely close to reality. Both proposals would provide health insurance for virtually everyone and would cover almost everything (including catastrophic and long-term illness) except for prolonged mental illness and nursing-home care. Both include a string of deductibles and co-insurance mechanisms, with CHIP so complex as almost to defy description. Both seek to hold down costs by giving individuals a financial incentive to limit use. Neither provides incentives for the medical community to contain costs, other than the importunings of insurance companies and state governments (CHIP) or the federal government (Kennedy-Mills), which have not been noticeably effective in the past.

CHIP would be financed largely through employer-employee contributions, with employees making a per capita payment; Kennedy-Mills substitutes a more (though by no means entirely) progressive proportionate tax. CHIP mandates insurance and gives a choice of private plans supervised through state agencies. Kennedy-Mills works largely through a special fund collected and administered by the federal government. The basic difference between them is that more of the cost of Kennedy-Mills shows up in the federal budget, while most of the cost of CHIP, as its acronym suggests, is diffused through the private sector.

The most likely consequence of both proposals would be a vast inflation of costs without a corresponding increase in services. Since medical manpower and facilities could not increase proportionately with demand, prices would rise. It would be Medicaid all over again, only worse because so many new things would be attempted and so many old things expanded. Almost before the ink dried on the legislation, efforts would be under way to delay this provision, lessen the cost of that one, introduce rationing in nonmonetary ways, find more forms for doctors and patients to fill out, and on and on. Cries of systemic crisis would be replaced by prophecies of systemic failure. But enough. My purpose is not to predict the medical consequences of these proposals but to analyze their political rationale.

Based on the political premise that some form of national health insurance was inevitable, CHIP sought to limit the government's liability. By joining the opposition, the Nixon administration hoped to control the apparatus so as to lessen its impact on the federal budget and bureaucracy. If people were determined to have something that wasn't going to help them, the government could at least see to it that the totals did not swamp its budget or overload its administration. The costs of failure would be spread around among the states, the various insurance companies, and innumerable individual and group medical practices. Just as revenue sharing was designed to channel demands to state and local governments, instead of the national government (here's a little money and a lot of trouble, and don't bother me!) so CHIP was devised to diffuse responsibility.

What the Republican administration did not foresee was that the rapid breakdown of the existing medical system would inevitably lead to demands for a federal takeover. When a company goes bankrupt, it is usually returned, not to its owners, but to its creditors. This insight belongs to the sponsors of the Kennedy-Mills bill. They seized on the Nixon plan to advance one that would load additional clients, services, and billions onto the shoulders of government. Wouldn't this proposal be too expensive and cumbersome? The worse the better, politically! For then the stage would be set for a national health service.

Under the Kennedy-Griffith (now Kennedy-Corman) proposal, which was the senator's original preference, every person in the United States would, without personal payment, be covered for a wide variety of services, thus replacing all public programs and private insurance with an all-inclusive federal system. Every public and personal medical expense would be transferred to the federal government, paid for half by additional payroll taxes and higher taxes on unearned income and half from general revenues. Obviously, as the sole direct payer, the federal government would have control over costs, but, by the same token, it would have to make all the decisions on how much of what service would be provided to which people in what way for how long.

The difference between Kennedy-Mills and the Kennedy-Corman Health Security Act (HSA) is that the latter would work directly on the Law of Medical Money by limiting the financial resources flowing into the medical system. Whatever the federal government allocated would be all that could be spent, except for the sums spent by those people choosing to pay extra to go outside the system. To put HSA in proper perspective, it is useful to contrast it with another proposal, one that would also limit supply but from a different direction. Senators Long and Ribicoff proposed to deal with the costs of catastrophic illness by setting individual-expenditure limits beyond which costs would be paid by the government. But Long-Ribicoff did not relate individual payments to income. For our comparison, therefore, it is more helpful to concentrate on Martin Feldstein's proposal for an income-graded program in which each person pays medical costs up to a specified proportion of his income, after which the government picks up the remaining (defined as catastrophic) expenses. Medicare and Medicaid are replaced, as all benefits are related to income. The poor pay less, the rich pay more, but everyone is protected against the costs of catastrophe. Although the catastrophic portion would rise in cost, especially for long-term disability, it would represent a relatively small proportion of medical expenditures. Total costs would be determined by overall financial inputs, which would be limited by the willingness of people to pay instead of inflated by using up their insurance or subsidy.

At first glance it might appear strange for national health insurance (whether through private intermediaries or direct government operation) to be conceived of as a method for limiting costs; but experience in practice, as well as deduction from theory, bears out that conception. The usual complaint in Britain, for example, is that the National Health Service is being starved for funds: hospital construction has been virtually nil; the number of doctors per capita has hardly increased; long queues persist for hospitalization in all but emergency cases. Why? Because health care accounts for a sizable proportion of both government expenditure and gross national product and must compete with family allowances, housing, transportation, and all the rest. While there are pressures to increase medical expenditures, they are counterbalanced by demands from other sectors. In times of extreme financial stringency, all too frequent as government expenditure approaches half of the GNP, it is not likely that priority will go to medicine.

So much for current trends. In the future, the nation will probably move toward (and vacillate between) three generic types of health-care policies: (1) a mixed public and private system like the one we have now, only bigger; (2) total coverage through a national health service; and (3) income-graded catastrophic health insurance. It will be convenient to refer to these approaches as "mixed," "total," and "income."

The total and income approaches have weaknesses. The income-catastrophic approach might encourage a "sky's the limit" attitude toward large expenditures; the other side of the coin is that resources would flow to those chronically and/or extremely ill people who most need help. The total approach would strain the national budget, putting medical needs at the mercy of other concerns, such as tax increases; on the other hand, making medicine more political might have the advantage of providing more informed judgment on its relative priority. The two approaches, however, are more interesting for their different strengths than for their weaknesses.

The income approach would magnify individual choice until the level of catastrophic cost is reached. Holding ability to pay relatively constant, each person would be able to decide how much (in terms of what money can buy) he is willing to give up to purchase medical services. There would be no need to regulate the medical industry as to cost and service: supply and demand would determine the price. Paperwork would be minimized. So would bureaucracy. Under- or over-utilization could be dealt with by raising or lowering the percentage limits at each level of income, rather than by dealing with tens of thousands of doctors, hospitals, pharmacies, and the like. The total approach, by contrast, could promise a kind of collective rationality in the sense that the government would make a more direct determination of how much the nation wanted to spend on health versus other desired expenditures.

How might we choose between an essentially administrative and a primarily market-oriented mechanism? Each is as political as the other, but they come to their politics in different ways. An income approach would be simpler to administer and easier to abandon. If it didn't work, more ambitious programs could readily be subsidized. A total approach could promise more, because no one under existing programs would be worse off (except taxpayers), and everyone with insufficient coverage would come under its comprehensive umbrella. The backers of totality fear that the income approach would preempt the health field for years to come. The proponents of income grading fear that, once a comprehensive program is begun, there will be no getting out of it—too many people would lose benefits they already have, and the medical system would have unalterably changed its character. The choice (not only now but in the future) really has to be made on fundamental grounds of a modified-market versus an almost entirely administrative approach. Which proposal would be not only proper for the people but good for the government?

Market versus Administrative Mechanisms

At the outset, I should state my conviction that doing either one consistently would be better than mixing them up. Both methods would give government a better chance to know what it is doing and to get credit for what it does. Expenditures on the medical system, whether too high or too low for some tastes, would be subject to overall control instead of sudden and unpredictable increases. Patients would have a system they could understand and would therefore be able to hold government accountable for how it was working. Under one system they would know that care was comprehensive, crediting government with the program and criticizing it for quality and cost. Under the other, they would know they were being encouraged to exercise discretion, but within boundaries guaranteeing them protection against catastrophe. Under the present system, they can't figure out what's going on (who can?); or why their coverage is inadequate; or why, if there is no effective government control, there are so many governmental forms. Mixed approaches will only exacerbate these unfortunate tendencies, multiplying ambiguities about deductibles and co-payment amid startling increases in cost. If we want our future to be better than our past, then let us look more closely at the bureaucratic and market models for medical care.

What do we know about medical care in a bureaucratic setting? Distressingly little. But there may be just enough collected from studies of HMOs and of systems in other countries, especially Britain, to provide a few clues. Doctors in HMOs work fewer hours than do doctors in private practice. This is not surprising. One of the attractions of HMOs for doctors is the limit on the hours they can be put on call. Market physicians respond to increases in patient load by increasing the hours they see patients; physicians working in a bureaucratic context respond by spending less time with patients. Two consequences of a public system are immediately apparent: more doctors will be needed, and less time will be spent listening and examining. Patients' demands for more time with the doctor will be met by repeated visits rather than longer ones. But will doctors be distributed more equally over the nation? The evidence suggests not. Britain has failed to achieve this goal in the quarter-century since the National Health Service began. The reason is that not only economic but also political allocations are subject to biases, one of which, incidentally, is called majority rule. The same forces that gather doctors in certain areas are reflected in the political power necessary to supply funds to keep them there.

Surely the ratio of specialists to general practitioners could be better controlled by central direction than by centrifugal market forces. Agreed. But a price is paid that should be recognized. The much higher proportion of general practitioners in Britain is achieved through a class bias that values "consultants" (their "specialists") more highly than ordinary doctors. (Consultants are called "Mister," as if to emphasize their individual excellence, while general practitioners are given the collective title of "Doctor.") The much higher proportion of specialists in America may stem in part from a desire to maintain equality among doctors—a nice illustration of the Axiom of Inequality. One result of the British custom is to lower the quality of general practice; another is to deny general practitioners access to hospitals. They lose control of their patients at the portal, leaving them without the comfort they may need in a stressful time and subjecting them to a bewildering maze of specialists and subspecialists, separated by custom and procedure, none of whom may be in charge of the whole person.

Would a bureaucratic system based on fixed charges and predetermined salaries place more emphasis on cheaper prevention than on more expensive maintenance, or on outpatient rather than hospital service? Possibly. (No one knows for sure whether preventive medicine actually works.) Doctors, in any event, do not cease to be doctors once they start operating in a bureaucratic setting. Cure, to doctors, is intrinsically more interesting than prevention; it is also something they know they can attempt, whereas they cannot enforce measures such as "no smoking." If it were true, moreover, that providing ample opportunities to see doctors outside the hospital would reduce the need to use hospitals, then providing outpatient services should hold down costs. The little evidence available, however, suggests otherwise. A natural experiment for this purpose takes place when patients have generous coverage for both in- and out-patient medical services. Visits to the doctor go up, but so does utilization of hospitals. More frequent visits generate awareness of more things wrong, for which more hospitalization is indicated. The way to limit hospital costs, if that is the objective, is to limit access to hospitals by reducing the number of available beds.

The great advantage of a comprehensive health service is that it keeps expenditures in line with other objectives. The Principle of Perspective works both ways: if an individual is not an aggregate, neither is an aggregate an individual. Left to our own devices, at near zero cost, you and I use as much as we and ours need. At the governmental level, however, it is not a question of personal needs and desires but of collective choice among different levels of taxation and expenditure. Hence, it should not be surprising that our collective choice would be less than the summed total of our individual preferences.

The usual complaint about the market method is money. Poor people are kept out of the medical market by not having enough. No one disputes this. And whatever evidence exists also suggests that the use of deductibles and co-payment exerts a disproportionate effect in deterring the poor from acquiring medical care. Therefore, to preserve as much of the market as possible, the response is to provide the poor with additional funds they can use for any purpose they desire, including (but not limited to) medical care. This immediately raises the issue of services in kind versus payment in cash. Enabling the poor to receive medical services without financial cost to themselves means they cannot choose alternative expenditures. A negative way of looking at this is to say that it reveals distrust of the poor: presumably, the poor are not able to make rational decisions for themselves, so the government must decide for them. A positive approach is to say that health is so important that society has an interest in assuring that the poor receive access to care. I almost said, "whether they want it or not," but, the argument continues, the choice of seeking or not seeking health care is neither easy nor simple: the poor—because they are poor, because money means more to them, because they have so many other vital needs—are under great temptation to sacrifice future health to present concerns. The alleged short-sighted psychology of the poor requires that they be protected against themselves.

The problem is not with the intellectually insubstantial (though politically potent) arguments that medical care is a right and that money should have nothing to do with medicine. The Axiom of Allocation assures us that medical care must be allocated in some way, and that, if it is not done at the bottom through individual income, it will be done at the top through national income. If medicine is a right, so is education, housing, food, employment (without which other rights can no longer be enjoyed), and so on, until we are led to the same old problems of resource allocation. The real question is whether care will be allocated by governmental mechanisms, in which one-man-one-vote is the ideal, or by the distribution of income, in which one-dollar-one-preference is the ideal, modified to assist the poor.

The problem for market men is not to demonstrate resource scarcity but to show that one of the essential conditions of buying and selling really is operating. I refer to consumer information about the cost and quality of care. The same problems crop up in many other areas involving technical advice: without knowing as much as the lawyer, builder, garage mechanic, or television repair man, how can the consumer determine whether the advice is good and the work performed properly and at reasonable cost?

The image in the literature is amateur patient versus professional doctor: the patient is not sure what is wrong, who the best doctor is, and how much the treatment should cost. Worse still, doctors deliberately withhold information by making it unethical to advertise prices or criticize peers. Should the doctor be less than competent or more than usually inclined to run up a bill, there is little the patient can do.

There are elements of reality in this picture, as all of us will recognize, but it is exaggerated. People can and do ask others about their experiences with various doctors; mothers endlessly compare pediatricians, for example. The abuses with which we are concerned are more likely to occur when patients lack a stable relationship with at least one doctor, and when there is no community whose opinions the doctor values and the patient learns to consult.

Nevertheless, it is obvious that patient-consumers do lack full information about the medical services they are buying. So, in fact, do doctors lack full knowledge of the services they are selling. How, then, might the imperfect medical market be improved? Would some alternative provision of medical services ensure better information?

Since all costs would be paid by taxpayers, government would have an incentive to keep the expenditures on a national health service in proportion to the expenditures for other vital activities. The very feature that has so far made a national health service politically unpalatable—it would take over about $50 billion of now private expenditures, thus requiring a massive tax increase—would immediately make the government financially responsible. Under a total governmental program, central authorities would have to determine how much should be spent and how these funds should be allocated to regional authorities. Basing the formula on numbers would put remote places at a disadvantage; basing it on area would put populous places at a disadvantage. How would regional authorities decide how much money to put toward hospital beds versus outpatient clinics, versus drugs, versus long-term care? There are few objective criteria. Would teams of medical specialists make the decisions? Professional boundaries would cause problems. Would administrators? Lack of medical expertise would cause problems. Administrative committees would have to decide who receives how much treatment, given the limited resources available from the central authority. Would their collective judgment be better or worse than that of individuals negotiating with doctors and hospitals? No one knows. But something can be said about the trade-off between quality and cost.

Suppose the question is: Under which type of system are costs likely to be highest per capita? The answer is: first, mixed public and private; second, mostly private; third, mostly public. Costs are greater under a mixed system because potential quality is valued over real cost: it pays each individual to use up his insurance and subsidy, because the quality-cost ratio is set high. Under the mostly private system, the individual has an incentive to keep his costs down. Under the largely public one, the government has an incentive to keep its costs within bounds. Because each individual regards his personal worth more than his social value, however, a series of individual payments will add up to something more than the payments determined by the very same people's collective judgment. At the margins, then, the economic market, preferring quality over cost, would produce somewhat larger expenditures than would the political arena.

Who would value a public medical system? Those who want government to exert maximum control over at least cost. The term "cost" here may be used in two ways—financial and political. Government does more, is able to allocate more resources, and has more of a chance of getting support for what it does. People who are more concerned with equality than with quality of care—though, of course, they want both—also should prefer public financing. It assures reasonably equal access, and it also places medical care in the context of other public needs. Doctors who value independence and patients who value responsiveness would be less in favor of a public system.

Who would prefer a private system, providing the effects of income were mitigated? People who want less governmental direction and more personal control over costs. These include doctors who want less governmental control, patients who want more choice, and politicians who want more leeway in resource allocation and less blame for bureaucratizing medicine.

I would prefer the income approach, because it is readily reversible; it means less bureaucracy and more choice. The total approach, however, could be infused with choice. Under the rubric of a single national health service, there could be three to six competitive and alternative programs, each organized on a different basis. There could be HMOs, foundation plans (under which individual doctors contract with a central service), and other variants. Patients could use any of these programs, all of which would be competing for their favor. The total sum to be spent each year would be fixed at the federal level, and each service would be paid its proportionate share according to the number and type of patients it had enrolled. Thus, we could mitigate the worst features of a bureaucratic system while maintaining its strengths.

Thought and Action

Let us summarize. Basically there are two sites for relating cost to quality—that is, for disciplining needs, which may be infinite, by controlling resources, which are limited. One is at the level of the individual; the other, at the level of the collectivity. By comparing his individual desires with his personal resources, through the private market, the individual internalizes an informal cost-effectiveness analysis. Since incomes differ, the break-even point differs among individuals. And if incomes were made more equal, individuals would still differ in the degree to which they choose medical care over other goods and services. These other valued objects would compete with medicine, leading some individuals to choose lower levels of medicine and thus reducing the inputs into (and cost of) the system. This creative tension can also be had at the collective level. There it is a tension between some public services, such as medicine, and others, such as welfare, and a tension between the resources left in private hands and those devoted to the public sector. The fatal defect of the mixed system, a defect that undermines the worth of its otherwise valuable pluralism, is that it does not impose sufficient discipline either at the individual or at the collective level. The individual need not face his full costs, and the government need not carry the full burden.

My purpose in writing this essay has not been to assess current political feasibility but to determine longer-lasting political virtue. The proposals I believe to be the worst for sustaining the legitimacy of government are at present the most popular. Proposals that deserve the most serious attention are ignored. The falsely assumed excessive cost of total care and the falsely believed inequality of the income approach have removed them from serious consideration. Perhaps this is the way it has to be. But I believe there is still time to change our ways of thinking about medical care. Medicine is by no means the only field where how we think affects what we believe, where what we believe is the key to how we feel, and where how we feel determines how we act.

If politicians did not believe that better health would emerge from greater effort, could they justify pouring billions more into the medical system? It could be argued that belief in medicine—doctor as witchdoctor—is so deeply ingrained that no evidence to the contrary would be accepted. Maybe. But this argument does not reach the question of what politicians would do if they believed otherwise.

Suppose the people were told that additional increments devoted to medicine would not improve their collective health but would give them more opportunity to express their individual feelings to doctors. How much more would they pay for this "caring"? Would it be as much as $10 billion? Would it be that high if the program contained no guarantee—and none do—that doctors would care more or be more available?

In any event, after the mixed approach fails, as it surely will, this country will be faced with the same alternatives—putting together the pieces administratively through a national health service, or dismantling what exists in favor of a modified market mechanism. But this is all too neat.

It could be, of course, that the future will find the worst is really the best. The three systems I have separated for analytical convenience—private, public, and mixed—may in practice refuse to reveal their pristine purity. What life has joined together no abstraction may be able to put asunder. A national health service, for instance, might quickly lose its putatively public character as numerous individuals opt for private care. In Scandinavian countries, even those in the professional strata who are convinced supporters of public medicine often prefer to use private doctors. They pay out to jump queues, so as to be treated when they wish, and to have private hospital rooms to carry on business or just to receive extra attention. By paying twice, once through taxes and once through fees for service, they raise the total cost of medicine to society. Would not a public system that was 20 or 30 per cent private be, in reality, mixed?

Consider an income-graded catastrophic system. It would, to begin with, have to pay all costs for those below the poverty line. As time passed, political pressure might increase the proportion of the population subsidized to 25 or 30 per cent. As costs increased, administrative action might be undertaken to limit coverage of expensive long-term illness. How different, then, would this presumably private system be from the mixed system it was designed to replace?

The present as future may be replaced by the future as future only to be superseded by the future as past. First the mixed system (the present as future) will be intensified by pouring billions into it (à la Kennedy-Mills). When that fails, an income-graded catastrophic plan or a national health service (the future as future) will be tried. Efforts to make the former system wholly private will be unfeasible, because public sentiment is against rationing medical care solely by money. Efforts to make the latter system wholly public will fail, because forbidding private fees for service will appear to citizens as an intolerable restraint on their liberty. Then we can expect the future as past. By the next century, we may have learned that a mixed system is bad in every respect except one—it mirrors our ambivalence. Whether we will grow up by learning to live with faults we do not wish to do without is a subject for a seer, not a social scientist.

Health policy is pathological because we are neurotic and insist on making our government psychotic. Our neurosis consists in knowing what is required for good health (Mother was right: Eat a good breakfast! Sleep eight hours a day! Don't drink! Don't smoke! Keep clean! *And* don't worry!) but not being willing to do it. Government's ambivalence consists in paying coming and going: once for telling people how to be healthy and once for paying their bills when they disregard this advice. Psychosis appears when government persists in repeating this self-defeating play. Maybe twenty-first-century man will come to cherish his absurdities.*

*I wish to thank Eli Ginzberg, Osler Peterson, Jack Fein, Lee Friedman, William Niskanen, Mark Pauley, Otto Davis, and Merlin DuVal for their helpful comments on various drafts of this paper. Responsibility for the final version, however, is mine.

SUGGESTED READING

Eugene Feingold, *Medicare: Policy and Politics, A Case Study and Policy Analysis* (San Francisco, 1966).

Martin S. Feldstein, *The Rising Cost of Hospital Care* (a publication of the National Center for Health Services Research and Development, Information Resources Press, Washington, D.C., 1971).

Elliot Friedson, *Doctoring Together* (New York, 1976).

Victor R. Fuchs, ed., *Essays in the Economics of Health and Medical Care* (National Bureau of Economic Research, New York, 1972).

Eli Ginzberg, "Preventive Health: No Easy Answers," *The Sight-Saving Review*, Winter, 1973-74, pp. 187-93.

Edward Hughes, et al., "Utilization of Surgical Manpower in a Prepaid Group Practice," *The New England Journal of Medicine*, October 10, 1974, pp. 759-63.

Herbert E. Klarman, "Application of Cost-Benefit Analysis to the Health Services and the Special Case of Technologic Innovation," *International Journal of Health Services*, 4:2 (1974), pp. 325-52.

Theodore R. Marmor, "Can the U.S. Learn from Canada?," in S. Andreopoulos, ed., *National Health Insurance: Can We Learn from Canada?* (New York, 1975).

Thomas McKeown, *Medicine in Modern Society* (London, 1965).

David Mechanic, *The Growth of Bureaucratic Medicine: An Inquiry into the Dynamics of Patient Behavior and the Organization of Medical Care* (New York, 1976).

Osler Peterson, M.D., "Is Medical Care Worth the Price?," *Bulletin of the American Academy of Arts and Sciences*, 29:1 (October, 1975), pp. 17-23.

Robert Stevens and Rosemary Stevens, *Welfare Medicine in America: A Case Study of Medicaid* (New York, 1974).

Alan Williams, "Measuring the Effectiveness of Health Care Systems," *British Journal of Preventive and Social Medicine*, 28:3 (August, 1974), pp. 196-202.

Warren Winkelstein, Jr., "Epidemiological Considerations Underlying the Allocation of Health and Disease Care Resources," *International Journal of Epidemiology*, 1:1 (1972), pp. 69-74.

IVAN L. BENNETT, JR., M.D.

Technology as a Shaping Force

IN SIMPLEST TERMS, A TECHNOLOGY is a way of doing things with objects that are not part of one's own body. Technological change or innovation is the application of a new way of doing things that results in the modifications of the products, services, or processes that support society. These definitions are important because their very breadth emphasizes the pervasive nature of technological change in modern American society, our dependence upon technologies, and the enormous scope both of the opportunities and of the problems associated with them.

The fears and concerns about technological developments are myriad: annihilation by the bomb, dehumanization, unemployment and displacement, pollution of air and water, urban blight, loss of natural beauty, and the extinction of plant and animal species, problems associated with the disposal of solid waste and radioactive by-products. The impact of technological change on industrial and urban society is also blamed for the deterioration of family life, insecurity, anxiety, alienation, boredom, and the escalation of drug use and the incidence of mental illness. Although technological development has not always been generated by scientific research, science is the major source for the knowledge required to generate technologic change, and technology is often defined as the translation into practical use of the results of scientific research. This definition begs the meaning of the word "practical," and, unfortunately, tends to focus public concern upon "science" as the sole culprit whenever the introduction of a technology creates problems.

Much of today's controversy over the role of technology in our society has to do with different opinions as to whether—in simplified terms—a given new product, service, or process represents an improvement or a liability, "progress" or "decline." To answer this question about any major technology cannot be simple: the introduction of any technological innovation leads to social costs as well as social benefits. Any answer, therefore, will depend upon the balance between these two (not calculated in monetary terms alone) and upon who is doing the balancing. For example, an apparent economic benefit in production costs may lose out against a loss of employee satisfaction in the repetitive assembly-line tasks that result. Taken as a whole, unanticipated, undesirable, and unwanted effects, direct or indirect, in our increasingly interdependent society have raised serious ethical, economic, emotional, ecological, and political questions about technological innovation. Indeed, a formalized process for anticipating the impact of new technologies, labeled "technological assessment," has been developed, and the establishment of a congressional Office of

Technology Assessment may provide the impetus necessary for making this type of anticipatory evaluation work.

New technologies can be classified roughly as *substitute* or *add-on*. A *substitute technology* provides a better, more efficient, or more productive way of accomplishing an existing task. Substitute technology, often taking the form of automation, requires fewer workers for the same unit of production or service, hence increasing productivity by substituting capital investment for labor costs. It can reduce costs for the consumer and increase profits for the provider, but it can also produce unemployment. Depending upon one's viewpoint (provider, consumer, worker), the cost-benefit ratio will be different; it will also be difficult to determine in any objective fashion. Agricultural technology in the United States is a prime example of the substitution of capital for labor with tremendous increases in productivity per worker and per acre. The unanticipated and unintended social and economic consequences of this substitution include (among others) rural unemployment, migration to cities, urban unemployment, and increased welfare rolls.

An *add-on technology* makes possible the accomplishment of something that was previously impossible or economically impractical. The wheel and the printing press are early examples, the automobile a more modern one. Clearly, automotive transportation has had, and continues to have, enormous economic and social value; if it did not, the direct costs of owning an automobile would never have been paid by the consumer. But the social costs have been equally high. One of them has been death and injury. Over 50,000 Americans die each year in auto accidents. The average age at the time of death is about 30 years, and at least 10 per cent of those killed are below the age of 15. These young people had long lives ahead of them, and possibly many things to contribute. The economic losses from the society's and the family's investment in their rearing and education are incalculable. A second set of costs are those associated with damage to health, vegetation, and structural material by exhaust pollutants; yet another, the human and environmental cost of the highway systems in terms of altered land use, invasion of private property, and destruction of countryside and wilderness.

The crude distinction between substitute and add-on technology is of particular importance in medicine because many—if not most—of the new medical technologies are add-on: they generate additional costs to accomplish something that was not previously possible. But they do not increase productivity in the health establishment, and they do not reduce health-care costs either to the consumer or to society in general. Hence the critical issue in arriving at judgments about them is their impact upon socially desirable goals such as preventing or shortening disability, lessening pain, or prolonging life.

Another characteristic of technological change is that it is stimulated by demand, that is, it grows out of the requirements of the market: someone will clearly be willing to buy the new products or services. The number of automobiles produced is related to the per capita income in most countries, because when people have enough disposable income, they will buy automobiles. This law of the marketplace—that consumer demand governs technological advance—appears to be essentially inoperative in medicine. As Lewis Thomas has put it, ". . . in medicine, it is characteristic of technology that we do not count the cost, ever, even when the bills begin coming in."[1]

There are two reasons for this state of affairs. The consumer of medical technology is, strictly speaking, not the patient, but the physician. He is the one who makes decisions about hospitalization, diagnostic tests, operative procedures, and use of drugs. When caring for the patient, the physician follows what many have called the "technological imperative," the belief that every physician in every hospital should have available for his patients all the technologies of medicine, regardless of cost, questions of priority, or the optimal allocation of resources: "There is no 'effective demand' among American consumers for a barium enema or a heart valve repair, and there is no 'free market' for hospital rooms as there is for hotel rooms. You don't get them at all without a physician's order: but when a physician orders them, you almost always get them. The suppliers control, even create, the demand."[2]

When this situation is coupled with the third-party payment systems of cost reimbursement for most medical care, the role of the physician as "purchasing agent" has led to a situation in which technological innovations in medicine are much less constrained by market forces than they are in other parts of the economy. The limit is simply the total amount of money made available for medical care by government, private health insurance, and direct payments by consumers. Attempts have been made by third-party payers to influence what the physician is able to prescribe, and these will undoubtedly intensify in the future. But efforts to limit expenditure simply by limiting total payment are likely to produce serious disruptions, because the present health-care-delivery system lacks any coordinated political process to ensure that the reallocation decisions in each institution as it adjusts to financial stricture will, in the end, add up to a total benefit to society. Nobody knows how to do this, for sufficiently detailed studies have not been made. The imposition of fiscal constraints on specific items, such as drugs, laboratory tests, x-ray procedures, and surgical operations, would obviously require an analytic and planning capacity that far exceeds the one we now have.

Another question common to technological development in all fields, but particularly critical to medicine, has to do with the compatibility of a proposed innovation with usage and with the existing organization of the system into which it will be introduced. Technologies require new housing, new technicians, and new bureaucracies and systems of organized behavior. The system of medical practice in the United States is changing, but slowly: it is not a system that heretofore has been distinguished by the rapidity with which it accepts structural reorientation or alteration in the traditional behavior patterns of its practitioners. Since it is still largely the individual physician who decides upon the use of new technologies, his professional judgment is interposed between the public and any proposed technological innovation. It is not surprising, then, that surveys have shown that, with the exception of the pharmaceutical industry, private investment in medical technology is relatively small; economic success depends upon a capricious market, controlled as it is by highly idiosyncratic physicians.

The situation was well summarized by Edward D. David, Jr., a former presidential science adviser:[3] "In the case of public health, we are dealing with a loosely organized network of private and public agencies, institutions, individuals, and industries. There are more than 300,000 individual physicians and 7,000 independent hospitals providing medical services to some 210 million consumers. This diversity is at once a strength and a weakness. It provides numerous opportunities for variety, competition, and for comparison of different methods of providing health care, but at the same time, it vastly complicates the research and development processes." The decision to exploit scientific advance by launching into technological development in the health field is, therefore, especially risky. The success of the innovation is dependent upon a disorganized series of decisions by individual physicians, and from the point of view of costs to the public, once an innovation is accepted, the "technological imperative" leads to an allocation of resources that rarely coincides with optimal social benefit. In addition, technological innovation in medicine must be reconciled with many other factors (common to innovation in any field), including obsolescence of existing equipment, the requirements and demands of labor groups, national distribution networks, compatability with existing systems, and even local building codes, and certificates of need. An important question, much studied but not yet answered, is how the coupling of the components in the chain of events that takes knowledge from the laboratory to the bedside is to be accomplished in our present, pluralistic health-care system. Clearly, there is need for a better system for choosing and allocating medical technologies.

In 1972, the Panel on Biological and Medical Science of the President's Science Advisory Committee (later abolished by executive order) prepared a report[4] which, although printed, was never officially released or widely circulated, possibly because it contained strong recommendations for generous and continuing federal support for biomedical research and research training, to which the Nixon administration would not have committed itself. This report emphasized the differences between *definitive technologies* for the prevention, cure, and control of disease, based upon scientific understanding of the disease process through research, and *half-way technologies*, described as techniques for palliation or repair. The important concept of the half-way technology has since been expanded by Lewis Thomas[5] to focus upon crucial issues of technological innovation in medicine, including the *scientific knowledge base* required for developing definitive technologies, the problem of *validation* or the effectiveness and safety of a technology before it is used in practice, and the need to choose among technological *alternatives* and to distribute them effectively in view of the finite resources available for health and the anticipation of increasing difficulties in obtaining these in competition with other vital human services.

There are numerous diseases where the knowledge and understanding generated by scientific research have made it possible to develop and apply effective methods for control, and which, without these technologies, would still be major sources of morbidity and mortality and heavy burdens upon the health-care system.

These past successes in medical technological development are exemplified by the control of infections through immunization and chemotherapy. As is true of many successful innovations, they are now taken for granted, and many have forgotten or, indeed, have never realized that these technologies did not arise accidentally. Both were made possible by knowledge painstakingly acquired through basic research that began in the latter part of the nineteenth century. Similarly, important and widespread diseases of non-infectious origin, including pernicious anemia, diabetes, gout, hyperthyroidism, and several severe nutritional disorders, have been controlled through technologies made possible only by basic research on their underlying biologic mechanisms. An incomplete list of additional lethal and disabling diseases that medical technology can now control so effectively that they need no longer represent major sources of suffering includes: epidemic meningitis, infantile diarrhea, epidemic typhus, trachoma, scarlet fever, cholera, yellow fever, bacterial endocarditis, typhoid, leprosy, syphilis, gonorrhea, lobar pneumonia, malaria, pallagra, rickets, scurvy, erythroblastosis fetalis, Addison's disease (adrenal insufficiency), juvenile diabetes, recurrent rheumatic fever, measles, rubella, whooping cough, diphtheria, smallpox, tetanus, puerperal sepsis, neonatal infection, and certain types of cancer.

This tabulation also illustrates the fact that when effective and definitive technologies for prevention, control, or cure of disease are developed, they are relatively inexpensive and simple. In addition to their social benefits they generate savings in manpower and money for the health-care system. Berliner[6] emphasized this point when he wrote: "The impression is widespread that advances in medical research only increase the demands for complex and manpower-intensive medical care. The most spectacular of current procedures—open-heart surgery, coronary intensive care, dialysis, transplantation—naturally attract attention. Less apparent are the patients who might have been hospitalized but are not because preventive and very simple therapeutic measures have made their hospitalization unnecessary."

Much of the complexity and burgeoning cost of present medical care results from the use of half-way technologies—measures which merely palliate the manifestations of major diseases whose underlying mechanisms are not yet understood and for which no definitive prevention, control, or cure has yet been devised. The recent history of medicine is replete with evidence that each time a major disease has been controlled, the definitive technology has been much cheaper and simpler than the technologies devised before the disease was understood. For example, the construction and operation of a specialized system of hospitals for the care of patients with chronic tuberculosis became unnecessary with the discovery of drugs that were specifically effective against the tubercle bacillus. The detection and control of this deadly disorder promptly became an insignificant factor in the cost of health care in this country. Similarly, until basic research distinguished three types of poliomyelitis virus and made it possible to grow them in quantity in tissue culture, all that medicine had to offer was palliation for the ravages of "infantile paralysis." The technologies included costly special facilities, iron lungs, intensive nursing care, hot packs, corrective orthopedic surgery, braces and other prosthetic and orthopedic devices, all technologically ingenious but expensive and by no means definitive. The bill for almost complete control of the disease today is the cost of vaccination.

Among the more conspicuous examples of today's half-way technologies are the surgical transplantation of kidneys and the use of the artificial kidney (renal dialysis) for the treatment of patients with severe kidney disease (renal failure). The underlying disease of the kidney in such patients is usually some form of chronic nephritis, whose mechanisms are not yet understood. Continuing research indicates that chronic nephritis may be an allergic or immunologic disorder. When understanding of the disease is complete and a specific "control technology" is devised, the need for expensive and only partially effective renal dialysis or transplantation will disappear.

In much the same fashion the enormous pressures to develop what appears to be "high" technology in the form of an implantable heart or continuing efforts to transplant human hearts are all that can be done until basic research improves our understanding of the mechanisms underlying disease of the heart muscle, heart valves, and coronary arteries. Present efforts represent, at best, expensive, half-way technologies.

There remain numerous important diseases for which no definitive technology is available: stroke, heart attack, congestive heart failure, most forms of cancer, atherosclerosis, cirrhosis of the liver, emphysema, glomerulonephritis, pyelonephritis, rheumatic arthritis, osteoarthritis, acute rheumatic fever, disseminated lupus erythematosus, asthma, multiple sclerosis, senile psychosis, schizophrenia, depression, genetic disorders of metabolism, mental retardation, muscular dystrophy, cystic fibrosis, many skin disorders, and many parasitic and viral diseases for which vaccines do not exist or are ineffective.

This list directs the future agenda of research and technological development for our health-care system because the diseases represent the major burden that the system must bear now and for the foreseeable future. This burden will not be lessened by more health workers or more clinic and hospital facilities. More effective and less costly controls will result from scientific understanding of the diseases, the development of truly effective technologies for their control, and the successful introduction and application of these technologies.

To emphasize the crucial need for definitive technologies of control is not to imply that medicine has nothing to offer patients with these diseases. There are virtually no diseases for which medicine cannot provide some type of treatment, but this often means "caring for" rather than curing or preventing them. It is a basic obligation of medicine to provide increased comfort, to relieve pain, and to alleviate anxiety. These efforts are often extremely time-consuming and expensive. Were it not for the effective technology which already exists for those diseases that can be promptly cured or prevented, the demand for the "caring" function of medicine would long since have exceeded the supply. The problem may be alleviated temporarily by increasing the number of physicians and other health workers, but for the longer run, the only sure solution lies in strengthening the national capacity in science and technology as it relates to medicine and the diseases that plague our country.

It is beyond argument that the resources which our country can invest in health care are finite. It is also beyond argument that existing policies have allowed for a disproportionate investment of these resources in technology and have demonstrated a lack of selectivity in its investment. Certainly, the investment has tended to be made on the basis of effectiveness for the individual patient rather than its benefit to society at large when compared with alternative investments. Fully as important as the economic problems are those of availability or access for all who might benefit from a new medical technology, particularly an expensive half-way technology. This introduces legal, social, and ethical considerations on which discussion has barely begun and for which little precedent exists. There is no sustained line of scholarly inquiry or body of knowledge upon which to draw.

The impact of a governmental decision making an expensive half-way technology available to all who need it is dramatically illustrated by the provision in the Social Security Amendments of 1972 (PL 92-603) for coverage under Medicare of individuals disabled by chronic kidney disease; they are provided under the act with the costs of treatment either by hemodialysis or kidney transplantation. The original cost estimates for this provision were $135 million for the first year up to, perhaps, $1 billion by the tenth. By the end of the second year, the costs were running 50 per cent above the estimates, and it is by now apparent that the program will eventually cost at least $2 billion annually. A panel of the National Academy of Sciences-Institute of Medicine reviewed the implications of this legislation and made these recommendations:[7]

Recommendation I. We urge the Congress and the Administration to follow closely the implementation of the hemodialysis and kidney transplantation provision of Public Law 92-603, noting the overall costs and impact on medical manpower and facilities.

Recommendation II. We recommend that the coverage of discrete categories of catastrophic diseases would be an inappropriate course to follow in the foreseeable future for providing expensive care on a universal eligibility basis.

Recommendation III. The following studies should be considered before additional diseases are considered for coverage:

(a) An assessment of technological advances that may be anticipated in the near future—how much they may cost, and how effective they may be in rehabilitating patients.

(b) An examination of the capacity of the private sector to take up the costs of treatment for certain catastrophic conditions.

(c) Comparison of the costs of various proposals for across-the-board catastrophic national health insurance with those of covering various specific catastrophic diseases on a categorical basis.

(d) A close examination of the problems of determining the most effective allocation of funds for research and for the delivery of health services, and the benefits of both to society.

These recommendations imply that the policy decision concerning the provision of half-way technology to all patients with chronic kidney disease who may benefit from it offers an opportunity to gain experience, to acquire information, to document, and to evaluate such a program. The call for systematic policy analysis and the examination of alternatives, largely on the basis of cost-effectiveness and economic feasibility, are most important. The *political* need to make this decision arose before the conceptual and intellectual base for a clearcut *policy* choice among alternatives existed, surely not a systematic way to make rational decisions.

The need for such a conceptual base is urgent. The problem can be highlighted by the dilemmas of the artificial heart—if one can be developed. Here, the relatively straightforward problem of estimating cost in dollars will be complicated by a set of legal, social, and ethical issues that fall within the term "distributive justice." The economic analysis demonstrates clearly that the resources to make it available to *all* who might benefit simply do not exist. How, then, will the choice be made among potential recipients? A panel chosen to carry out a "technology assessment" of the artificial heart wrestled with the problem and concluded that there should be a random selection which would take the form of a lottery, as contrasted with a first-come, first-served method. The panel was not unanimous in this view, and the tone of the report and a number of dissenting views included in footnotes and appendices indicate unhappiness over the results of the deliberations. In an excellent discussion of the ethical dilemma posed by such a technological development, Jonsen stated: "Behind both difficult problems—availability and selection—stands the thesis that every person has a 'right to health care.' Neither indigence nor 'social unworthiness' are sufficient reasons to bar a person from care needed to sustain health and life. This thesis is presently more a political slogan than a philosophical truth. Its further definition and argumentation remains an indispensable task for medical ethicists."[8]

The report of the panel on the totally implantable artificial heart is an important document—not because it offers an acceptable solution to the problem of distributive justice and medical technology, but because it represents an attempt to define and to sharpen the array of problems that must be confronted. It could, and should, serve as one basis for further consideration of the policy alternatives.

It is important that debate and discussion of these issues continue and expand so that some conceptual framework, some sustained stream of critical thought, on the nature and purpose of medical technology assessment, particularly when it involves ethical judgments, can be developed. The time is growing short because the "experiment" with hemodialysis and kidney transplantation is underway, and the extension of coverage to hemophilia (possible annual cost: $150 million) and the artificial heart (possible annual cost: $1.75 billion) is very much on the horizon. It is earnestly to be hoped that the next several years will see a more coherent and open confrontation of these issues. It is an absolute social necessity, lest we bankrupt ourselves in a sea of artificial hearts, while other more pressing issues, such as epidemic venereal disease, are neglected.

One further aspect of technological advance in medicine deserves mention. Medical technologies have often unwanted, harmful side effects, the best example being iatrogenic illness caused by untoward reactions to drugs. Less obvious, but fully as important, are the risks involved in diagnostic procedures on the heart or the brain. Coupled with the fact that this is an increasingly litigious society (a fact not to be minimized), technological advance in medicine has contributed significantly to the problem of growing numbers of malpractice suits against physicians and hospitals.

Public expectations for medicine are much too high, partly because of the failure of the medical profession properly to inform the public, partly because of the "pop medicine" stimulated particularly by television shows, where doctors and hospitals must always produce a happy ending in thirty or sixty minutes (less time out for the commercials). This "Marcus Welby syndrome" is responsible for much of the current and growing malpractice crisis. Unfortunately, neither the public nor the courts seem to distinguish between true malpractice and unsatisfactory therapeutic results. Medical technologies are neither perfect nor risk free. Unfortunate complications of illness may have nothing to do with negligence, carelessness, incompetence, or clumsy techniques. The fear of litigation has created an unhealthy adversary situation between physician and patient. The doctor practices defensive medicine: he orders more technology, such as extra tests and x-rays, to protect himself or the hospital against future law suits. He may shy away from complex or difficult procedures that could benefit the patient but that also entail risk. Defensive medicine leads to overuse of diagnostic technologies, which in turn escalates health costs. "Malpractice," to a very large degree, is a result of technological advances in medicine. This is not meant to imply that the public does not deserve or need to be protected from negligence or incompetence, but that one of the tasks of medicine and society must be to set limits "to the boundless hopes and expectations, constantly escalating which technology has engendered. Advanced technology has promised transcendence of the human condition. That is a false promise, incapable of fulfillment. Human desires are infinite and cannot be achieved by the finite means of technology."[9]

Advances in the scientific understanding of disease will make possible the development of definitive technologies for the control, cure, or prevention of diseases that can now only be "cared for" or palliated by expensive half-way technology. The major problems that we face for the remainder of this century are to find out how to choose between alternative technologies, how to allocate scarce resources equitably, and how to deal with the ethical, moral, and legal problems as well as the untoward effects of technology to the benefit of society as a whole.

REFERENCES

[1]Lewis Thomas, *Aspects of Biomedical Science Policy: An Occasional Paper* (Institute of Medicine, Washington, D.C., November, 1972).

[2]H. J. Geiger in the *New York Times Book Review*, March 2, 1975.

[3]*Improving Health Care Through Research and Development: Report of the Panel on Health Services Research of the President's Scientific Advisory Committee*, Appendix F (U.S. Government Printing Office, Washington, D.C., 1972).

[4]*Scientific and Educational Basis for Improving Health Care: Report of the Panel on Biological and Medical Science of the President's Science Advisory Committee* (U.S. Government Printing Office, Washington, D.C., 1972).

[5]*Ibid.*

[6]R. W. Berliner, "The Relevance of Medical Science to Medical Care," *Archives of Internal Medicine*, 125 (March, 1927), p. 510

[7]*Disease by Disease Toward National Health Insurance* (Institute of Medicine, Washington, D.C., June, 1973).

[8]A. R. Jonsen, "The Totally Implantable Artificial Heart," *Hastings Center Report*, 3:5 (November, 1973).

[9]D. Callahan, "Science: Limits and Prohibitions," *Hastings Center Report*, 3:5 (November, 1973).

WALSH MCDERMOTT, M.D.

Evaluating the Physician and His Technology

I. Evaluating the Physician

OUR NATION HAS ANNOUNCED ITS COMMITMENT to work toward an equitable distribution of satisfactory health care. To accomplish this requires mechanisms both for ensuring universal access to care and for ensuring that, once obtained, it will be of high quality. To say this, of course, implies that quality can be measured, which in turn implies the existence of some absolute standards. Unfortunately the development of such standards in medicine is in fact at a very primitive stage, and as a consequence we face a large number of problems all of which arise from our inability to measure quality with any accuracy.

The need to find these methods stems from the need to determine accountability and be assured of quality care. To begin with the second, it is widely believed that the level of health in a given community will constantly improve if the shortcomings of health care can be identified, measured, and reported back to those providing it. These findings could also become the basis for corrective training for professionals and improvement of curricula for students of medicine. Taken together, these constitute "quality assurance." Included among the first—accountability—are a number of issues, such as the need for methods to evaluate returns on public investment in health, professional-standards legislation, the possible certification and recertification of specialists and generalists, a demonstrated ability of medicine to contribute to the solution of the malpractice problem, and some basis for comparative studies of the effectiveness of the health care delivered by health workers.

To find methods for the measurement of the quality of health care is, then, undoubtedly desirable, but to be useful they must not require so much effort as to rival that needed to deliver the care itself. And this is no trivial danger: many of the issues involved provide a rich fuel for abstract intellectual exercise. A short-term effort to find some method has been undertaken in what is virtually a "crash program," made necessary when Congress passed the Professional Standards Review Organization (PSRO) legislation in 1972. This legislation mandated some system of review for those physicians receiving fees via the Social Security mechanism; it got well under way in 1976.[1]

But what might be called the long-range effort in quality methodology is a search for methods that might prove useful in the nineteen-eighties and -nineties. If we are to have these methods at hand by the time we need them, we must begin now. It is by no means certain that a collection of satisfactory methods can even be

135

developed, or at least developed within the range of reasonable effort. It may also turn out that the more important of the two goals—that of quality assurance—can more readily be attained in some unforeseen and simpler fashion.[2] Be that as it may, the stakes are so great and success so vital that it seems appropriate to take a look at how we might best proceed.

Quality has several meanings, each of which tends to shade into the others. One is that the quality of something is identical with its nature. Another is "rank order" or "degree of excellence." The adjectival form, "qualitative," is the antonym of quantitative: whatever quality is, therefore, it cannot be quantitated. There is also a somewhat elusive connotation of wholeness in its meaning, wholeness in the sense of being greater than the sum of the parts; if one removes a component of quality, the quality itself is lost. From all this, one might reasonably conclude that quality cannot be quantitated or fragmented, but it can provide a basis for a rank order. In other words, it can be measured, though without any degree of precision.

How about health or health care? Health can also not be defined very precisely because its presence is so largely a matter of subjective judgment. About as precise as one can be is to say that health is a relative state that represents the degree to which an individual can operate effectively within the particular circumstances of his heredity and his physical and cultural environment. What can be measured is disease, and in a particular society the pattern of disease closely reflects major features of that society. As there are only some four or five disease patterns, it is possible to classify different societies by level of health, i.e., by their particular disease pattern.[3]

Health care is to some extent performed by oneself, but it is for the most part performed by others. These "others" are found in one of two systems: the public health system, which embraces the activities of a wide range of health professionals serving with various degrees of autonomy and only loosely and indirectly related to the physician, and the personal-encounter-physician system, in which a considerably narrower range of health professionals works in a much more direct relationship to the individual doctor. The biomedical influence of these two systems affects us all. We are also affected by a third factor—the style of living permitted by our socioeconomic or technological status. The impact of this last and of the public health-care system are closely intertwined, but they can be analyzed separately in a fair number of instances, so that it then becomes possible to relate their functioning to outcome. Thus, for at least one of the two health-care systems, that of public health, we can measure the disease pattern of a community, and therefore its level of health, and rank it in these terms with other communities.

With the personal-encounter-physician system the situation is quite different. Here we are measuring the activities of individual physicians and their various associates rather than the diseases present in a community, a much more difficult undertaking. Everything the physician does is some combination of technology and what we might call "samaritanism." Technology includes all those products of medical science that are useful in preventing or altering disease in a specific fashion. "Samaritanism" is the collection of acts that provide reassurance, or at least support, to someone troubled by disease or illness. These two functions—the technological and the samaritan—are separable in theory but not in practice. A doctor cannot get a passing grade by being proficient at one but not the other; he must be good at both, for they are to be regarded as opposite sides of the same coin.

We can then ask ourselves whether these two components can be evaluated separately, even if they are not in practice separable. In the case of the samaritan function the answer is probably no; we simply lack satisfactory methods for the task. In the case of the technological aspect, however, evaluation is possible at least in those instances where we can measure with a fair degree of precision the fitness or appropriateness of the choice of a particular technology and the effectiveness of that choice in operation. Let us turn, then, to possible methods of evaluating appropriateness of choice and the effectiveness of the technology, in that order.

There are several methods that might be used to measure an individual physician's performance with regard to the appropriateness of his acts.[4] One is to select a consecutive series of hospital cases and review the performance of the physicians as a group, an indirect method since it focuses on the appropriateness of hospital usage for the health condition involved. The usual procedure for that method is to select some commonly encountered malady—for example, urinary-tract infection—and, by reviewing the records, determine how well it was managed. Such a review is conducted by physicians who make judgmental decisions sometimes with, sometimes without, preset criteria, i.e., with or without using standards of care that were decided upon in advance. Some idea of the crudity of various ways of measuring these can be found in a study by Brook (1973),[5] which uncovered considerable variation in measurement when different methods of review were applied to the very same data.

Another system is to review the performance of individual physicians one by one. But before we consider this system we must first ask what we mean when we say that someone is a "good doctor." We mean, I think, that he can be trusted. As he cannot reasonably be expected never to make a mistake, we mean by "trusted" that it is probable he will provide care of a high quality in a roughly determinable set of circumstances in his declared area of expertise. To determine this probability we could look at how he has performed in the past, his general reputation among his peers, and especially reports about him obtainable from his closest colleagues. However, since this judgment is highly subjective and the information upon which it is based limited to a small number of people within his immediate professional circle, we shall need to find a more systematic procedure for assessment.

Such a systematic assessment could conceivably be conducted, but the effort necessary would resemble that required to conduct a serious biographical study. Experts would have to review random samples from among the physician's patients, using preset standards and a sample large enough to include a number of serious challenges to his skills. Such an evaluation would tell us a great deal about the physician, but it would have little value for comparison with the performance of another physician because the disease problems presented by a series of individual patients would differ so widely from one doctor to another. To get around this, one might use an examination where all physicians were faced with the same challenge; to do this, however, one would need to choose an illness that occurs very commonly, and its very frequency would have the effect of negating the value of the procedure— even a rather poor doctor can be expected to recognize and adequately to treat an illness commonly encountered.

The diseases that really test a physician's skill are not the common but the unusual ones; it is also the ability to manage the rare disease that distinguishes the physician from the physician's assistant or nurse practitioner. Examples of a single specific rare disease, however, are not very apt to be present in any one physician's recent practice, and, when conducting a review, it is precisely the recent practice that must be examined. This means once more that only the commonplace diseases or conditions will be used for testing. If a physician mishandles, in terms of prerecorded standards, a commonplace condition, it tells us something we need to know; but if he manages the condition in an acceptable fashion, it really does not tell us much about his capacity to perform: his ability to handle the technology, or his ability to handle crises, or to identify rare, potentially serious situations. It would only tell us whether a minimal standard of effectiveness had been met, and little, if anything, more.[6]

One recurrent theme in the literature on performance measurement is the call to develop methods that emphasize "outcome" rather than "process." Process-outcome linkages are feasible for reviewing the performance of the public health system, because what is being measured is the presence or absence of particular diseases in a designated group and not the performance of a function. Moreover, there is no personal element involved in the application of the technology which might alter its reception. With the personal-encounter system the situation is quite different. This gets us into the question of what it is that the encounter physician can do and what he cannot do in terms of altering disease or illness by his intervention. In today's world, the separation of the good doctor from the bad doctor is probably seen much more often in the management of nonsurgical, chronic disease than in nonsurgical, acute illness. Many acute conditions are self-correcting within a few days. In those that are not, the failure of initially incorrect management is frequently so apparent that even the bad doctor will probably correct it. There is seldom a straight-line traceable relationship between what the doctor does and the outcome in an illness of any complexity. Broadly speaking, those components of the physician's performance that permit process-outcome linkage are again the easy things. As a result, if we try to focus on outcome on an individual basis, we once more end up with detecting minimal performance, but nothing more.

Much, perhaps most, of what a physician does must be categorized as process, and process not even calculated to affect outcome.[7] Indeed, in many cases, whether or not a particular process was initiated is the only true "outcome" that can be measured. In addition, to determine whether a particular disease is present is itself a question of judging probabilities, and there are many times when a second therapy must be started in addition to the main treatment in order to cover a particular, but relatively remote, possibility.

To give one example, the rational selection of an antimicrobial drug cannot be made until the physician knows precisely what infection is present, but to determine this may take hours or even days. Otherwise it is simply a case of great technologic power wielded in ignorance. In the meantime, however, the physician must "correct" for this situation by making decisions based on his experience and knowledge of the probabilities. Given a patient with the syndrome of bacterial pneumonia in its severest form, the physician will choose penicillin as the best drug for the most likely infection, that due to pneumococci. However, he might also give another drug as a temporary measure until the technology-based diagnosis can be made. This other drug would be for the control of one or two other microbial agents not affected by penicillin but with only a remote chance of being present. If he were to await the technologically based report before subjecting the patient to the risks of this second drug, he could easily allow the pneumonia to pass beyond his powers of treatment. The "outcome" in this situation in the overwhelming majority of cases will be recovery from pneumococcal pneumonia by administering penicillin. But the physician who had given only penicillin, even though in the end it proved to be the only drug necessary, would still not have been providing the best care for his patient. In such a case, it is administering an irrelevant remedy that marks the superior physician.

A great deal of the best use of current biomedical science and technology ends up with a negative "outcome." Extensive investigations undertaken to establish that a particular equivocal finding is not caused by severe disease are cases in point. To diagnose a small lump in a woman's breast involves the discriminating use of a great deal of complex technology (mammography, xeroradiography, thermography, tissue microscopy). Having used it all, the result is that the patient turned out not to have cancer.

And how can preset standards be used to judge performance when the physician's decisions must take into account the risks and benefits of a course of remedy for three separate diseases, each of which in itself and in its treatment can react with the other two? Take the not infrequent occurrence of a patient with Hodgkin's disease who has a positive skin test for tuberculosis. If corticosteroids are administered for the Hodgkin's disease, the patient should also receive the anti-tuberculous drug isoniazid to prevent the hormone from reactivating latent tuberculosis. The subsequent appearance of jaundice in the patient could then either represent a manifestation of the Hodgkin's disease or a potentially fatal reaction to the isoniazid. Judging a physician's performance on the basis of preset criteria in decisions such as this one is obviously risky.

As a measuring methodology, the practice of using preset goals is not objectionable, but it does carry with it a serious potential danger in the tendency to forget that the preset goals are simply a handy guide: by a subtle process they become commandments to be violated at the physician's risk. This has the obvious effect of stifling innovation and perpetuating archaisms in the system. The physician begins to practice "defensive medicine"; he departs from the conventional wisdom at his peril. Then preset goals serve as a dead hand on medical progress. For a thousand years European medicine followed without deviation the medical practice originally set forth by Galen: too great a preoccupation with preset goals could usher in another era of "Galenic" medicine.

It seems amply clear that individual-performance evaluation based on chart or record review, while it can be done, can only be done at great cost in time, effort, and money, and can only measure a portion of the physician's act. At this considerable cost, we simply discover whether or not minimal standards are met. By contrast, the same costs might be acceptable for the monitoring of a few experimental programs on a research basis.

The difference between the two forms of performance review can be shown by comparing two different publications by Brook.[8] The first report—the one on urinary-tract infections by Appel and Brook—was retrospective, as a review necessarily has to be. It presented characteristics of the orthodox performance review discussed above. But his second study[9] was quite different. It was an actual experiment and thus necessarily prospective; the results were therefore unpredictable. A particular intervention—the "briefing" of interns on the chemotherapy of hypertension—was followed by a measurable improvement in the effectiveness of their performance. The "outcome" was a predetermined range of blood-pressure measurements.

This study has three important implications, quite apart from its actual results: first, it begins to approach an analysis of the physician's act rather than simply a monitoring of it; second, it indicates how our training programs could beneficially be modified; and third, although the methodology actually used was the conventional individual-performance review, it calls to mind the possibility of a community or group review rather than one for each individual physician. Speaking only to the first two points, in one or two medical centers monitoring efforts might be set up to serve as a basis for intensive analysis of the physician's act. The same unit could also provide appropriate changes in the educational program as results become known. Costs in time and money that are quite unacceptable when employed simply for monitoring individuals on a routine basis might prove a wise investment when employed for a sustained analytic effort. For such an effort might be useful not only for the training of health workers but also for comparative studies of their effectiveness in different situations.

When review methods are applied to the technological component of medicine in a hospital or in a community as a whole, the drawbacks—for example, the fact that the method is able to detect only minimal competence—become less important because the method is widely applied before the result is obtained. Moreover, as noted before, what is being measured is actually different. In the community or institutional review, what is being measured is the status of certain illness-producing diseases, not the performance of learned acts, and the entire health-care system is being examined, not just the judgment of individual physicians.

The tracer-disease technique[10] is one conceivably suitable for such community evaluations. It is based on the assumption that the management of a small number of diseases in a community is indicative of the "quality" of medical care in that community more generally. A good example can be found in the incidence of ear disease (otitis media) in young children. All suffer from earache at the initial infection, but those who go untreated, or are improperly treated, are far more apt to end up with perforated eardrums and draining ears.[11] It should be possible by appropriate sampling to determine the presence of this disease in a community and to determine the extent to which conventional medical care is being made available and is being used. Other common ailments that could be checked in this manner are high blood pressure and respiratory insufficiency.

While recognizing that the method is limited to the technological component and to the minimal standards connected with it, it can probably still serve a useful function. At the very least, it has the great advantage of being aimed squarely at the problem, namely, ready access to continued care with acceptable standards. Reasonable success, however, would require a degree of social organization that is probably too much to expect from our current health authorities, both governmental and non-governmental.

But even if it has no real prospect of widespread usefulness in the foreseeable future, its logic is so compelling that one or two experimental programs[12] would seem to be a sound investment. They would tell us what we really wish to know: not how Dr. Jones is doing, but whether the medical care being received by a community of people is satisfactory. It is conceivable that one or more hospitals might be willing to cooperate in a continuing review that would list the status of all patients with a particular readily identifiable condition, e.g., hypertension, and assume responsibility for ensuring satisfactory care. The hospital theoretically has that responsibility now, but it is generally loath to exercise it, especially for the patients of a private practitioner, unless the breach of acceptable care is gross.

Today's examinations can measure cognitive skills but have no way of measuring the ability to deal rationally and wisely with the problems encountered in clinical practice. Two varieties of other testing are needed: one for identifying the most suitable candidates for clinical practice from among medically experienced personnel, such as nurses, mid-level health workers, and foreign medical graduates, and from among those without clinical experience, such as the customary medical-school applicant. Computers have been suggested as useful for this purpose. Whether a computer-based examination would be helpful in identifying students with potential clinical aptitude is, in my judgment, unlikely. Evidence that it could be developed for identification of potentially competent clinicians among allied health personnel or FMGs (foreign medical graduates) is more persuasive. Without question a number of people who would make first-class physicians are present in each of these quite different pools; *the problem is we have no real way of identifying them*. Because the tests would be based on ability to perform in one who has actually performed rather than in one who has merely expressed a desire to do so, the prospects of identifying those with potential clinical ability seem good. The principle involved here is a simple one.

The most direct method of testing would require each of the candidates to examine seriatim, say, one hundred patients with various diseases and illnesses, the essential details of which are known. Obviously, such a procedure would not be feasible, but with a computer-based program as a substitute, something very like this situation could be simulated and a valid comparison made. To be sure, the actual observations and the detection of the anatomic and physiological derangements essential in a physical examination would not be tested directly, although a certain amount could be examined via audiovisual techniques. However, the medical history, the physical examination, and the laboratory data would all be recorded, and their interpretation probably represents the more important part of the physician's act. The development of such a system would still be a very large order, but the need for such clinical assessments is so great that the possibility should nevertheless be considered.[13]

Roughly three-quarters of the nonsurgical physician's care today (both general and specialist) is not curative but supportive. This fact is known but is frequently misunderstood by the non-physician student of medical care. To say that the principal contribution is "supportive" is not to say that it is unimportant, nor that it does not require mastery of the technology. On the contrary, the pattern of disease that has been shaped by our economy and our public health measures has created a situation in which supportive therapy that is largely, though not exclusively, technological becomes the physician's major function.[14] Involved here is quite sophisticated management of the deranged physiology of ultimately fatal disease. Whether a particular patient was entered into the vital statistics as a death from heart disease in 1972 or in 1975 makes little difference to the demographer's curve, but it may have represented three years of effective life to the individual. These years were made possible through this physiologic management component of "supportive" medical care. Thus far, we lack indicators by which to measure the impact of this care. The situation is the same for measurement of the samaritan function of supportive care.

In sum, what is *not* being measured in today's efforts at quality control is considerably more important than what is or what can be, a point that has obvious implications for the future of the field. Quality, we recall, is a property of the whole, and the whole of medicine is an inseparable blending of the science and the spirit. The quality of the physician's act in its entirety could conceivably be measured, but to do so would require a Boswell for every doctor—surely a grossly magnified effort for what would be quite limited results.

From the nature of these problems, therefore, one suspects that satisfactory direct measurements of physician performance (i.e., those based on observation or record review) are unlikely to be forthcoming. But this need not exhaust our possibilities. There are at least two other avenues to quality assurance that seem worth exploring. The first is a critical review of the many indirect methods for measuring physician performance, e.g., such devices as the hospital "tissue" committee, where pathologists examine surgical or post-mortem tissues to verify diagnoses, and the weekly "history meeting," where records are examined. The second is a multifaceted research attack on the complex of phenomena involved in samaritanism. Some studies on the latter have already been done, but the effort they represent falls far short of the need. Still, those attempts should not be discouraged on the grounds that "the compassionate physician is born, not made." Clearly some of us are less immediately lovable than others. Conceivably, however, systematic study might reveal some ways of doing things, especially of communicating things, that are likely to give patients support. And if such studies are to be fruitful, it is important that experienced physicians as well as social scientists be members of the research group.

II. Validating the Technology

The physician's performance is only one part of determining how effective treatment will be; validation of the physician's tools is the other. What is meant by "validating" a technology? In the case of medicine, the term "technology" embraces everything based on science that a physician does—the learned acts he performs on the patient, the diagnostic aids, the drugs, and the vaccines. By "validation" is meant the verification that any one of the items comprising this technology works—that it can be counted on to perform predictably in a certain set of definable circumstances. The need for such validation is obvious, and the problem of obtaining it lends itself well to the quantitative approach.

To say that methods for validation are easier to develop than measures for individual performance, however, is not to say that the task is simple. On the contrary, there are many difficulties. One of the major ones is that, generally speaking, the work requires considerable expertise, but does not provide much excitement; hence recruitment for the task is difficult. Another involves the ethics of conducting studies on the validity of an intervention; how does one do this without violating important principles that underlie the ethics of human experimentation? In order to consider the validation problem in greater detail, certain characteristics of medical practice must first be recognized.

Medicine's capacity for decisive intervention employs three skills—the diagnostic, the therapeutic, and the preventive—and the key decisions to the use of any of the three depend in large measure on a fourth skill—namely, the capacity to make accurate prognoses. Taken together, they comprise the physician's technology, which includes not only such things as computerized x-ray scanners and fiberoptic endoscopes but also learned acts such as the ability to listen to hearts or to choose and administer the appropriate anti-microbial drug.

It is important to remember that medicine is the one science which had a delivery system, in the form of the physician, for several centuries before it had a technology. Ordinarily one has the technology first, which then gives rise to institutions for its management and delivery—for example, an AEC for atomic energy. The pre-technological personal-encounter physician employed a great many remedies, but none—or very few—were interventions that were decisive in any way. They were based on a combination of dogma, superstition, empiricism, habit, and personal foible.

The period of decisive intervention has really been the past fifty years. Within that period one development followed upon the other with extreme rapidity. But as each intervention was introduced, it did not necessarily displace its predecessor: even if the "old" treatment was not as good as the "new" treatment, it was not automatically pushed aside; medicine based on science did not replace medicine based on dogma in a single day. Consequently the shift from interventions based on precedent to intervention based on science was gradual. One might well ask whether a period of fifty years is not sufficient to throw out the non-rational and leave us with a fully validated technology. Had it been possible to validate all the new interventions as they came into use, fifty years would certainly have sufficed. But very little of today's technology is even fifty years old, and very little of what is new has been validated.

At any one time, therefore, the body of knowledge that forms the practice, especially the therapeutic practice, of medicine is a curious mixture of a highly effective technology interspersed with islands of dogma, empiricism, conventional wisdom, and, at times, superstition. With the exponential growth of "interventions," however, this situation can no longer be tolerated. The persistence of unvalidated technologies leads not only to serious diagnostic error but to waste of skilled services and of money; it also contributes to the increasing load of medically induced, i.e., iatrogenic, disease and, by perpetrating untruths about serious chronic diseases, can give rise to untold human anguish and misery. An abundance of examples can be mustered in support of these statements, a few of them follow.

A. DIAGNOSTIC TECHNOLOGY

Chest x-rays were introduced early in this century, became standard procedure in the twenties, and had come to be considered a most exact diagnostic technique for tuberculosis by the early nineteen-thirties. Solely on the finding of an abnormal density on the x-ray or a change in the appearance of a density in serial films, momentous decisions were made that profoundly altered the lives of individuals. A young wife living in Brooklyn would be made to leave her husband and small children and be hospitalized in the Adirondacks for periods of a year or more; medical students would have to quit; young physicians, to change careers; school teachers, to abandon teaching. Moreover, these things happened *frequently* because, until the end of World War II, tuberculosis was the greatest cause of death and invalidism in the 15-to-35 age group. After the war, in the nineteen-forties, in one of the first attempts at "validating" a technology of medicine, Yerushalmy et al.[15] found that, in making this x-ray interpretation, in one out of three cases the physician would not only disagree with a second or third "reader" but in 20 per cent of the cases would not even agree with himself. That is to say, when confronted on two different occasions with the same pair of x-ray films, he would give diametrically opposing answers. Yet it was on this supposedly "decisive" technology that decisions radically affecting the lives of people were made.

During roughly the same time a serologic diagnostic test for syphilis was introduced by Wassermann. The test proved extraordinarily sensitive in that few patients with untreated active disease yielded negative reactions. What was not realized was that the test was overly sensitive. Of all those people yielding positive reactions, only about one-half were actually syphilitic. But this "validation," so to speak, of the test, this characterization of its inadequacies, was only performed decades after large-scale public health campaigns (including laws governing pre-marital examinations) had brought thousands of people under treatment. Quite aside from the mental anguish brought on by a diagnosis of syphilis, the antisyphilitic treatment of the time carried considerable risk for those thousands of people, not the least of them the fact (discovered even later) that the treatment was an important source of hepatitis. These four or five decades, during which thousands of patients who did not have syphilis were subjected to the shame and dangers of antisyphilitic therapy, are not from the medical era of bleedings and leeches, but from the modern era of interventionist technology. It was science-based medical practice. The physician would choose and carefully administer the science-based technology, an arsphenamine derivative known to have a high degree of effectiveness in definable circumstances, specifically the presence of the microbes of syphilis. But those definable circumstances—the presence of the spirochete—were not actually there, or rather they were not always there, or even there with a high degree of probability. Yet the particular bit of unvalidated technology that led to this massive 40-year-long unfortunate mistake represented the practical application of basic principles of the new science of immunology.

This story also illustrates another reason why validation of the technologies of medicine can be such a difficult task. Throughout much of the world of nonmedical technology, the circumstances in which a new item—a new tool or machine—is to operate are obvious. One does not have to try out a new tool blindly, under circumstances that may or may not be appropriate for its proper functioning. But in "the physician's act" these all-important "appropriate circumstances" must be sought in a living setting capable of extraordinary and rapid changes. Consequently, we have to have an elaborate diagnostic technology simply to detect the presence of the circumstances in which our interventionist technology would predictably work. Thus, in validating a technology for its medical value, i.e., in determining the probabilities as to whether its introduction will have the predicted outcome, we must not only establish its degree of effectiveness in definable circumstances, but also determine whether those definable circumstances are actually there.

B. THERAPEUTIC TECHNOLOGY

So much for diagnostic technology; the situation with therapeutic technology is even worse. Surgical therapies are extremely difficult to validate; an innovation can therefore gain quite a foothold before suspicion of its inadequacies becomes prevalent. A major part of the problem here is that, unlike many other interventions, the new surgical procedures tend to be aimed at chronic disease. Virtually all cardiac surgery, gastric surgery, and lung surgery are performed on conditions in which the initial surgical procedure can be shown to produce some tangible effects, but the overall success or failure of the intervention cannot really be judged until the patient's status some months later can be determined. Today, tonsillectomy is probably the most obvious example of an operation performed on a large scale for decades, yet one now considered to be seldom, if ever, of value. Controversies arise as to the value of radical versus less radical surgical approaches for conditions such as breast cancer. These are extremely important issues to the patient, but they are difficult to resolve.

The validation situation is no better with nonsurgical therapies; indeed, in many ways it is worse, for the very nature of surgery provides a set of barriers against casual innovation. Even new therapies introduced with great care, however, can attain long-term acceptance and wide use without necessarily being effective. A case in point is the use of anticoagulant drugs for acute myocardial infarction (heart attack). Acceptance of the value of this procedure became so widespread that for a time it was conceivable that a physician could have been found guilty of malpractice if he had not employed it. Then followed a period in which the value of the treatment was widely questioned; most expert opinion was that it had small benefit. This "small benefit" was obtained through a treatment that required a weekly laboratory procedure at high cost and that subjected the patient to risk of serious bleeding, either spontaneously or following minor trauma. At present, the pendulum seems to be swinging back toward more limited use. A significant feature in this case was that the spread of anticoagulant use was undoubtedly facilitated by the fact that validation studies, large-scale, so-called "controlled clinical studies," were conducted that were interpreted as showing it to be beneficial. Apparently, the validation procedure has not been regarded as entirely convincing.

C. PREVENTION TECHNOLOGY

Unlike the diagnostic or the therapeutic technologies, prevention technology, for example, vaccination, can at least theoretically be subjected to some sort of validation before it is generally introduced. As further experience is gained, information about possible drawbacks might conceivably emerge, but the advantages, i.e., the fact that the vaccine is effective to some extent, will have been established before large-scale use is undertaken. Generally speaking, this is true; it is definitely true for the most recently introduced vaccines. However, the effectiveness of the three major antibacterial vaccines—antityphoid, antituberculosis, and anticholera—has repeatedly been brought into question by responsible students of the subject over the years.

In order to validate a vaccine, it is necessary to set up multiple-year field studies involving hundreds or thousands of people, the number depending on the attack rate of the disease that is supposed to be prevented by the vaccine. Ethical considerations enter the picture because, in order to prove the point, it is necessary to leave a considerable number of people unvaccinated in a locality chosen specifically because the disease attack rate is high. This is the familiar and poignant moral dilemma of Sinclair Lewis's *Arrowsmith*.

This issue was particularly powerful in the case of these three antibacterial vaccines because no means were known whereby the immunizing effectiveness of the vaccine could be tested in laboratory animals. It was therefore not realized, first of all, that in the case of the vaccines against typhoid and tuberculosis, the individual lots varied in potency all the way from the fully effective to the completely valueless. Large numbers of people and hundreds of thousands of dollars were employed in large-scale field studies, some of which portrayed the vaccine as ineffective simply because, unknown to the testers, the particular vaccine lot used was no good. It finally became evident that the effective lots of the typhoid and tuberculosis vaccines had to be chosen by methods essentially the same as those used by an expert on wines. When this was done and only the lots of established effectiveness were used, both vaccines were found to afford valuable protection. The old killed-bacteria anti-cholera vaccine was ultimately judged to be of little value, but a new one based on the use of inactivated cholera toxin (toxoid) can probably be made effective in the future.

D. PROGNOSTIC TECHNOLOGY

The above examples reveal some of the harm that can occur when poorly validated or unvalidated technologies are employed. As we have seen, all three forms of intervention—diagnostic, therapeutic, and preventive—can be involved. Technologies are also involved in the fourth form of intervention—the formulation of a reasonably reliable prognosis. For the proper use of the diagnostic, therapeutic, and preventive tools depends in large measure on the degree of accuracy by which the dangers to the patient are perceived. On the samaritan side, the ability to forecast with reasonable accuracy is one of the most important things a doctor can do, for it allows the patient, the physician, and any others involved a chance to adjust to—or cease to worry about—what lies ahead. Obviously, when any of these four technologies—diagnostic, therapeutic, preventive, or prognostic—is invalid, the resulting health care even in the best of hands will be low in quality, if not positively harmful.

The natural history of disease, i.e., its behavior in the absence of treatment, serves as the basis for both prognosis and for one of the two major ways of validating a therapy. The reliability of the prognosis is of obvious importance in the thoughts and affairs of the patients and those close to them. Moreover, as noted above, the reliability of the prognosis is of great importance for the choice of interventions: it acts as a weighty, frequently the determining, factor in the choice of the particular diagnostic or therapeutic technology. One can easily visualize, therefore, how a mistaken idea of the natural history of a disease could lead to false interpretations about a therapeutic intervention. What is less often noticed is that such a mistaken notion can be the cause of extreme mental anguish lasting many years. Probably the most dramatic example is again the natural history of syphilis mentioned above.

Until past the midpoint of this century, for people to hear that they had syphilis produced a shock only exceeded by hearing that they had inoperable cancer. At the outset the very fact that syphilis had been diagnosed would raise questions of trust between marital partners. Then to the one afflicted came the image of a serious, potentially fatal disease transmissible to one's spouse, children, and grandchildren, a disease that could destroy one's brain or spinal cord, drive one blind, and damage the heart. While these thoughts were going through the patient's mind, the physician's thoughts were only a little less gloomy. He might well be convinced, on the basis of the first validation for any long-term therapy, that treatment, particularly treatment early in the disease, would prevent a few of these events and that a few others (e.g., transmission to grandchildren) would probably not occur at all. Nevertheless, in view of the range of possibilities and the fact that so many of them were so serious, all the physician's reassurances usually gave little comfort.

The terrible threats of this major catastrophic disease were suddenly reduced drastically by a study published twenty years ago by Gjestland of Norway.[16] He was able to show quite convincingly that if a patient with syphilis received no treatment whatsoever, the chances of the development of a truly serious late form of the disease were only about 15 in 100. This meant two things: (1) that even if penicillin should prove relatively ineffective in preventing late forms of the disease (which from other evidence is almost certainly not the case), 85 of 100 patients with untreated syphilis would go through life virtually unscathed. (2) The unlucky fifteen would really be no worse off than their contemporaries who suffered a myocardial infarction or a stroke in late middle age. Thus for half a century thousands of people had had to live with a devastating fear of a disease that turned out to have been largely a paper tiger, simply because we had little precise knowledge as to its natural history.

How could this curious state of affairs have come about? Why did the doctors not know the natural history of syphilis? In fact, they did know quite a lot about it in the sense that they knew all the lesions of which the disease was capable, all the organs that could be involved, and all the various types of serious or fatal outcomes. What they had no way of knowing was whether the outcomes they witnessed were the usual occurrence, which they assumed they were, or relatively rare occurrences, as they actually turned out to be. In short, physicians had no notion as to how syphilis behaved in a defined population—a fixed number of people. One reason for this, though not the only one, was that an interval of one to three decades commonly elapsed between the initial and the late manifestations of syphilis. Thus, to determine its natural history would require finding a population every member of which was clearly shown to have early syphilis, keeping them from receiving any anti-syphilitic therapy, and having the opportunity to examine them forty or fifty years later.

Wildly improbable as it may seem, eventually this formidable set of requirements was actually met. By a curious coincidence, Boeck and Gjestland, two physicians who never knew each other, in effect collaborated over a sixty-five-year period.[17] During the first twenty years (1890-1910), Boeck meticulously diagnosed all the early syphilis in the city of Oslo and hospitalized all those infected until the surface lesions had healed. He did this because he believed that mercury—the existing treatment for syphilis—had no therapeutic value. When arsphenamine was introduced in 1910, he adopted its use and thus ended his part in the "experiment." During the nineteen-forties in this same relatively stable Scandinavian community, Gjestland undertook a study of the disease. He was able to trace most of the recipients of Boeck's turn-of-the-century "no treatment" therapy. He was also able actually to examine most of the survivors and to obtain reasonably detailed and apparently quite reliable information about those who had died. It was from this careful delineation of the natural history of the disease that he was able to determine that roughly 85 per cent of syphilitics go through life essentially unharmed.

The Boeck-Gjestland story is an important lesson for our studies regarding the effectiveness of health care. For the effectiveness of the health care for the patient with syphilis was radically altered and immensely improved not so much by the new drug, penicillin (for the old drug, arsphenamine, was quite a good one), but by acquiring new information about the natural history of the disease at a level of precision that made that information useful. Obviously, it was a wildly fortuitous set of circumstances that made it possible to acquire this knowledge. Could it have been acquired in any other way? Clearly not by the customary methods of clinical investigation. One could hardly set up a study in which for twenty years all patients with early syphilis in the city of Oslo were hospitalized but kept untreated and then examined thirty or forty years later. Conventional clinical investigation obviously cannot give us that kind of information to store in our textbooks.

At first glance one might say that, after all, syphilis represents an extreme case in view of its long chronicity. A moment's reflection, however, reveals that syphilis with its decades-long interval from first lesion to clinical illness is much more a prototype of today's problems than an exception to them. Indeed, with our present gross lack of useful information on the natural history of diseases, we are not even fully aware that we are dealing with an entirely new situation that will require entirely new approaches.

So long as the pattern of illness faced by the practitioner in the United States was almost always that of an obvious microbial disease among the younger members of the population, the knowledge on which his ability to forecast was based was reasonably adequate. With most microbial diseases, individual cases all tend to be alike, and the period from onset to full clinical illness is only a matter of days or hours. Under these circumstances, the data supplied in the disease descriptions in textbooks is quite satisfactory. But the United States' pattern of illness faced by the practitioner today is no longer mainly a matter of obvious microbial disease among the young, but of highly diverse hidden structural diseases, frequently with several decades between actual (undetected) onset and outcome. Textbooks of medicine, which can easily communicate the prognosis of measles or rabies with accuracy, can provide only the most general sort of information about such maladies as coronary heart disease, rheumatoid arthritis, or cancer of the prostate that today claim the physician's attention. Although a particular chronic disease may be common, its individual expressions may be so diverse as to afford a single physician encounters with only one or two examples of each expression in his professional lifetime.

Even that statement assumes that the physician will be aware of the encounter and will be able to enter it into his experience, which may not, in fact, be the case unless he happens to have access to the full range of diagnostic technologies appropriate for the disease in question. On careful scrutiny, therefore, "the recorded medical experience" about our major chronic diseases will be found sufficient to permit forecasts on a community-wide basis, but will be of little help, and may even be distressingly misleading, in the individual case, especially when the chronic disease has been detected in an early, asymptomatic, stage.[18] Generally speaking, only symptomatic diseases get into the hands of the specialist early on, and it is the specialist's observations that form most of our "recorded medical experience." Furthermore, this same "recorded medical experience" is so lacking in precision that it frequently permits the introduction of new therapeutic procedures on the false grounds that their use will produce results better than those attained in the past.

Thus, the technological evolution that has shifted the disease pattern in the United States from the acute microbial toward the chronic non-microbial or degenerative diseases has had the paradoxical effect of appreciably reducing the physician's ability to forecast and has created formidable problems in establishing the value of new therapies.

E. METHODS FOR VALIDATING TECHNOLOGIES

The discussion thus far has been concerned with the disastrous effects that can ensue and long endure when our diagnostic or therapeutic technology is not validated or when we lack information of sufficient precision to yield meaningful prognoses in cases of chronic disease. The question now arises whether the available methods for such validations are sufficient and can be counted on to do a reasonably adequate job in the future.

Broadly speaking, there are two ways to validate a technology: one approach provides only a portion of a carefully studied group with the technological intervention, the individuals in the total group having first been selected randomly; the other approach provides the technological intervention to a consecutive series of persons with the disorder, and the nature and extent of change in the disorder from its previous characteristic behavior serves as the basis for evaluation. In the first method, the assumption is made that enough is known about the disease to allow significant particulars to be identified for ensuring the comparability of "experimental" and "control" groups.[19] Its efficacy, therefore, depends on the state of our ability to detect individual instances of the disease across its full range of expression. The second method depends upon the accuracy of our knowledge concerning the natural history of the disease in question.

The usual procedures for the control-group technique consist in setting up a group of cooperating investigators who will agree on such matters as a common set of criteria defining the disease and its proper general management, and who will agree to submit all patients meeting the criteria to chance selection, e.g., by flipping a coin, as to whether or not a particular intervention is to be introduced. At first glance, this seems like an excellent way to go about things, and any results obtained should be decisive. In fact, however, there are a number of constraints limiting the usefulness of this procedure and at least one internal defect in the method itself.

Ideally, a new intervention—let us say, a new therapeutic agent—should be subject to chance selection from the start. The difficulty is that, in the initial stages of the drug trial, no data are available concerning its toxicity for humans, or at least toxicity from its continued administration. In such circumstances, it would be grossly improper to use chance selection to determine the first subjects to receive the drug. Accordingly, the initial experience has to be on a selective basis. Attempts are usually made to start with those instances of the disease that carry a poor prognosis due to failure of all previous treatment or to the nature of the underlying process. In such cases, the trade-offs of potential drug toxicity versus potential drug effectiveness are clearly in favor of the patient's receiving the untried therapy.

It is only after the overall usage of the drug has been determined in this way that it is possible to proceed to cooperative random selection. But by that time, even with this limited clinical experience, physicians have already formed some notion of the value of the new drug. If they think it might have some effectiveness, they will obviously be reluctant to submit their patients to a process of chance selection which risks their ending up without the drug. This dilemma dampens enthusiasm for a cooperative study; when it does take place, the same dilemma leads to fatal compromises. For example, in each cooperating institution, someone has to decide whether a particular patient is to be "included in the study," i.e., have his treatment decided by chance selection, or whether the disease is to be managed "outside the study." The more seriously ill tend to be excluded from the study, a decision that already will affect its final results.

In short, it is not ethical to give a drug by chance selection until some notion of its safety for humans has been established. By the time this occurs, judgment has also usually been made regarding its therapeutic value. At that point, it may seem equally unethical to withhold it. To give an example: Let us say that a one-year study is regarded as necessary to determine efficacy. At the end of six months, the individual investigators have frequently made up their minds about it—from their own observations, if it is not a double-blind study, and from the work of others, if it is. Now as a result of the assignment of some of their patients to a "control" group for a drug they perceive as effective or to a treatment group for a drug they suspect of being ineffective, they find themselves in a position of providing what they have come to regard as a less than satisfactory treatment. Few physicians would be willing to put themselves in this position for any length of time. And for today's major diseases (the chemotherapy of hypertension, for example), extraordinarily long trials—much longer than our hypothetical year—are necessary before efficacy can finally be determined.

The costs of chance-selected control studies tend to be high because, in order to include enough cases to produce significant results, it is necessary to enlist the cooperation of hospitals geographically distant from one another; special systems may have to be created to transport specimens; additional personnel employed at the various hospitals to perform the necessary administrative or laboratory work; and the evaluation team must travel frequently and usually over long distances. Above all, there must be a central, and frequently traveling, directorate keeping a close watch so that each group will continue to make with care the detailed observations that are necessary, but that soon become dull and routine.

The design of the cooperative clinical study is crucial, and it is essential that the designers fully comprehend the variables in the situation under study. It is by no means uncommon that a result reported from a long-term, chance-selected study fails to be confirmed by another study because of faulty design or faulty understanding of the disease variables in one or the other of them. Because this method of study does not always yield the same answer when applied to the same question, Cochrane has maintained[20] that, before a particular result is accepted, the chance-selection study must be undertaken twice. He said this with reference to a study of the results of treating patients with myocardial infarctions at home rather than in a hospital. Although he did not go into its ethical aspects, they could be staggering. If a large-scale cooperative study had results that, when interpreted by the experts, revealed that procedure X was superior to procedure Y in the treatment of an acute coronary attack, a cooperating group of physician-investigators would then be asked to submit their patients to a chance-selection procedure whereby about half would receive only the now clearly judged inferior procedure Y!

Obviously, then, the weakness of this so-called "double blind" clinical trial is that, if responsible ethical standards are to be met, the instrument can be employed only on questions that are not really matters of deep concern or that have already been tacitly decided. If a physician believes anticoagulants stand a real chance of helping his patient, he is loath to put that patient at risk of not receiving them; once he has decided that anticoagulants probably have little or nothing to offer, he is willing for his patient to take that chance. For a physician to submit his patients to random decisions regarding their therapy, he must be genuinely undecided on the value of that therapy. Few physicians are truly that undecided, or, if they are, they are in that state for only short periods. It is not sufficient for the individual physician to know that "the experts" are undecided as to the value of a particular intervention or that some experts take one position and others take another. It is what the physician himself feels and thinks about that particular intervention that determines the ethical propriety of his participation.

We have already noted that a basic assumption of the large, chance-selected clinical trial is that our knowledge of the entity in question allows us to identify it in its various forms. The very success of the method requires that this be done, otherwise, the two groups of subjects, the control and experimental, will consist not of people with the same disease in the same stage, but of people whose disease appears to be the same but is actually different in highly significant particulars. When this occurs, one may have a splendid study design in terms of epidemiologic and biometric principles, but one will also have a faulty experiment.

An example of this phenomenon may be seen from studies of the value of coronary-by-pass procedures. In a recent analysis[21] of what was thought to be two comparable groups of patients, all with essentially the same forms of coronary disease, the intervention (surgical by-pass) was found to be of no value. When more detailed knowledge was brought to bear, it was found that the total group of some thousand or so patients in reality contained three subsets, each with a quite different prognosis. Instead of finding that the procedure was of no value, it was found that in one group it was harmful and in one group of no benefit, but that in a third group it was of definite value.

The instrument of the large scale clinical trial is thus not only of limited usefulness on ethical grounds, it also contains built-in defects that originate in our lack of sufficiently precise knowledge about the individual subsets of a particular disease. The reason we do not have such detailed knowledge is that its accumulation is painfully slow, and until now it has had no special usefulness.

If the usefulness of the random clinical-trial method is sharply limited, the situation with the so-called "natural history" method is little better. By this method the post-intervention and pre-intervention illnesses are compared in a significant number of people all having the same disease. Everyone receives the treatment; there are no concurrent controls; theoretically each person serves as his own control. Imperfect and relatively primitive forms of this process represent the way virtually all our present interventions have been evaluated. Drug A is administered to patients with a particular disease. The results attained are considered to be unprecedented. If the results are truly without precedent, the case is strong that they represent effectiveness of the intervention, particularly if they occur with some consistency and within a relatively short time after the intervention.

What we have here is a controlled experiment in which "precedent," i.e., the documented behavior of the disease, is the control. The word "documented" is used because having something in an individual physician's memory is not sufficient. It might be enough to convince *him*, but even in so personal a case he would wish to consult his own records. If he had no records, his "memory" of precedent would be classified as something that gave him an opinion about the intervention, nothing more.

To use precedent as a control thus requires very solidly established data. As we stated above with respect to prognosis, the data available for the acute microbial diseases are sufficient for use in this method. The individual variations or "subsets" of a particular microbial disease do not differ markedly from the prototype. If a disease progresses rapidly and is almost uniformly fatal, as, for example, is the case with bacterial infection of the heart valve or tuberculous meningitis, the subsets formed by its individual variations are less important because they are easily identified, and their significance is now well characterized. Death or recovery occurs within a reasonably predictable period. Our textbooks provide the "data bank" which can serve as a control against which the effectiveness of the new intervention can be measured. But with the chronic diseases that are the major features on today's scene, the situation is altogether different. As mentioned above, for most of these disease conditions, we have no such carefully documented data bank of past experience.

If periods of months or years customarily elapse between the start of the disease process and the "outcome" in terms of death or permanent disability, a range of outcomes is possible. The outer reaches of that range can be very different: for example, survivals of fifteen or twenty years for some people are to be contrasted with survivals of one or two years for others. Yet all have the same disease. To be sure, the disease manifestations form patterns that can be refined into subsets. With chronic disease, the question then arises whether and how many subsets are sufficiently different from each other to have different outcomes, and how many of them are sufficiently different to be diagnosed in the living patient. Then the rather common situation of a complicating factor such as hypertension or diabetes can greatly expand the total number of possible outcomes, thus producing a still larger number of subsets each with certain characteristics all its own.

A total listing of these subsets is not to be found either in textbooks or in the scientific periodical literature. There are several reasons why. First, it is probable that for the major chronic diseases, i.e., the neoplastic diseases and disease of the heart, kidneys, and brain due to atherosclerosis, the listings would be far too long to be encompassed in a textbook. The purpose of a textbook article is not to be encyclopedic about a disease but to enable the physician to cope with the forms most frequently encountered. The periodical literature does contain (although considerably less so than in days gone by) individual case reports of unusual instances of a disease, and every now and then someone attempts to analyze these reports collectively. Only a rather limited amount of information is obtainable in this way, however, because the observations, both clinical and laboratory, have been made in many different clinics, each with its own somewhat differing practices. In such reviews of the literature, as with the textbook, the object is to detect patterns of similarities rather than of differences in order to help the physician cope with those forms of the disease he is most likely to see, and provide him with a guide whereby he might pursue the unusual. One of the major reasons why there is no such body of knowledge is that to assemble it from the recorded literature even for a single condition would be an enormously detailed and tedious task.

To summarize, then, the quality of medical care depends not only on how well the physicians and other health workers perform their tasks, but also on the reliability of the technologies available to them for diagnosis, therapy, prognosis, and prevention. Those technologies that have long been in use presumably can by now be considered reliable, especially those used in the treatment of acute microbial diseases. For less acute conditions there are methods in widespread use for decades that are of clearly demonstrable unreliability, and it is precisely those subacute and chronic conditions that pose the problem today. In the meantime, new methods are constantly being introduced over the whole range, from blood antibody tests for the presence of cancer to new therapies and vaccines. It is essential that these be validated if a satisfactory level of health care is to be maintained. Yet the methods for doing so have been rendered inadequate in two important ways, viz., the shift of the major disease pattern toward chronic conditions and a growing sensitivity regarding the ethics of human experimentation. In the future, therefore, it appears that medicine will soon find itself overwhelmed with new and unvalidated technologic interventions and be without feasible methods to validate them. The major lacuna will be inadequate knowledge regarding the various expressions of the major chronic diseases.

As indicated above, because of ethical constraints, comparison with past experience will probably be the only method we will have to validate new therapies, especially those for the chronic diseases. The technical problem—the differing outcomes of an almost infinite variety of different manifestations of the same long-lasting disease—is one eminently suited to the methods of computer technology. It is illusory, however, to believe that this can or will be done, for to accomplish the task requires extensive knowledge about a disease and a constantly renewed supply of patients carefully examined and seen in a sufficient number over a sufficient time. Storing this information so it can be retrieved for application to the problems of some future individual represents an enormous project, and one that only a few would be both capable and willing to attempt. Finding a group with the experience and knowledge, the volume of patients, and the patience for what would be at most times a very dull and tedious job would be of the greatest importance, but also the most difficult to achieve. Yet if such a data base could be built and fulfill its anticipated promise, it would have as much impact as a major therapeutic breakthrough.

For these reasons, it is unlikely that a usable data base will be constructed for perhaps half a century, although a few groups might assume responsibility for carrying out the task earlier for some major disease area of a particular body system. One such effort over roughly ten years might even be sufficient to determine whether the approach itself had merit. While failure for one disease would probably discourage the effort altogether, a sufficiently clear-cut positive result would represent a major technological breakthrough. Without such a convincing demonstration, however, it is unlikely that society will organize itself so that its actual medical experience can be turned into a precise instrument for future medical and health care.

Assuming, however, that electronic data processing will some day be helpful, the question remains how the data bank could be used as the "control" or "precedent" by which to establish the effectiveness of interventions. Rather than collecting patients with a certain pre-chosen form of the disease, the intervention would have to be made in whatever patients were available. The various subsets of the disease present in those patients would have to be identified and the patients' postintervention course compared with the corresponding disease course recorded in the data base, a process that would have to be continued for several years. Unlike the random-selection method of validation, no "control" subjects could be maintained over such a long period. It must also be conceded that a procedure that uses past experience as a control, no matter how well documented, risks being misled by some unperceived environmental factor that was contemporary with the intervention but not with the cases forming the data base.

III. Conclusion

It is widely assumed today that if we had the methods to measure physician performance, the "quality" of that performance could be sustained at a higher level. The physician, knowing that his practice may be subjected to systematic review, might be more likely to adhere to standards than at present, when the sole review is his own conscience. In addition, a frequently repeated "error" found through the review process could be analyzed and corrected, and solutions could be fed back into professional training.

The term "quality" in this context really means the appropriateness with which the technology is used and the degree of effectiveness it has been possible to attribute to it—how good is the doctor in his use of tools, and how good are his tools? While, in theory, methods for measuring these could be developed, the initial efforts have concentrated on the appropriateness with which the technology is used, as measured by record review and results. As a practical matter and for a variety of technical reasons, these tests can measure only minimal technological performance. Only rarely can what the encounter physician does be clearly related to outcome, and the substitute—using preset goals as "outcome"—carries with it real dangers of stifling medical progress by rigidly institutionalizing the current systems of diagnosis and therapy.[22]

At present we are far less capable of approaching measurements of health care effectively than one might think. Just how far we are away from a large productive effort can be seen by the following:

> Whether the more detailed quality criteria and the increased cost of data require-
> ments are justified by improvements in the quality of care *is a major evaluation issue*. To
> assess the impact of review in terms of changes in the quality of care, measures such as
> compliance rates with criteria, validation of the process criteria by outcome methods,
> and changes in preventable deaths *must be evaluated* [italics added].[23]

The statement is clear: the concepts on which the present "quality assurance" movement is based are unproved propositions. Nevertheless, these methods are undergoing serious study because of the urgent need to find ways to satisfy the intent of the PSRO legislation. In my judgment, they are basically temporary mechanisms, and eventually either or both of two developments can be anticipated. Performance review of individual physicians will become a *pro forma*, minimally challenging affair, and ways for evaluating performance based largely on community- or group-linked indicators will be developed. With the latter, the status of key elements in the disease pattern of a community, or even in the "constituency" that has happened to be served by a large medical center, can be measured, an approach that has the advantage of involving the measurement of *disease* rather than the measurement of *performance*.

This method has the further advantage of touching on all elements of the health-care system rather than just the physician's performance. As in the case of physician review, however, the community approach could easily eliminate its usefulness by striving for a degree of precision inappropriate for its central purpose—in short, it could become too academic. With that caveat, however, it is believed that already existing tools, notably in epidemiology, could be used to create a feasible set of community-evaluation procedures.

Most important of all, however, it is only through the development of such "total group" approaches that the impact of the personal-encounter-physician system on health can be measured. For it is quite wrongly, but very often, stated that the personal-encounter physician has very little influence on health. What he lacks influence on is not health but those *indicators* of community health devised in the eighteenth, nineteenth, and early twentieth centuries for quite a different purpose. The great achievement of today's personal-encounter physician—the ability to modulate the deranged physiology of ultimately fatal chronic disease—is something for which we lack measures. Today's often repeated cliché that what the physician does has relatively little influence on health is more correctly stated that what the physician does has relatively little influence on those indicators of health that are largely irrelevant to what he does.

As we have said, the word "quality" in the context of the measurement of physician performance means the appropriateness with which biomedical technology is used and the degree of effectiveness it has been possible to attribute to it—how good is the doctor in the use of tools and how good are the tools. Methods for measuring this would be handy to have, and we face a multitude of problems because we lack them. Developing them appears at first glance to be an easy enough task, but when the issues are examined in detail, the difficulties become apparent. Indeed, what is *not* capable of measurement is considerably more important for quality assurance than what is, at least at an acceptable cost.

These methodological defects may reflect inherent problems: we may never be able to develop direct measurements and may always have to rely on indirect methods to ensure quality. But if we fail to develop even indirect methods, efforts to ensure quality using today's methods by the systematic review of physician performance are likely to devolve into *pro forma* logrolling or into thinking up ways for managing costs. This situation is unlikely to change without a thoughtfully focused, long-range effort.

Of the main issues involved, the several that stand out are: (1) The great difference between measuring quality in the public health system, in which it can be reckoned by changes in disease pattern, and in the personal-encounter-physician system, in which it is a matter of the appropriateness of a human act: so-called "outcome" results are obtainable in the former, but, as a practical matter, are seldom helpful in the latter. (2) The emphasis to date on technological measures because of inability to evaluate the samaritan function. (3) The ethics of clinical investigation and the predominance of the chronic, *non*microbial diseases. The first limits the usefulness of that much-talked-of technique—the randomized clinical trial—to the study of relatively minor questions; the second markedly curtails the usefulness of recorded medical experience, either for forecasting or as a "control" against which to measure post-intervention disease behavior. (4) Devaluation of the technology of prognosis, which is of particular importance because it is the overriding technology. Each decision on the use of an item from the diagnostic, the therapeutic, or the preventive technologies depends on the physician's estimates of the future consequences of alternative courses of action. The compromising of his ability to forecast has come from the shift in disease pattern. When the major critical problems were acute microbial disease, the individual instances were essentially similar, while with the "new" disease pattern, a relatively few chronic nonmicrobial diseases contain unknown but apparently large numbers of significantly different subsets of manifestation, each with its own natural history. (5) The need to intensify study of the samaritan function, i.e., attempts to analyze the interpersonal function of the physician's act. Considerable knowledge relevant to the subject has come empirically in medical practice and from work in clinical psychology and other social sciences. However, the subject appears to lend itself to a systematic attack with the goal of obtaining knowledge useful in measuring the quality of care or of obtaining ways to teach the interpersonal or samaritan skills to health workers, and it should be. (6) The need to develop indicators of the effects of the physician's physiologically based supportive therapy on a community's health. (7) A need to intensify the present efforts to develop examination systems whereby the most promising of the clinically experienced non-doctors could be identified and granted credit so that they might pursue a shortened course toward the M.D. degree.

It seems reasonable to assume that if we could measure the competence of physician-delivered health care, we would be in a greatly improved position to assure care of acceptable quality. But, in our dedication to this cause of assuring quality, it is essential to realize that the particular approaches used today of attempting *direct* evaluations of physician performance and validation of his technologies contain serious defects and may well prove to be failures. Other methods that follow quite different lines of approach will almost certainly have to be devised, and it is essential that we start now to create them.

It is equally certain that we are entering an era in which it will be increasingly important to validate each element of our technology as it is introduced; but we will be unable to do so unless we can find ways to record a sufficiently detailed supply of knowledge of the various expressions of the major chronic diseases.[24] A computer-stored data bank that could serve as a simulated clinical "experience" against which to test new possible interventions appears to represent the best available prospect, but trying it out is a task that almost certainly will never be done if it is left to the laissez-faire system and its present pattern of choice and support of subjects for medical research. Nonetheless, it must be started now, when its returns will be of little value, if it is to be available when the need becomes pressing some twenty-five years hence. If it is managed successfully, we might conceivably find ourselves in a situation where recorded medical experience can once again become a major tool in health care.

REFERENCES

[1]*PSRO: Organization for Regional Peer Review*, ed. Barry Decker and Paul Bonner (Cambridge, Mass., 1973).

[2]For example, the "Quality Assurance Monitor" of the Commission on Professional and Hospital Activities (CPHA) gives mortality rates for the common operative procedures in one's own hospital. Also provided for comparison are the corresponding values from a 200-hospital system. Thus, individual hospital staffs can readily rate their own performance with that of a spectrum of hospitals across the nation. With a properly organized surgical staff, this information might be all that is necessary for a hospital to have to feed back to its surgical staff to ensure maintenance of quality.

[3]Walsh McDermott, "Demography, Culture, and Economics and the Evolutionary States of Medicine," in *Human Ecology and Public Health*, ed. E. D. Kilbourne and W. G. Smillie (New York, 1970), pp. 7-28.

[4]The methodology for measuring physician performance is set forth in: R. F. Goldstein, J. S. Roberts, B. Stanton, D. B. Maglott, and M. J. Horan, "Data for Peer Review: Acquisition and Use," *Annals of Internal Medicine*, 82 (February, 1975), pp. 262-67; Robert H. Brook and Francis A. Appel, "Quality-of-Care Assessment: Choosing a Method for Peer Review," *New England Journal of Medicine*, 288 (June 21, 1973), pp. 1323-29; a policy statement by a committee of the Institute of Medicine, National Academy of Sciences, *Advancing the Quality of Health Care: Key Issues and Fundamental Principles* (Washington, D.C., 1974); Robert H. Brook, "Quality of Care Assessment: The Role of Faculty at Academic Medical Centers,"

Clinical Research, 22 (April, 1974); Avedis Donabedian, "Evaluating the Quality of Medical Care," *Milbank Memorial Fund Quarterly*, 44 (July, 1966), pp. 166-202.

[5]See Brook, "Quality of Care Assessment," cited above, note 4.

[6]A possible exception to this is a panel review with the use of specially prepared manuels. See J. Fine and M. A. Morehead, "Study of Peer Review of Inhospital Patient Care," *New York State Journal of Medicine*, 71 (1971), p. 1963.

[7]It is for this reason that I find inacceptable the last (underlined) portion of the "operational" definition of the quality of care recently published (February, 1976) by the nine Experimental Medical Care Review Organizations (EMCRO). The definition reads: "Quality of care is operationally defined by the EMCROs as the extent to which scientifically established procedures in diagnosis and management are properly applied to the *patients who can benefit from their application*." In actuality the proper use of the technology is frequently its application to those who conceivably *might* benefit rather than those who *can*. See "Data for Peer Review," cited above, note 4.

[8]Brook and Appel, "Quality of Care Assessment: Choosing a Method"; Brook, "Quality of Care Assessment, the Role of Family," both cited above, note 1.

[9]*Ibid*.

[10]David M. Kessner and Carolyn E. Kalk, *A Strategy for Evaluating Health Services, Contrasts in Health Status*, 2 (Institute of Medicine, National Academy of Sciences, Washington, D.C., 1973).

[11]Walsh McDermott, Kurt W. Deuschle, and Clifford R. Barnett, "Health Care Experiment at Many Farms," *Science*, 175 (January 7, 1972), pp. 23-31.

[12]An example of what I have in mind is the long-term study of heart disease made in Framingham, Massachusetts, in which the majority of the population continues to participate.

[13]A study of such computer usage has recently been completed (with Carnegie Corporation and Commonwealth Fund support). A major conclusion from this study is that: "It is feasible to use computer programs to simulate patient problems for presentation to large numbers of physicians for interactive workup and solution. Interactions may take place at terminals located close to home but may be processed and recorded by remote computers connected via telecommunications networks. Within present technical capability and reasonable cost, it is possible to assess solutions to ten or twelve standardized clinical problems in a six-hour period of testing. The recorded interactions can be scored objectively to distinguish with reasonable confidence between candidates in high or low criterion groups." John R. Senior, *The Development and Validation of a Computer-Based System for Testing and Teaching Clinical Competence* (a research project supported by the Carnegie Corporation and the Commonwealth Fund, 1971-1973 [January 31, 1974]).

[14]Walsh McDermott, "General Medical Care: Identification and Analysis of Alternative Approaches," *The Johns Hopkins Medical Journal*, 135 (November, 1974), pp. 292-321.

[15]J. Yerushalmy, L. H. Garland, J. T. Harkness, H. C. Hinshaw, E. R. Miller, S. J. Shipman, and H. B. Zwerling, "An Evaluation of the Role of Serial Chest Roentgenograms in Estimating the Progress of Disease in Patients with Pulmonary Tuberculosis," *The American Review of Tuberculosis*, 64 (September, 1951), pp. 225-48.

[16]T. Gjestland, "The Oslo Study of Untreated Syphilis: An Epidemiologic Investigation of the Natural Course of the Syphilitic Infection Based upon a Re-Study of the Boeck-Bruusgaard Material," *Acta Dermatology and Venereology*, 35, Supplement 34 (Stockholm, 1955).

[17]*Ibid*.

[18]Walsh McDermott, Ralph R. Tompsett, and Bruce Webster, "Syphilitic Aortic Insufficiency: The Asymptomatic Phase," *American Journal of the Medical Sciences*, 203 (February, 1942), pp. 202-15.

[19]It appears that the first large-scale, randomly selected clinical trail was carried out by J. Burns Amberson, B. T. McMahon, and M. Pinner, and reported in 1931 in the *American Review of Tuberculosis*, now the *American Review of Respiratory Disease*. The study showed that it was not possible to detect beneficial effects from the gold therapy (Sanocrysin) of pulmonary tuberculosis. See J. B. Amberson, Jr., B. T. McMahon, and M. Pinner, "A Clinical Trial of Sanocrysin in Pulmonary Tuberculosis," *American Review of Tuberculosis*, 24 (1931), p. 401.

[20]A. L. Cochrane, "The Feasibility of Relating Quality Control to Medical Outcomes: A Critical Appraisal," talk given at the annual meeting of the Institute of Medicine, National Academy of Sciences, Washington, D.C., November, 1974.

[21]R. A. Rosati, J. F. McNeer, C. F. Starmer, B. S. Mettler, J. J. Morris, and A. G. Wallace, "A New Information System for Medical Practice," *Archives of Internal Medicine*, 135:8 (August, 1975), pp. 1017-24.

[22]This issue has recently been discussed by Paul J. Sanazaro, "Private Initiative in PSRO," *New England Journal of Medicine*, 293 (November 13, 1975), pp. 1023-28.

[23]"Data for Peer Review," cited above, note 4.

[24]Institute of Medicine, Panel on Health Services Research, *Assessment of Medical Care for Children* (*Contrasts in Health Status*, 3), (Washington, D.C., Institute of Medicine, National Academy of Sciences, 1974); Eugene A. Stead, Jr., "The Way of the Future," Presidential Address, *Transactions of the Association of American Physicians*, 85 (Atlantic City, New Jersey, May 2 and 3, 1972).

DONALD S. FREDRICKSON, M.D.

Health and the Search for New Knowledge

THE EXTRAORDINARY GROWTH in biomedical research and development of the past quarter-century seems now to have ended, and it is likely to be followed by a period of reassessment and adjustment. The choices made regarding the support and direction of the now vigorous research apparatus over the next decade will be critical for the future health and productivity of the medical sciences. And biomedical research today determines medical practice tomorrow. From results of research come the means of improving the quality of health care and, ultimately, of reducing its costs.

Yet the ready translation of the findings of health research into benefits for patients is limited. A great deal of research cannot be coupled directly to the solution of health needs, and only a small fraction of the yield at any one time is convertible to useful technology. Moreover, the application of new medical technology is far more tedious and complex than is generally realized. In contrast to the relative ease with which many infectious diseases are controlled by immunization and antibiotics, the use of drugs and devices to combat chronic diseases can be costly in both time and resources. In addition, the price of technology is often too high in the short term, or too high in terms of its benefits.

The last quarter of the twentieth century will find scientists, health-care providers, and consumers drawn into a much closer community of interests. These will include: (1) field trials to examine, in statistically valid terms, the potency and safety of new medicines, instruments, and techniques; (2) far more extensive health education, emphasizing individual responsibility and the relation between benefit and cost; and (3) an increasing awareness of environmental hazards, and an increasing ability to assess genetic differences among individuals in their adaptation to the environment.

Because innovations in the system can only be evaluated through sensitive measurement of changes in the health of populations, data about people and the results of their encounters with the health system will have to be gathered on a vastly larger scale. The health of Americans is much affected by social and economic factors and by the choices people make in the way they live. These are now beyond the realm of conventional biomedical research; should they be included, debate about the ethical and moral aspects of such research is likely. By the nineteen-eighties, competition for resources can be expected to decrease that part allocated to science, threatening the pursuit of new research at a time when revolutionary techniques such as cell hybridization and fast-reaction measurements (among others) are reducing the gene, the cell, and even the brain to molecular terms.

In the next decade the research community must demonstrate its ability to

159

improve the health of the population, while displaying a due regard for the costs of health-care procedures and the competition for finite resources from other social imperatives. This carries with it a degree of responsibility for the substance of medical practice never previously sought or accepted by the research community. It is vital that these new demands not be allowed to interfere with the free-ranging inquiry which is still the most critical element in biomedical research.

The United States can take particular pride in its support of the biological sciences and their adaptation to medicine, because there was no established tradition for it in this country's origins. The Declaration of Independence is silent on the subject of science, and the Constitution mentions it only with reference to patents. During the first century of the republic, we were therefore simply the passive heirs of the biomedical tradition of Western civilization. The outstanding advances of the nine-teenth and early twentieth centuries, such as those dealing with respiration, metabo-lism, homeostatis, the Roentgen ray, bacterial causation of disease, and the life-saving possibilities of vaccination and asepsis, were products mainly of Western Europe. The contributions of American medical science accelerated, however, during the first decades of this century. Important advances were made in microbiology, immunolo-gy, tissue culture, nutrition, and chemotherapy. But the United States did not take the lead in the field until after World War II, when it did so with explosive force. Its contributions were especially notable for their richness of detail in exposing the complexities of biomedical subjects, and they were made possible by an intensive, large-scale effort unstintingly supported by a high level of technology.

This dramatic growth is attributable to the acceptance by the public of responsibil-ity for research financing. As late as 1945, the only significant support was provided by the Rockefeller Foundation and a handful of other private philanthropies, pharma-ceutical firms, and the modest endowments of a few hospitals and universities. Government funding was limited essentially to military medicine and a small National Institute of Health (NIH). The latter, established through the National Cancer Act of 1937, was expanded when university contracts were transferred to it at the termination of the wartime Office of Scientific Research and Development. While originally this move was meant to be a step toward the phasing out of wartime activities, its research soon revealed how scientific knowledge could be stimulated by national support and this led to its continuation and expansion. This far-reaching decision forged strong ties between academic science and the federal health missions.[1]

Congressional authorization to pluralize "Institute" in the NIH title came in 1948, when programs to explore heart and dental diseases were added to the existing program of cancer research. The growth of the National Institutes of Health after that date has been much documented elsewhere.[2] Between 1950 and 1975, United States expenditures for health research and development increased from about $160 million to more than $4.7 billion, with the government providing almost two-thirds of that amount. The country, once committed, has also been generous in its support of biomedical-research training and the institutions that conduct it. The National Science Foundation was created in 1950. Its provision for broad federal support to both the natural and social sciences included a relatively modest but important contribution to the vitality of the basic biological disciplines. Although the data are inadequate for valid comparisons among nations, we may safely say that no other country has shown greater public concern for these endeavors.

The expanded federal support of biomedical research had three principal aspects. The first was the development at Bethesda, Maryland, of a scientific center, which was to become the largest biomedical research facility in the world, with a diversified program in the major disease categories. NIH laboratories and clinics soon contributed a steady flow of talented investigators to the nation's medical schools and other research institutions. The research undertaken directly by NIH and other federal agencies probably represents about a tenth of the full-time scientists, floor space, clinical beds, and money devoted to biomedical research in America.

The second aspect was represented by the emphasis placed, from the earliest expansion of federal funding in the post-war period, on the support of scientists outside government. This led to the development of a national research effort that was extraordinary for both the excellence and the variety of the research conducted and for the number and broad distribution of institutions and scientists participating in it. In this development, a special role fell to the medical schools, which from the outset had received about half of the awarded funds.[3] Here a dual purpose was served: the research which the government paid for not only advanced knowledge, but significantly enhanced teaching programs to the eventual benefit of medical practice.

The third aspect—and the one ultimately supporting the quality of all these efforts—was the adoption of a policy supporting projects that were initiated by an investigator but evaluated through a system that ensured objective selection by a committee of peers. This system was, and basically still is, at the heart of federal biomedical-research policy, although minor modifications have been made to reflect current trends in research support and organization.

In 1975 about $4.7 billion was spent nationally on health-related research and development. Of this, 60 per cent came from the federal government and 12 per cent from state governments, voluntary health agencies, foundations, and other sources. The rest was derived from industry. It was nearly all used by its donors for explorations ranging from basic research to the development of new commercial products, and was concentrated in the pharmaceutical industry. While industrial concerns are not presently eligible for Department of Health, Education, and Welfare grants, they did receive $270 million in federal contracts for health research in 1975.

A lack of precise knowledge about these industrial activities forces us to concentrate here on nonindustrial developments. There, it is clear, the American public is the major supporter and the university the major performer. In 1975 about $1.4 billion flowed from federal agencies to academic institutions (and to the hospitals they own) in support of health research. The NIH supplied about three-quarters of this sum. The rest came mainly from other HEW agencies, the Energy Research and Development Administration (formerly the AEC), NSF, NASA, and the Department of Agriculture.

The principal federal agency responsible for behavioral science is HEW's Alcohol, Drug Abuse, and Mental Health Administration (ADAMHA), which has been independent of the NIH since 1967. Its research expenditures for fiscal 1975 were $139 million. In that year the NIH spent an additional $25 million for behavioral and social research. We may expect to see both agencies increase their support for, and conduct of, such research, for there is evidence that psychosomatic illness, the role of human motivation in health needs, family planning, aging, and other sociobiological phenomena will become progressively more amenable to biological description. The President's Biomedical Research Panel is considering whether ADAMHA's research program, some of whose activities are now conducted in NIH facilities, might not benefit from being returned to the full responsibility of the NIH.

Between 1965 and 1975 the federal government met almost two-thirds of the nation's health-research costs, and the NIH budget steadily accounted for between 55 and 65 per cent of the federal share. The proportion contributed by private, nonprofit donors declined slightly, while industry's share rose from about 23 to 28 per cent.

Several economic trends in recent years are important to biomedical-research support. For example, the enterprise has not escaped the impact of recession and inflation. Unlike the research in industries based on advancing technologies, biomedical research cannot be justified through profits from the sale of products. And the "market" of total health cost, to which research is often linked, has the anomalous property of inspiring general regret at its unremitting growth. It would seem that research should be increased as the market expands and should ultimately reverse the trend as total health costs are reduced by new technologies, particularly as a consequence of disease prevention. However, a relative decline in research expenditure has even now actually occurred. Total health costs in America rose more than threefold between 1965 and 1975 ($39 billion to about $120 billion), while the percentage of the total represented by health research declined from 4.8 to less than 3.9 per cent. This shrinking of the proportion of the health dollar spent on research is likely to continue. Not only can the rise in health costs be expected to accelerate, particularly if national health insurance is introduced, but the federal share of these costs will probably grow, greatly increasing competition for uncommitted public funds.

The reduction of life in all its complicated forms to certain fundamentals that can then be resynthesized for a better understanding of man and his ills is the basic concern of biomedical research. Although increasingly complex technology is utilized, biomedical research, like all scientific work, is dependent upon human creativity. That ideas, curiosity, hard discipline, and effort are essential is reflected in the application of about 70 per cent of the total direct cost of research to the payment of the individuals involved.

Research is the making of observations under conditions designed to establish relationships with exacting requirements for proof. Substantial knowledge and experience, some of it learned only by apprenticeship, are required. The sophistication of modern research demands that more and more of it be done by full-time professionals. If they are also trained as practicing physicians, they must choose between scholarly recognition and the larger income gained in private practice.

The American supply of biomedical-research manpower comprises about 90,000 doctoral scientists—six times as many as in 1950.[4] About 60 per cent are academic scientists (i.e., Ph.D.s) and most of the rest are medical doctors (1971 ratios). About half of these latter are on medical-school faculties, and about 70 per cent of the former are on the faculties of either medical schools or other educational institutions. A little more than a tenth of the total supply is employed by government.

While the location, number, and kinds of scientists can be reasonably estimated, there is no fully satisfactory description of the more general task in which they are engaged. It resembles the construction of a vast mosaic comprising myriads of tiny pieces. Whole areas are still blank and if they are to become accessible must be worked upon by the most capable artisans, who are at the same time often the most independent ones. With time, certain areas of knowledge are developed to a point where exciting patterns become visible and the gaps can be filled. The heightened effort of the last quarter-century has revealed large portions of the grand design. Proof has been found that a fundamental unity exists among the biological systems in most living things and that concurrent and coordinated research in biology and medicine is therefore essential. Many patrons, with quite different perceptions of need and opportunity, take a lively interest in influencing the distribution of labor and the resources applied to the pieces of the unfinished mosaic, but it must be added that these well-meaning efforts are nearly all concentrated at points of high clinical visibility—that is, they relate to the problems of human disease.

From the beginning, federal support—through NIH—has been categorical, that is, its interests have been subdivided principally into organ systems or diseases and administered by institutes bearing their names. These subdivisions have steadily increased over the years, partly because highly specific legislative mandates have resulted from political pressures on the Congress. Some more recent examples are those calling for intensified investigation, detection, and treatment of sickle-cell anemia, diabetes, arthritis, epilepsy, and orthopedic disabilities. In the early nineteen-seventies, legislation was passed that singled out cancer and cardiovascular, lung, and blood diseases to receive larger shares of the federal research budget. Indeed, provision was made for developing the budget for cancer studies independently of all other biomedical research. The impulse came primarily from outside the scientific establishment, though its proponents also included scientists and aficionados of science. The result was an unfortunate subordination of technical to political judgment or to emotion in the orchestration of the major biomedical-research efforts.

The effects have been mixed. There is no longer much question that the maximum utilizable funds are being devoted to research on cancer, a set of particularly dread and noxious diseases, that the quality of cancer research has risen, and that the vigor of the total research enterprise, whose expansion in constant dollars was leveling off prior to the National Cancer Act of 1971, is now being maintained. Moreover, a quality of "imbalance" is inherent in the support of research, for technical opportunities and needs are never evenly distributed.

There is a troublesome side, however, to this increased support: in only five years it has risen from about 17 per cent to 33 per cent of the annual NIH expenditure. Cancer research is by no means at a stage comparable to that supporting the engineering feat of placing a man on the moon. Knowledge is not yet adequate to "program" a certain decline in cancer mortality or morbidity, and viable leads are limited. Indeed, what we need to know could just as easily end up coming from research in some other, more basic disciplines whose support might well have been diminished because of budgetary constraints. Annual outlays for cancer research may soon reach $1 billion and must increase at least $100 million yearly just to keep pace with inflation at its current rate. At present the nation does not spend even half of that *increment* on population control, to give but one example for comparison. Attempts to accelerate research in this one quarter have perhaps been so vigorous as seriously to upset momentum of the general research movement. In the long run, the adjustment of support for research to retain the vitality of the whole is more desirable than is excessive dedication to one disease problem.

Interesting and controversial changes have also been made in the methods by which public funds have been provided to biomedical researchers between 1950 and the present. Initially, nearly all NIH funds were awarded to individual scientists in institutions of higher learning to pursue their research ideas in operations of relatively small scale. These awards soon became the "project grant," an instrument of "free enterprise" the acquisition of which was dependent upon two important conditions: one was that it was subject to renewal in three to seven years; the other, that it pass the judgment of the researcher's own peers. Powerful sentiments and persuasive logic speak for maintaining the project-grant system as the primary vehicle for research support. Many important advances can be traced to the adaptation, extension, and successive refinement of discoveries supported by such grants. Indeed, there is little question that, if some disaster were to reduce biomedical-research expenditure to a fraction of its present level, the wisest course would be to commit it entirely to support in the form of project grants of the best and brightest scientists.

Over the years, NIH obligations to the traditional project grant have continued to increase, even allowing for inflation. The awards totaled $327 million in fiscal 1965 and $680 million in fiscal 1975 ($393 million in constant dollars). Indeed, in any given year, a steady 10 per cent of the investigators thus supported are entering the system as grantees for the first time.

But the main increase in NIH support of research has been absorbed by larger units: the "program project" and the "center grant." These require the performing institutions to coordinate individual research projects in ways intended to enhance the national research effort more generally. However, the central, competitive, peer-review mechanism is still in operation for the components as well as the total of most of these operations, allowing individual initiative to survive even in these larger programs.

Another trend has been to increase the programming, or "targeting," of research. The desirability, and even inevitability, of this trend has escaped many of its detractors, who view the use of one of the instruments, the contract, as a steal from the traditional mode. The contract is often more useful than the grant in these highly focused activities; it is a tool, not an issue. Contracts constituted one-fifth of the $1.8 billion awarded by all NIH for research and development in 1975. The major use of contracts has been for programs supporting cancer, heart, and lung research. In these and other areas, however, grants as well as contracts are now being applied increasingly to specific health problems. In this kind of programming, identification of the appropriate questions to be answered by the research is more important than the choice of funding device. The distinctive feature of the contract, in contrast to the grant, is that it throws greater responsibility for the details and strategy of the research concept on the staff of the supporting agency.

A corollary of both programming and aggregation is an increase in coordination among research centers. Both the information exchange and the competition that have resulted are no doubt beneficial to the acquisition of knowledge; but the consolidation of the research network may also have other effects on educational institutions, the consequences of which are not yet clear. Biomedical research will forever be intertwined with the educational process. Institutions of higher education continue to receive the major part of federal health-research funds—for example, about 70 per cent of all NIH awards in 1975. At the same time, medical schools conduct other research which is primarily designed to maintain the quality of teaching and which may be in conflict with the utilitarian approach to biomedical research that lies behind the awarding of federal funds. This duality of interest is a potential source of conflict. The increasing sophistication and size of research operations and the growing demands for external coordination inevitably pull the medical-school scientist in one direction, while rising demands upon him for teaching and other services to his institution are pulling the other way. How the nation's medical schools will adjust to the current pressures for reform in the health care system will have far-reaching effects upon how much, and how well, biomedical research will continue to be conducted in intimate relation to the education of physicians.

Between 1938 and 1972, the NIH contributed to the training of approximately 94,000 scientists, a number that constitutes a major part of the nation's biomedical-research personnel. Funding peaked in 1969, when obligations totaled $168 million, and declined to about $155 million in 1975. Meanwhile, support for research training had been phased out in most federal programs, while the administration in the previous five years had been questioning the NIH training programs with increasing intensity. On January 29, 1973, the president's budget proposed an abrupt termination of all new NIH training grants and fellowships, on the grounds that it was time to reduce a potential oversupply of scientific personnel. In addition, the awarding of fellowships solely to biochemists and clinical investigators was viewed as unfair discrimination against other disciplines. Members of Congress also thought it improper that some of the subsidized research trainees were subsequently turning to clinical practice for the sake of its much higher remuneration.

Fortunately for the biomedical research community, the cessation of training programs has been averted, at least until the issues can be better sorted out. As of 1975, the training authorities of the NIH and the Alcohol, Drug Abuse, and Mental Health Administration (ADAMHA) remain intact, though curtailed. Provisions are being instituted to recover the federal investment from any trainee who fails to remain in research, teaching, or other specified activities for a prescribed period. And the National Academy of Sciences has been commissioned to conduct annual studies to identify areas warranting future federal training support.

We lack information about the national pool of biomedical research personnel. In the present period of selective growth, roughly 3,000 new scientists are believed to be entering the profession each year. About two-thirds have received federal stipends for some stage of their training. The rate of turnover is uncertain, and the calculations are complicated by the changing roles scientists play in the system, depending upon their age and experience. That a continuous infusion of the young and talented is essential cannot be challenged. What is in question is the amount of financial risk and sacrifice that these individuals are willing to accept to enter and stay in research. An abrupt and complete termination of support would be a disastrous way to find the answer: determining research manpower needs will therefore be on the agenda for the coming decade.

As the nation's biomedical research programs have expanded, so has public interest in their conduct. Administration and congressional inquiries on the subject have tended to be addressed to the agency rather than to the discipline or the problem. Since the nineteen-fifties, the NIH has been examined by at least ten federal and non-federal commissions, most notably the Wooldridge Committee (1965),[5] and the President's Biomedical Research Panel which reported in the spring of 1976. Congress has also conducted hearings. More recently, statutory mandates with time and dollar limitations in designated areas reflect an extraordinary congressional interest in specifying the substance of certain programs.

The passage of broadened freedom-of-information legislation has exposed to public scrutiny most of the mechanisms for the research advisory process. Aside from threats to certain delicate aspects of peer review and to the still contested proprietary rights of scientists in their ideas, increasing public audit of biomedical research is generally salutary. It demonstrates clearly that research is susceptible to public direction and is in no sense the exclusive province of an unmanageable elite.

The "accountability" of biomedical research for the dysfunction of the present-day health-delivery system is difficult to assess. For the most part, research programs have been kept free of activities directed at regulation and delivery of health care. Attempts to reform health care through government intervention, however, have enlarged the several agencies of the Public Health Service. And debate has tended to clarify the point that NIH and ADAMHA, the principal federal supporters of medical research, are not *science* agencies but *health* agencies. ADAMHA combines missions of service and research. NIH has focused on its research mission, but has for years engaged periodically in "control" or "demonstration" activities designed to improve the translation of research findings into health practice. The relations between the research agencies and the health agencies of the federal government are poorly defined and are in need of periodic adjustment, particularly to ensure that health-service research and preventive activities are not neglected. Far greater discontinuities exist between the government and the private health sector; they have not yet achieved an entente capable of controlling some major deficiencies in health care.

While it is unlikely that biomedical research *per se* will produce further dramatic effects on, for example, infant mortality or the mean survival of those who have reached three score and ten years, it will continue to have considerable influence on decreasing premature death among those under age 65 and on improving health at all ages. These are not the only arguments, however, for retaining a powerful capacity to improve biomedical knowledge and its related technology. Biomedical advances are essential to the survival of the species. If we are to regulate our numbers in a rational way, we will have to control fertility by more effective biochemical or physiological methods than we now have. In the endless search for new sources of energy, food, and economic growth, we will continue to tamper with our ecology. Our ability to keep those environmental changes within the limits of human tolerance and adaptation will mean forever pushing forward the limits of our knowledge. Although the whole world will be at risk, it is the most affluent and advanced countries that must continue to bear the cost of such research and development.

In this perspective, the apparatus for effective conduct of biomedical research that has been created in North America, Western Europe, and the Soviet Union is a world resource. It must not be allowed to fall into disrepair, for once lost, it may well be impossible to replace. Furthermore, the "mosaic" of knowledge is becoming extraordinarily refined in certain areas. If continuation of the present pace is maintained, we will assuredly have a return on this investment in a mastery of most of the stubborn, chronic health problems we recognize today. In some respects, the growth of knowledge in biology and clinical research in the last decade alone has been breathtaking, and this momentum may be expected to increase if support is reasonably steady and wisely allocated, and if there is sufficient growth at least to accommodate young investigators and fresh ideas.

In the decades ahead, then, research will have to be carried out in a world made suddenly aware that its resources are finite and are shrinking under inexorable population pressures. For the developed nations, there may be an end to affluence; for developing nations, there may no longer be any hope of acquiring it. One need not subscribe totally to the bleakness of this vision to perceive that competition for resources of all kinds and at all levels is likely to intensify.

Some thought should therefore be given to the goals chosen for the decades ahead. Highest priority should not be given to the extension of the normal life span. There is little evidence that an even longer life means a better one, and a cure for aging is one of the least likely products of biomedical research. On the other hand, the aging process and its relation to diseases must be studied, for this approach offers promise of improving the quality of life. Limiting premature death, with maximum narrowing of current differences in life expectancy based on sex and race, should be given priority, as should minimizing the impact of physical and mental disability, and augmenting the positive aspects of health and well-being. Scientists must also supply the effective knowledge needed to make decisions in several critical areas of long-term social policy. These include efforts to provide a means for matching population levels with anticipated resources, to achieve the quality of environment sought, and to move toward a reduction of the burden of deleterious genes.

Finally, the scientific community must assume a greater degree of responsibility for the quality of the health care delivered, particularly by developing ways for applying research findings to the health-care system. This must include achieving consensus on what is ready and developing mechanisms for passing applicable findings from the community of research to that of health practice.

A corollary problem is presented by palliative technologies, such as renal dialysis, applied at exorbitant cost in present-day clinical settings. The mounting demands that these be extended to every patient in need of them suggests that science has some obligation to anticipate the fruits of its research, although it is not reasonable to expect inquiry to cease simply because it might lead to expensive therapies. A formula for compromise, incorporating both human and scientific values, is needed.

One of the perennial questions in biomedical science, particularly in public-policy discussions, is what constitutes an appropriate level of support. Philosophically, the question, How much research is enough?, has no objective answer. Subjective perceptions of its needs and opportunities must compete with assessments of needs and opportunities in other social areas. Yet, decisions on funding must be made.

The federal policy for the decade that began in 1956—that all meritorious research proposals should be funded—appears no longer to be feasible. Even at the time, the expansive policy attributable to HEW Secretary Folsom and endorsed by congressional action was only possible because of the relatively limited number of acceptable research proposals. Research support can probably never be increased rapidly enough to meet the infinite pressures generated by scientific opportunities, social needs, and public expectations. Yet it seems that any major advance in reducing disease and controlling health costs must derive from research; continued investment in research therefore becomes a *sine qua non* of public-health policy.

We are now at a plateau in federal biomedical-research support, during which increases will be modest and will not permit a significant expansion of the national enterprise. But what of the future? A breakthrough toward control of any one major disease might lead to a short-term spurt in research appropriations, with perhaps later reductions or reallocations of funds to other areas. A major (or continuing) financial crisis for the government might depress prospects for research funding even at its present level in the decade ahead. If Congress takes a strong stand in support of its own overall budget ceilings, this might greatly reduce the competitive advantage now enjoyed by more popular federal programs including biomedical research. If national health insurance is adopted, this might strengthen the case for additional research, but it might also diminish research resources by making ever greater claims on the total health dollar. In the face of these unpredictables, the biomedical-research community would do well to propose a basis for setting some reasonable level of support. Perhaps the strongest case could be made for linking research expenditures to the cost of health problems to the nation, starting with the present ratio—about one dollar spent for every twenty-five of medical cost—and striving to maintain it.

The funding of health-related research by industry has grown erratically in recent years, increasing by about 5 per cent from 1969 to 1970 and about 9 per cent from 1974 to 1975. We can reasonably assume that there will be a modest expansion in constant dollars for the next few years, constituting a prudent investment in the development and testing of new and improved technologies for a steadily expanding world health market.

Private philanthropy has not quite kept pace with inflation in its support of health research. A decline in the share from private foundations has been largely compensated in recent years by voluntary-health-agency gains, but there is no reason to believe that private support can replace public support to any degree. The best hope is that a steady level (in constant dollars) of private funding will fill needs inadequately met by federal programs, provide seed money in areas where federal policy or public opinion inhibits federal support, and complement federal support in areas of common interest.

Research funding grows increasingly more unstable. In recent years, late appropriations have been further delayed by impoundment, release of impoundment, rescission, deferrals, and supplemental appropriations. One can learn to live on "continuing resolutions," but individual scientists and their institutions, not to speak of program managers, are ill-served by excessive uncertainties that may compromise continuity or lead to hasty commitments.

There are a number of possible ways to moderate these cyclical swings in the annual budget process, but no immediate prospect of implementing any of them. One would be to change from annual to multiple-year appropriations, with levels set for two, three, or five years ahead. But this is not likely to occur unless it is government-wide. However, if the Congress cannot meet its schedules under the new congressional budgeting act, such a change may be forced upon the system.

An alternative method would provide stable multi-year support for a basic core of research activity, with additional funds supplied through the annual appropriations process to handle special programs, such as expensive clinical trials. Through this system the predictable long-term needs of medical schools and other key institutions in the research process could reasonably be accommodated.

A third possibility is that of assigning an arbitrary support level for biomedical research (in constant dollars) for a specified period—say, five years—with that level determined by the activities under way at the time of decision, coupled with an assessment of additional opportunities and a frank exercise of bargaining power. The level of funding could be set through the usual political and budgetary process, but should include a panel of experts providing advice. A survey on the Wooldridge model at the end of the first four years would assess the program issues (including how well the money was being spent) and provide recommendations for levels of support during the next five years.

If we could choose among these alternatives we would not fail to improve conditions by opting for the first two- or three-year funding of the major enterprise, with compensation for rising costs and supplemental funding for projects of great promise. Periodic review of programs and needs conducted by experts through mechanisms ensuring objectivity and social responsiveness should be included.

A final problem, partly one of funding, partly of organization, concerns the distribution of appropriations for research. Is it preferable to concentrate such support in one or two agencies or to disburse it more widely throughout the executive branch of the government? Concentration provides visibility, which some contend would make budget cuts unpopular. It also permits the protection of vulnerable basic research by making its extension into application more obvious. On the other hand, diffusion of support provides for interagency competition, a healthy way to see that the public will is done, especially in areas of need that engender less professional enthusiasm.

It is this last consideration—how best to answer the needs of the public—that probably should prevail over a search for mere efficiency. And so it does. The organization of both the NIH and ADAMHA reflects the pragmatic orientation of this country (we are more interested in solving disease problems than in solving science problems) and the political strength of each of its categories—for diseases and disciplines both have political constituencies.

A new development that will affect the orientation of the health-research agencies and shift the boundaries between them and their sister federal health agencies concerned primarily with manpower, service, and regulation (Health Resources Administration, Health Services Administration, Food and Drug Administration, Communicable Disease Center) is the need to hold down federal health expenditures, driven upward by factors that not only increase the cost of health service but also expand the role of government as its purchaser. Where these costs can be laid to deficiencies in medical or psychiatric care, the biomedical and behavioral research communities must expand their activities to include more clinical trials of new interventions. The substantive issues here are scientific and technical, and the answers sought result from research. The scientific community cannot shun these practical responsibilities, nor would it be expedient for the government to create a "third force" to deal with this important dysfunction in the health system. There are many methodological problems in health-care delivery, however, for which answers, some of them extremely technological, must be found. Agencies other than the NIH and ADAMHA are equipped to deal with some of these problems, at least to a limited extent. Their competence should be strengthened and attached more closely to the other scientific forces; but health care will benefit by their retaining separate organizational identity and receiving separate appropriations.

We have all come to recognize another feature of health-care delivery which is not confined to America, nor, for that matter, to any social or political system. As the rate of change in technical content is increased by research and development, an intrinsic inertial lag in response to change becomes more prominent, partly because the delivery system is still relatively decentralized and unregulated. Some see a solution in combining research and health care. For example, there is a widely held belief that adequate treatment of certain forms of cancer can be obtained only in centers of cancer research. A large proportion of NIH support for cancer research is devoted to the establishment of these centers and to their extension into the community. This is laudable as an attempt to put research into practice and as a means of broadening access to the best health care. To the extent, however, that the health needs of today and tomorrow will be different, they cannot be served by a complete fusion of research and service. The goals are the same, but the processes and people involved are not. Understanding and preserving the differences will continue to be essential.

In ways that insist upon responsible performance and permit the achievement of difficult ambitions, the search for knowledge underlying man's physical and mental health must continue to be publicly supported and encouraged. It remains one of the brightest sources of light and hope for improvement in the quality of our lives and those of our children.

REFERENCES

[1] J. W. Shannon, "The Advancement of Medical Research: A Twenty-Year View of the Role of the National Institutes of Health," *Journal of Medical Education*, 42 (February, 1967), pp. 97-108.

[2] *Basic Data Relating to the National Institutes of Health, 1976*, Division of Legislative Analysis, Office of Program Planning and Evaluation, NIH, February, 1976.

[3] *DHEW Obligations to Medical Schools, Fiscal Years 1967-69*, Division of Resources Analysis, Office of Program Planning and Evaluation, NIH, June, 1971. *DHEW Obligations to Institutions of Higher Education and Selected Non-Profit Organization, Fiscal Years 1965-72*, Division of Resources Analysis, Office of Program Planning and Evaluation, NIH, December, 1974.

[4] Derived by Division of Resources Analysis, Office of Program Planning and Evaluation, NIH, from data maintained by the National Academy of Sciences and the Association of American Medical Colleges.

[5] D. E. Wooldridge, Chairman, NIH Study Committee, *Biomedical Science and Its Administration: A Study of the National Institutes of Health, Report to the President, February, 1965*, The White House (U.S. Government Printing Office, Washington, D.C. February, 1965).

ROBERT H. EBERT, M.D.

Medical Education in the United States

PREOCCUPATION WITH THE PHILOSOPHY OF EDUCATION amounts almost to an obsession in this country, and that makes it impossible to have a discussion of medical education without quoting the Flexner Report of 1910 and referring to the "Flexner model." The Flexner model is that of a medical school totally integrated into the university, and so powerful has it become that the reality of what exists today and, indeed, what has existed for a very long time, is often obscured by its influence. Because medical schools and medical centers, according to the interpreters of Flexner, are supposed to be integral parts of universities, they are described as being so, even though it should be apparent to the most casual observer that the relationship of the medical school-medical center to the university bears no resemblance to that of any other school, faculty, or division in it. A dominant theme of this essay will center on the tension that arises from the often artificial attempts to give this belief credence by describing non-university activities as being university ones.

Medical education is a continuum which begins in college, progresses through medical school, and ends with the postgraduate years of internship and residency training. These three phases—college, medical school, and residency—are convenient divisions of the educational process, since the conclusion of each is marked by an academic degree or certification. But there is also another way of describing the phases—as a university phase and a non-university or hospital phase. This division will be viewed with disfavor by those who adhere to the Flexner model, yet it may be a more accurate description of the educational environment than are the traditional distinctions based on the granting of degrees. The university phase comprises the collegiate or premedical portion of the education of the physician plus the so-called preclinical portion of medical school. The hospital phase includes the clinical clerkship during the last two years of medical school together with internship and residency training. In whatever way the education of the physician is viewed, it is remarkable how little change has taken place in the fundamental organization of medical education over the past half-century. The most significant modification has been in the non-university or hospital phase of the educational process, and this change has occurred predominantly in the internship-residency period of hospital training.

The University Portion of Medical Education

University departments of medicine were created in the latter part of the

171

eighteenth century at the College of Philadelphia (now the University of Pennsylvania), King's College (which became Columbia University), and Harvard. These were in fact departments rather than separate schools, and they did not immediately set the pattern for medical education in this country. The dominant force during the nineteenth century was the proprietary medical school. Baltimore was the setting for the first proprietary school, established in the early nineteenth century, and, judging by the number of imitators, it proved to be a remarkably successful model. During the century after the Baltimore school was established, 457 medical schools were founded in the United States and Canada, and the majority of these were proprietary. Many did not survive, but they often represented lucrative business ventures for the physician-entrepreneurs who started them. Teaching was didactic, with little or no laboratory work; consequently, expenses were low and profits high. In addition, the clinical professors were usually chosen because they controlled hospital services, and it was customary for graduates of the proprietary schools to refer patients to their professors once they were in practice. Clinical professorships in proprietary schools became so profitable that it was not unusual for them to be bought and sold. Little attention was paid to the educational backgrounds of students applying for admission to proprietary schools; it has been claimed that the abilities to read, write, and pay tuition were the only requirements in many of them.

Obviously, the educational standards in proprietary schools were exceedingly low, and the Flexner Report was scathing in its indictment of them. Flexner recommended that all proprietary schools be closed and that only medical schools associated with universities be certified for the education of physicians. Even medical schools attached to universities came in for their share of criticism: only Johns Hopkins was singled out as the model of what an American medical school ought to be.

Flexner did his undergraduate work at Hopkins, but it was not the loyalty of an alumnus that caused him to praise the Johns Hopkins Medical School. The medical school was designed to be an integral part of the university, and the Johns Hopkins University and the Johns Hopkins Hospital, although created as separate corporations, were meant by their founder to be closely associated for the purpose of medical education. Funds were not sufficient to open the new hospital and the medical school simultaneously, but an additional gift from a Miss Gannett permitted the medical school to open in 1893—four years after the hospital. One condition of Miss Gannett's gift was that students be required to have the baccalaureate degree as a prerequisite for admission to the medical school. Accepting this condition was an important decision, for it formalized what had become a significant difference between the American and European approach to medical education. In the European university, medicine was considered an undergraduate discipline; any student entering the university could study medicine if he wished. In the United States, medicine became a graduate discipline, with separate admissions standards and procedures and a separate curriculum.

Undoubtedly there were other reasons for the differences in medical training between the United States and Europe. One may have been that many American students, particularly those from rural areas, attended small liberal-arts colleges, and they might have been excluded from medical school had the European model been adopted. Another may have been that in some ways it was more efficient to make medical education a graduate subject: the quality of secondary education was uneven in this country, and a college education was apt to be remedial for students who were poorly prepared in high school. College could also be used as a trial period to determine which were the students sufficiently qualified and properly motivated to become doctors.

Following the submission by Flexner in 1910 of the report to the Carnegie Foundation on the state of medical education in the United States and Canada, many of the reforms recommended by its author were implemented. Proprietary schools were closed in the course of the next few years, licensing of physicians was made much more stringent, and the general pattern of medical education for the next sixty-five years was defined. The university phase of medical education was divided into two parts—a premedical portion for the undergraduate and a preclinical portion for the graduate student. While most medical schools did not follow the Hopkins lead and require the baccalaureate degree for admission, it gradually became a de facto requirement through the pressure created by the large numbers of students applying for admission to medical school. Following World War II, only the exceptional student could be admitted without a college degree in the majority of medical schools.

Why did medicine become such a popular career? Why has the number of qualified students always exceeded the number of places for students in the entering classes? The practice of medicine has a number of attractions which distinguish it from other vocations: the physician can choose where he works and with whom. He can, if he wishes, work alone, or he can, if he prefers, work with other physicians in a group. He can choose the field of medicine he wants to practice, and his services will always be needed—for to some extent he creates his own demand. The practice of medicine is probably the most secure vocation in this country, and it is very well paid. It is not surprising, then, that it has become progressively more popular in recent years.

Premedical requirements are reasonably standardized today; they include several courses in chemistry (inorganic and organic chemistry and, in some cases, physical chemistry), usually college-level courses in physics and elementary calculus, and possibly a college course in biology. These few requirements can be fulfilled in two or three semesters, making it obvious that four years are not needed to prepare for medical school. If that is the case, how is the time used up, and how do educators continue to justify the four years of undergraduate education they require?

The majority of students hoping to enter medical school have either taken a prescribed "premedical" course which is heavily oriented toward the sciences or they have majored in one of the sciences, most often biology or chemistry. A minority have pursued degrees in the humanities or the social sciences. The justification for the continued separation of the undergraduate phase of medical education from the preclinical phase is the desire of college faculty members to keep the baccalaureate period "unprofessional." In other words, the undergraduate phase is supposed to be a time for general education, and any attempt to combine it with a part of the medical school or to shorten it is thought to adulterate the experience. This is a curious argument, since students majoring in physics, chemistry, economics, or history and planning to go on to graduate school might as easily be regarded as pursuing a "professional" education at the undergraduate level. Certainly they are at least specializing to the same extent as the students taking those courses in the sciences that are basic to medicine.

The preclinical phase of university education, which occurs in the first year and a half to two years of medical school, has remained remarkably constant in its subject matter despite a number of modifications in the manner in which it is taught. The subjects covered include anatomy (both gross and microscopic), physiology, microbiology, biochemistry, pharmacology, pathology, and some aspects of neurobiology. These may be taught as separate or as "integrated" disciplines, but, whatever the approach, the ultimate knowledge required of the student is the same. One significant change, however, should be noted: most schools have abandoned much of the traditional, rigidly didactic instruction for clinical medicine and have substituted so-called pathophysiology, an approach that attempts to explain disease in terms of altered biology rather than in terms of distinctive sets of particular signs and symptoms.

But the most profound change, perhaps, is one that has nothing to do with the way in which medicine is taught. This is the enormous scientific progress that has been made in the field of biology itself. Modern molecular biology and cell biology have blurred the boundaries among the various biological disciplines and have become the common scientific language of all biology. In fact, it would be fair to say that biology as a science has "arrived"; now even physical scientists view it as a respectable field. One consequence of its success is that some of the disciplines traditionally belonging to the medical school are now of concern to the faculty of arts and sciences. Biochemistry, once considered a "cookbook chemistry" that belonged only in medical school, has now become one of the most exciting areas of modern chemistry. The bacteriologist turned into the microbiologist, and his attention shifted from disease to the fundamental understanding of bacterial physiology and molecular genetics. The bacterium *E. Coli* became the experimental tool for even those biologists who had no-interest either in classical bacteriology or in medicine.

The blurring of boundaries among the various biological disciplines has made the separation of premedical from preclinical education even more difficult to justify. At one time, the various disciplines taught by the basic-science faculty in medical school were distinct, and one could easily justify a faculty totally separate from the faculty of arts and sciences. But this is no longer the case. The scholarly work done in medical-school departments of biochemistry, microbiology, anatomy, physiology, and even pathology can be quite similar to work going on in arts-and-sciences departments of biochemistry and biology. It would seem to be a relatively simple proposition, therefore, to revolutionize the university phase of medical education. Why not teach all the necessary biology as an undergraduate subject using the biochemists and biologists on the faculties of liberal-arts colleges or universities? The difficulty is that, while the language of molecular biology and cell biology is universal, the fields of anatomy, physiology, and microbiology do not represent the exciting cutting edge of the science. But the physician must still know something about them (for example, gross and microscopic anatomy, organ physiology, and the bacteriology of disease), and these are not areas that the fundamental biologist can teach.

This does not mean that the present separation of undergraduate and graduate teaching of those sciences that are basic to medicine need persist. It is obvious that departments of physiology, anatomy, and pharmacology could just as well be departments in the faculty of arts and sciences as departments in the medical school. At Oxford University all the basic medical-science departments are included in the general organization of the university faculty, and subjects such as anatomy, physiology, and pharmacology are taught to undergraduates. Why should the separation persist if the basic medical sciences are as interesting to undergraduates as any other course available in biology? The answer includes a number of reasons but the central one is the integrity of the medical school as presently organized. It is claimed that separating the basic medical sciences from the medical school would emasculate it and make it little more than a hospital medical school. Here the English provide us good do the example of what could happen. There is some apprehension that the standards of science teaching in the clinical departments would be lowered if the preclinical and clinical departments were separated.

Another argument concerns the integrity of the basic disciplines which now exist in medical schools. Would the classical disciplines of anatomy, physiology, et al., be lost if they were to be absorbed in the faculty of arts and sciences? Scientific disciplines appear to be less stable in American universities than in their British counterparts. Some are apprehensive lest all the traditional medical disciplines become departments of molecular biology and cell biology. Who would then be available to teach medical students what they need to know in preparation for the clinic?

Another reason, not often mentioned but very real, is the pecking order that exists in universities. In the past, the medical-school basic-science departments were considered more "applied" and less "intellectual" than their opposite numbers in the faculty of arts and sciences. This is in fact no longer true, when one considers the quality of the science in medical schools, but some residual feeling remains that an appointment in a medical-school department may somehow be less prestigious than a comparable appointment in arts and sciences.

In some universities, the basic medical sciences are considered to be an integral part of the general faculty and not a separate faculty. The University of Chicago can be taken as the best example of this organization: the Division of Biological Sciences comprises all biology, including the clinical and preclinical components of the medical school, and the faculty teaches both undergraduates and medical students. Yet the separation of the medical school persists, and the two phases of education are not integrated—as they are, for example, at Oxford. An experiment being supported by the Commonwealth Fund in the teaching of biology to medical students and general students of biology is still in its early stages; we cannot tell yet whether any truly new definition of medical education has been found. It already seems apparent, however, that the medical school as it exists today will persist, although now with two groups of students—those who enter the experimental program and those who are admitted from other colleges.

This is the likely outcome because efforts—at Hopkins, Northwestern, and Boston University—to shorten the educational process by combining undergraduate and medical-school education, while successful for selected groups of students, have never managed to modify the overall approach, even at the universities carrying out these experiments. Each of those three universities developed a program that combined general education with medical education and granted the M.D. degree at the end of six years, rather than the usual eight. Students graduating from these programs have done as well as, or better than, graduates of traditional programs, but these "fast tracks" have neither been expanded nor have they replaced the regular M.D. program at any one of the three universities that use them.

In summary, one can argue that the premedical and preclinical experiences could be combined and presented to undergraduates wishing to pursue careers in medicine. For a variety of reasons, however, including the most formidable—inertia—it is unlikely that any significant change in the organization of medical schools will occur.

The Hospital Phase of Medical Education

Flexner was critical of all phases of education in proprietary medical schools, but in those associated with universities he pointed the accusatory finger primarily at the clinical services. He felt that clinical teaching in American medical schools was unscientific, dominated by successful practitioners, and inferior to the teaching in the rest of the university. It was his recommendation that a full-time clinical faculty should be recruited and that the teaching of medicine should be in the hands of clinician-scholars rather than practicing clinicians. His model was the German university.

What was the German medical school really like, and was the teaching hospital an integral part of the university? Some teaching hospitals were owned by the state and were designed as university hospitals, while others were municipal. No matter how the teaching hospitals were owned and operated, however, they had one characteristic in common. All were organized on the basis of *Kliniken*, while the basic medical sciences were organized as *Institute*. Each *Institut* or *Klinik* was headed by a professor, who was not only the academic head of the department but also the director of the *Institut* or *Klinik*. Each *Institut* had its own lecture rooms, preparation rooms, library, museum, and research laboratories, so that it was essentially an autonomous unit within the university. Similarly, each *Klinik* had its own laboratories, teaching amphitheater, library, and record room. The staffing of each *Klinik* with assistants at various levels was entirely controlled by the professor, and there was little or no relationship among the various *Kliniken* or *Institute*. The teaching of medical students was largely by lecture and lecture demonstration; the German medical student received little direct instruction in the care of the patient.

This is a rather different concept of a university from the one that evolved in this country, for each of the departments in the German medical school, whether in the basic medical sciences or in the clinic, was organized essentially as an autonomous institute. There is little question that it was a successful model in terms of research and advanced training in scientific medicine. But it was a poor model for the education of medical students, and it produced a large number of rather badly trained general practitioners and a relatively small number of very well trained specialists. It is probably fair to conclude that the German teaching hospital was an integral part of the German university, but this statement must be qualified by the observation that the entire structure of the German university was highly decentralized; the university was little more than a loose federation of autonomous departments.

Whatever the merits of the German teaching hospital, it could not be adopted as the model in this country for a number of reasons. American universities were organized in a pattern different from that of German universities, and the structure of the hospital system in the United States was equally different. German hospitals were government owned, whereas hospitals in the United States were almost all privately owned. Nevertheless there were attempts to adopt parts of the German system and to bring about a closer relationship between the teaching hospital and the university. Some medical schools adopted the Hopkins model, building university hospitals with the purpose of providing an environment for teaching and research. State medical schools built teaching hospitals with the added purpose of providing referral centers for practicing physicians in their states. Municipal and voluntary hospitals developed teaching services in association with medical schools and, after World War II, the Veterans Administration developed a close working relationship between its major hospitals and the nation's medical schools. All these hospitals differed in organization and relationship to the university but they also all had one characteristic in common—the presence of at least some salaried full-time clinical faculty. The dominance of full-time faculty did not occur immediately; it evolved over a period of decades, although accelerating markedly after World War II. Between 1950 and 1968 the National Institutes of Health poured money into American medical schools, which facilitated the rapid expansion of full-time faculties. American medical schools had arrived. American medicine became as dominant a force in the world as German medicine had been during the latter part of the nineteenth century and the first part of the twentieth.

But had the teaching hospital in fact become a part of the university? There were many who would note the predominance of full-time faculty, the high quality of research, and the commitment to teaching, and would say "yes." They would claim that clinical departments—or at least some clinical departments—were every bit as academic as the basic-science departments. And there would be some truth to these claims. But do any or all of these claims make the teaching hospital an integral part of the university? Not necessarily, for a fundamental difference between the teaching hospital and the rest of the university always remains. The hospital must provide a service—namely, the care of the sick—which is unrelated to the primary role of the university, and it must provide that service day in and day out, year in and year out, whatever the requirements may be for teaching and research.

The hospital-service role creates an environment quite different from that of the university. Complex technology, both diagnostic and therapeutic, is required, as are radiology departments, operating rooms, intensive-care units, emergency rooms, and all the expensive machinery and manpower needed to operate them, because service to patients must be provided. The physical resources needed by the modern teaching hospital are vast, and the manpower requirements for services alone are often greater than the manpower needs of all the rest of the university put together. Similarly the hospital budget may be as large or larger than the total remaining university budget. By far the largest part of the hospital budget is for service, not for teaching and research, and its income is derived from quite different sources than those of the university. Most hospital income comes from third-party payers, whether government (Medicare and Medicaid) or private insurers, and reimbursement is for service. Unlike the university, the patients served—not the students—represent the primary constituency of the hospital.

A popular aphorism frequently quoted by medical educators in the nineteen-fifties and -sixties was that teaching, service, and research comprised an inseparable triad. One can, of course, argue that it would be impossible to teach clinical medicine without patients and to pursue clinical research without patients, and that to this degree teaching, service, and research should indeed be viewed as inseparable. But what was ignored in this argument was the growth in commitment to service by all teaching hospitals, a growth that greatly exceeded the requirements of teaching and research.

Why should the very people who claimed that the teaching hospital was an integral part of the university wish to expand its non-university function? The reasons are complex. First of all, the teaching hospital by its very nature provided expertise in the various specialties of medicine, and it therefore naturally became a referral center. Referrals were encouraged, for they soon became an important source of income for the clinical faculty as well as of "teaching material" for the groups of students whom the clinical faculty valued most—the interns, residents, and fellows committed to specialty training. The more dominant the teaching hospitals grew, the more detached they became from the university. In the United States today the largest and technologically the most advanced hospitals are teaching hospitals; they have become an integral part of the nation's health-care system. They control the training of specialists in all areas of medicine and therefore also the specialist mix that enters practice. They are more dependent on the federal government for financial support than is the rest of the university. Federal funds not only support patient care, via Medicare and Medicaid, but hospital training programs and research as well. It is not uncommon for a single large clinical research program to have a budget in excess of a million dollars a year. There are few research programs in the rest of the university with federally supported budgets anything like that size. In addition, clinical faculties, whether entirely salaried or partly salaried and partly supported by funds collected as professional fees, are far better paid than other members of the university faculty. The teaching hospital is certainly academic, but it represents the part of the educational system devoted to the training of physicians. It works with the university, but it is not an integral part of it.

The American medical student enters the hospital phase of his medical education after one and a half or two years of preclinical work. He then experiences an education totally different from the one he has had in the past. He becomes a member of a team assigned to care for patients in the hospital, and he learns by working on clinical problems in the real world. The clinical clerkship is adopted from the British system and is totally unlike the didactic training of clinical medicine which dominated German teaching. Indeed, the American medical student is given a substantial responsibility for the care of patients—even more than his British cousin. He has clerkships in medicine, surgery, pediatrics, and obstetrics, as well as some of the other specialties of medicine.

The major change which occurs between the granting of the M.D. degree and the first year of graduate training comes with the student's selection of his major specialty. As he proceeds through the residency, he assumes greater and greater responsibility for his patients, but the general character of his education remains much the same.

The Rise of Specialty Training

Prior to World War I, the majority of physicians entered general practice. Only a few major medical centers, such as those in Boston, Baltimore, New York, Chicago, and Philadelphia, trained specialists. It was common for American specialists to conclude their training abroad, especially in Germany, which was the major center in the world for postgraduate training. It was also common for the medical-school graduate to enter practice after a year of internship, sometimes returning to a medical center for specialty training after some years as a general practitioner. Others developed special interests and trained themselves as specialists simply by restricting their practice to particular ills. Then, as today, specialty practice carried with it greater prestige and greater financial rewards. Specialty societies already existed in the nineteenth century, suggesting that specialty training was not unknown in the United States. But it was not until the early part of the twentieth century that the specialty boards were established to provide certification for practitioners. The boards developed appropriate examinations for specialist certification and defined the number of years of training and specialized practice required before the physician could be certified. It is significant that these specialty boards were organized *outside* the university, even though they were to define what was to become the most important part of the physician's training.

World War II represented a turning point in the training of specialists. Physicians entering the armed services immediately discovered the value of specialization— board-certified specialists were given higher rank, better assignments, and additional pay. This lesson was not lost on those young physicians who entered the service after a year of internship. Many on returning from the service sought additional training, and the number of residencies expanded rapidly. Because of the sudden increase in demand, many community hospitals were able to develop residency training pro- grams; their success was short-lived, however, for after the bulge in specialty applicants immediately following World War II, the numbers leveled off, as more and more of the training of residents was carried out in teaching hospitals. The number of teaching hospitals, including Veterans Administration hospitals (staffed by full-time clinicians, salaried by the Veterans Administration, but holding faculty appointments in medical schools) also expanded.

The pattern of education now changed. The majority of graduates took a minimum of two to three years of hospital training after graduation and then usually proceeded immediately to specialized training, eliminating the customary period of general practice. The number entering general practice consequently dwindled; family physicians who retired or died were rarely replaced.

Specialization did not result purely from social and economic factors, however. Rapid advances in medicine had occurred after World War II, and medicine had consequently become far more complex. The recent graduate followed the example of his specialist teacher: he set out to master one field of medicine rather than become superficially familiar with many. He was often also quick to note that his teachers were really "subspecialists," that it was more prestigious yet to become a thoracic surgeon or a neurosurgeon than a general surgeon, better to be an endocrinologist or gastroenterologist than a general internist.

Subspecialization was further encouraged by training programs developed by the categorical institutes of the National Institutes of Health (e.g. Cancer, Heart and Lung, Arthritis, and Metabolic Disease). Their purpose was supposed to be to train clinical investigators, but many trainees entered practice after the conclusion of their fellowships in order to practice their subspecialties. It is sometimes forgotten that the federal government with the strong support of the Congress had its part in encour- aging the rapid specialization of medicine in the United States.

The Students and Faculty

Until relatively recently medical students were predominantly white, male, and middle class. Now more women and minority students are entering medical school:

the percentage of women has increased from 5.7 in 1960 to 18.1 in 1975. The percentage of blacks has risen from 0.9 in 1969 to 6.3 in 1975. But the majority of students remains a relatively homogeneous group.

European universities spend far less time than we do in selecting medical students, preferring to weed out incompetents on the basis of examination. In contrast, American medical schools devote an enormous amount of time to the admissions process with the expectation that everyone accepted will receive the M.D. The procedure is reasonably successful; at least the attrition rate is less than 1.5 per cent. There is an unfortunate by-product, however, and that is the intense competition that has developed among students to gain admission: in the neighborhood of 45,000 of them are applying for 15,000 places. An individual from a populous state has a less than one-in-three chance to gain admission because most state schools require that state residents be given preference. Thus a resident of New Mexico has a better chance of gaining admission to medical school than does a resident of New York. The aspiring physician begins to worry about his or her academic record in high school, and the pressure increases as the college years progress.

There is almost always a psychological letdown during the first year of medical school, partly in reaction to the race for admission and partly because the first year is not so very different from a year in college. It is quite possible that this letdown could be avoided if admission to medical school were earlier and the premedical and preclinical experience were combined.

The professionalization of the medical student begins with the hospital phase of his education and continues through the internship and residency. It is difficult to define precisely what this means, but the process is very real and it is probably more intense than in any other profession, with the possible exception of the military. At its best, professionalization imbues the physician-in-training with an intense commitment to the welfare of his patients, even to the point of personal sacrifice. At its worst, it makes him arrogant, unwilling to believe that anyone outside the profession has anything useful to say about the practice of medicine.

Perhaps it is this process of professionalization that distinguishes the clinical faculty from other members of the university. Members of the clinical faculty are physicians and specialists first and faculty members second. They have been through intense study and training, which includes research experience as well as clinical training, and they are by and large older than their non-clinical colleagues by the time they have attained academic rank. They tend to be more single-minded than their non-clinical colleagues in their devotion to their own specialty. While they might value the university, they usually feel greater allegiance to the hospital and as a group are little interested in university affairs. The hospital is where they work and where most of them (whether or not they are salaried) earn a significant part of their income.

The young instructor or assistant professor in a clinical department has another distinction; he knows that, unlike his non-clinical colleague, he is not committed to a university career. If he tires of the academic life or if an appropriate university position is not available, he can always practice medicine, and he may even be able to continue his association with the teaching hospital. In fact, his life need not change dramatically, for he may still involve himself with teaching clinical clerks and residents. The ease with which the academic physician can enter a lucrative practice has played its part in inflating the salaries of academic physicians above those for the rest of the faculty.

The Government and Medical Education

The President's Biomedical Research Panel was established early in 1975. It was charged by Congress to review and assess the conduct, policies, and management of the biomedical research in this country that was being supported by the National Institutes of Health and the Alcohol, Drug Abuse, and Mental Health Administration. It commissioned a number of studies, among them one by the American Council on Education, the Association of American Medical Colleges, and the Rand Corporation on the impact of federal health-related research expenditures upon institutions of higher education. One purpose of the study was to determine the extent of academic medical-center[1] dependence on federal funding for research and whether the pattern of this funding had changed in any significant way between 1965 and 1974. They found that the total operating budgets of all academic medical centers (exclusive of patient care) had increased from $783 million to $2,409 million in those years, that federal research funds had increased from $280 million to $493 million, but that as a proportion of the budget they had *decreased* from 36 per cent to 21 per cent. Total federal support of academic health centers, including research funds, federal teaching and training funds, indirect costs, and federal capitation,[2] increased from $425 million in 1965 to $1,022 million in 1974 but as a proportion of budget they decreased from 54 per cent to 42 per cent. Even though the proportion of federal support of academic medical centers decreased, it still represents the largest component of support for academic medical centers. It is particularly striking as compared with the proportion of the budget derived from student fees (4-5%) or endowment and gifts (3-4%).

Two other sources of funding changed significantly between 1965 and 1974: state and local government funds increased from $100 million to $471 million and increased from 13 per cent of the budget to 20 per cent. The other changes were in professional fees and service programs, which increased from $31 million to $522 million and increased from 4 per cent to 22 per cent of the total revenues for all academic medical centers. Thus, academic medical centers derive over one-fifth of their support from patient fees, that is, from funds generated by the clinical faculty. No other part of the university relies on service to the general public for a significant proportion of its revenues.

The health-manpower legislation that has been debated for the past two years has aroused considerable concern among the universities, for it appears to them that precedents are being set that will affect the entire system. State and private universities are equally worried about the possibility that university education can be regulated through certain recommendations governing the clinical education of medical students and residents. One version of the House Health Manpower Bill set a six-week clinical experience at a site remote from the medical school as a requirement for capitation payments to medical schools. This was regarded as an invasion of the right of universities to define their own curriculum requirements, as well as a dangerous precedent that could spread to other parts of the university. Another provision in the Senate version of the legislation would have set percentages for the number of residents required to enter the primary-care specialties in each medical school, in effect restricting the number of residents trained in fields other than general internal medicine, general pediatrics, and family medicine.

Do these really represent precedents that could be extended to the rest of the university? Probably not. It is more likely that they would remain regulations solely for the hospital phase of medical education. If a precedent is being set it is more apt to be one that presages further regulation of the teaching hospital and the hospital phase of medical education.

Nor is it surprising that the Congress and the executive branch should show such interest in medical education, for the federal government represents the single largest source of funding for academic medical centers. The federal establishment is also aware that teaching hospitals and academic medical centers control the national output of specialists; if there is maldistribution among the specialties—as there is—what better way of dealing with it than to regulate the institutions that control the supply? Regulation will not stop there either, for teaching hospitals are also a major resource for the provision of tertiary care, and much of the new technology introduced into medical practice is conceived in the teaching hospital. There will be more federal regulation, not because Congress particularly wants to regulate universities, but, on the contrary, because it wants to regulate those many things that go on in teaching hospitals which have nothing to do with a university education.

Conclusion

American medical education has been remarkably successful in many ways. It attracts some of the ablest college graduates, and the level of competence of the physicians it educates is generally high. It has produced too few primary-care physicians and too many specialists, but the resulting maldistribution is remediable, and does not constitute a criticism of the quality of the training provided. Many feel that not enough attention is paid to the particular educational requirements of the primary-care physician, but this, too, is a soluble problem and does not require any radical modifications of the educational approaches used. The research output of medical faculties has been high, and the practice of medicine promises to be increasingly scientific. At first glance, it would appear that everything Flexner wished for and asked for has come to pass.

Where, then, is the Achilles heel of medical education—if, indeed, there is one? Probably it can be found in the failure to recognize that the teaching hospital is *not* an integral part of the university, for this misapprehension has adversely affected the relationship of the teaching hospital both to the university and to the community. The sheer magnitude of the hospital operation makes it difficult to develop a comfortable relationship with the university. In addition, the differences in sources of funding, in function, and in management make hospital and university an incompatible mix. Conceptually, the medical-school experience turns out to be only one aspect of a physician's education: there is no longer any particular logic to the division between premedical and preclinical education, on the one hand, and the clinical portion of medical-school education and residency training, on the other. A redefinition of the several components in the education of the physician might make possible different approaches to medical education. If the premedical and preclinical portions of medical education were accepted as the fundamental province of the university, perhaps they might be joined in ways that would make better educational sense than the system prevailing today. Similarly, if the clinical training of the physician both at the medical school and graduate level were recognized as the primary responsibility of the teaching hospital, there would be further opportunities to experiment with clinical education. The teaching hospital should remain affiliated with the university, but even in its teaching function it should no longer be regarded as an integral part of it.

Still more important, we must recognize that the teaching hospital has a vital community role which is quite different from that of the university. Many teaching hospitals are situated in communities where the level of general medical care is poor and the only medical resources available are their outpatient departments. Too often this role has not been considered important, since it is regarded as a service obligation rather than an academic function. And, of course, it is, but it is one that is difficult to ignore if the teaching hospital is the only medical resource available to the surrounding population. More recently, a growing interest in primary care has encouraged teaching hospitals to respond less reluctantly to social pressure for service to the community, but even more could be done if they would admit that one of their functions was to provide that service.

In part, the teaching hospital has been reluctant to assume a primary-care role because it looks upon its functions as being those of a referral center and an institution for tertiary care. But it has not provided a notable degree of leadership in tertiary care either, at least not to the extent one might expect from an institution that should have the capacity for considering policy issues larger than the immediate welfare of individual clinical departments. New and expensive technologies have been produced by many clinical departments in teaching hospitals, but rarely is any thought given to the ramifications of their introduction into practice. Almost no analyses have been made to determine the marginal value of new technologies, and no systematic examinations have been made regarding how new technologies should be evaluated once the initial clinical trial has been concluded.

Finally, teaching hospitals have provided very few innovations in the provision of health services, although they represent a major health resource of the nation. In part they have failed because the scientific qualifications that make department heads and senior full-time clinicians are not those directed toward service. Too often teaching hospitals are so intent on being "academic" that they ignore the need for individuals expert in the problems of health-care delivery.

The present organization of medical education allows neither the university nor the teaching hospital to fulfill its proper role. Perhaps a first step might be to recognize that the teaching hospital is not now, and cannot be, an integral part of the university and that attempts to force the teaching hospital into this mold are damaging both to the university and to the hospital. The recognition that the university and the teaching hospital are equal but separate institutions would facilitate their relations with one another, with the government, and with the public in the years to come.

REFERENCES

[1] Academic medical center is a term which includes a medical school, at least one and often several teaching hospitals, and one or more semi-autonomous research institutes; its largest component is the teaching hospital.

[2] Federal capitation grants, first provided in 1971, are formula grants based on the number of enrolled medical students and the number of graduates.

SUGGESTED READING

Commission on Medical Education, A. Lawrence Lowell, Chairman, *Medical Education: Final Report of the Commission on Medical Education* (New York, 1932).

John A. D. Cooper, "Undergraduate Medical Education," *Advances in American Medicine: Essays at the Bicentennial*, I (Josiah Macy, Jr., Foundation, 1976).

Robert H. Ebert, "The Medical School," *Scientific American*, 229:3 (September, 1973), p. 139.

Abraham Flexner, *Medical Education in the United States and Canada. A Report to the Carnegie Foundation for the Advancement of Teaching*, Bulletin 4 (Boston, 1910).

Abraham Flexner, *Medical Education: A Comparative Study* (New York, 1925).

John H. Knowles, ed., *The Teaching Hospital* (Cambridge, Mass., 1966).

Report of the President's Biomedical Research Panel, Appendix C, Impact of Federal Health-Related Research Expenditures upon Institutions of Higher Education, U.S. Department of Health, Education, and Welfare, Public Health Service, DHEW Publication No. (OS) 76-503.

MERLIN K. DUVAL, M.D.

The Provider, the Government, and the Consumer

HUMAN BEINGS HAVE VALUED GOOD HEALTH since their appearance on this earth, a value no doubt based on their instinctive will to survive. To achieve it, they have resorted to practices varying from witchcraft, exorcism, and punishment for transgressions to the invocation of elements drawn from the supernatural and the cosmic. Only in the comparatively recent past have knowledge, philosophy, and reason displaced these earlier practices. But whether one believes that the source of good health is to be found in mysticism, religion, or science, what is important is the good health itself, for its absence can absorb the mind to the exclusion of the many other things that are also important in our lives.

Not long ago, when the World Health Organization attempted to define health, it could do so only in negative terms—that is, it spoke in terms of the absence of physical or mental disease. In my opinion, it is preferable to consider health in positive terms, that is, to define it as a state that permits one to achieve an acceptable accommodation to one's environment and circumstances and to be able fully to join with others in being productive and useful members of society.

When defined in these terms, health is only marginally affected by medical care; indeed, much of contemporary, scientific medicine is almost irrelevant to good health. Those medical professionals who are franchised by society to render medical care have been neither ethically nor professionally prepared to address the important factors that ultimately have impact on the health of the majority of the people, because they have been trained to focus on disease. Consequently, a serious imbalance exists today between public expectations regarding health and the capacity of the professional community to meet them. Those who provide health services may affect the degree to which their services are accessible, and they clearly determine the costs. In the final analysis, however, the individual's behavior, his environment, and his living habits have a far greater impact on his health than anything medicine might do for him.

Whether in spite or because of the remarkable scientific achievements that we can attribute to modern medicine, many of the fruits of these advances are not equitably distributed. Heightened expectations for real benefits have been matched by barriers to their acquisition, whether financial, geographic, or due to ignorance regarding their value and availability. Increasing concern for those of our fellow citizens who have not been in a position to receive the benefits of new procedures and rapid changes in society demand that we solve the problems of equity. These issues force us to consider alternative ways of organizing, financing, and delivering health services. It

185

seems clear that the notion of a "right" to health care will play an important part in the way these newly emerging patterns and arrangements develop.

The idea that health care is a "right" has been proposed, assumed, debated, and postulated as a political expectation for many years in the United States. President Franklin Roosevelt included it in the economic bill of rights he proposed in the thirties. Its existence was a premise of a study commissioned by President Truman in 1945. That such a right exists has been discussed in Senate hearings. In 1968, Senator Edward M. Kennedy suggested: "All Americans have come to expect health care as one of the basic rights of citizenship."

In many ways, the idea that health care should be a "right" is a curious and puzzling phenomenon. Historically the conception of individual rights conveys the implication that governments or other authorities have a clear duty to refrain from interfering with an individual's freedom. The primary thrust of the American Bill of Rights, for instance, is to limit the power of the government over the people. In a sense, such a conception of rights is negative in that it prohibits others from frustrating or preventing the exercise of the enumerated rights. The contemporary concept of a right to health care, however, takes a decidedly different tack. It suggests that someone has a positive duty (derived from an unwritten social contract) to provide an explicit service to the holder of such a right, and the scope of the service depends not only on the existence of the right, but on economic and other considerations as well. It necessarily follows, if the basic premise is correct, that medical care is only one small part of the maintenance of health. It would be easy to miss the mark by limiting our focus, and our future choices, to the field of medicine alone.

These issues and the choices that lie before us as we address them become clearer when we examine the three basic elements in this imbalanced equation: the provider, the government, and the patient himself.

The first century of American medicine can best be characterized as practitioner-oriented and practitioner-dominated. The establishment of the American Medical Association in 1847 for the dual purpose of advancing both the education for and the quality of medical practice reflected this emphasis: it permitted the dominance of professional education and professional politics—incidentally, an international rarity even today. The subsequent establishment of the university as the academic and scientific underpinning of medicine was another outgrowth of American Medical Association efforts, and it has come to characterize the profession in the second century of American medicine.

While this movement generated the development of an increasingly strong scientific and technological base for medicine, it also exaggerated the separation between the interests of those who practiced medicine and the interests of their patients and the public at large. As a consequence, the profession became increasingly autonomous; its members selected their own students, determined their education, and set the criteria for licensing (and subsequently certification). Free choice of specialty practice and geographical location was never questioned. Because there was little external regulation or control, further independence and autonomy of the component parts of the medical establishment, such as practitioners, nursing homes, and hospitals, were fostered, culminating in what is now described as a medical "non-system." Medicine thus came to be perceived by many as having been organized primarily for professional convenience and for serving professional and personal purposes.

This development was hardly surprising in view of the simultaneous emergence of a political system in the United States that recognized the individual as, at least theoretically, supreme. While the Constitution of the United States speaks to the form and structure, rather than to a philosophy, of government, the first Congress set the tone for the development of an American philosophy when it adopted the first ten amendments prescribing the rights and privileges reserved to the people themselves. In some respects, the philosophy behind the American government and the political attitudes of its people are more accurately traceable to the Bill of Rights than they are to the original Constitution. The American physician, as citizen, enjoyed the same freedom as the rest, and he seized this opportunity to become totally autonomous. He had the advantages of status and a specialized knowledge that dealt with matters of life and death. Society could scarcely afford not to grant him even greater freedoms than it gave to ordinary citizens.

The orientation of the provider of medical services in the United States today is thus so strongly embedded in the private-enterprise system that it exerts an extraordinary influence on both the conduct and the performance of the contemporary health-care "non-system." Few would question the remarkable strength that has derived from this development. It was so striking that not until the past decade or two have some weaknesses become apparent. The first of these was that public expectations of the profession began to outstrip the capacity of the profession to meet them; the second that, through its own self-determination, the profession had relied on others, principally the governments, to fill the gaps it had left, and the third that a profession organized for its own convenience and performance was ill-equipped to meet ever greater demands for universal access to all forms of medical care.

Because both the educational and the practical aspects of American medicine had evolved from an earlier necessity to concentrate on the identification and treatment of specific diseases, it was not surprising that other factors influencing people's health were either neglected altogether or dealt with by other means. Since many of these other factors were communal, it was logical that they would be attacked through governments. Three levels of governmental medicine arose as a consequence, each of which tended to serve a somewhat different function.

At the most local level, the county, or in a few specific instances the municipal government, by law has some responsibility for public health matters. There are over 1,600 full-time local health departments serving approximately 2,500 counties and over 300 cities. Irrespective of their jurisdiction, the customary approach of these units has been to establish a board of health, appointed by the local governing authority, to oversee the activities of the local governmental health units so that they would not impinge on the private sector of medicine. The organized medical profession made sure of this. Local health units ordinarily assume responsibility for six functions: (1) the collection of vital statistics; (2) the control of sanitary conditions; (3) the control of communicable diseases; (4) the provision of laboratory services; (5) the care of mothers and infants; and (6) the general education of the public on health matters. In fulfilling these obligations and responsibilities, the local governmental health unit often undertakes to provide both ambulatory and general medical and surgical care for the poor, as well as to operate programs of preventive medicine and public health, including immunization, sanitation, and environmental control. Financial support for these activities may derive from the local governmental unit, from the state, or from grants from federal agencies.

On the next level, the state through its constitution or, in some instances, statutes defines the responsibility that is to be undertaken for the protection of the general health and welfare of its citizens. These laws differ substantially among the fifty states. A few have detailed public-health laws, codified and classified to form a clear legal basis for health functions; in other states, only broad principles are laid down, and specific laws are then enacted to meet specific situations. In all states, however, there is provision for some kind of supervisory board of health whose functions may be both advisory and quasi-legislative.

In general, the role of the state government is primarily complementary to the services otherwise provided by the county government or the private sector. In many instances some overlap results. Thus, at the state level one usually finds an administrative unit that is responsible for communicable-disease control, vital statistics, environmental sanitation, maternal and child health, public-health laboratory services, public-health nursing, health education, mental hygiene, and industrial hygiene. The state may also operate facilities to manage problems for which adequate financial support is not forthcoming at the local level. Thus, the state is also involved in the direct provision of medical services: for example, custodial and treatment centers for individuals with chronic disabling diseases such as tuberculosis and mental illness. Recently, in response to new federal legislation, states have enlarged their roles in licensing and accreditation of local institutions, the determination of needs for services at the local level, review (and, in some instances, control) of institutional costs, the support of education of health manpower, and, in general, a broader role in health planning to rationalize local systems of health care.

The third level comprises the activities of the federal government. For approximately 150 years the government has been making its contribution to public health but, until quite recently, its role was directed primarily at meeting the requirements of designated federal beneficiaries. In 1798, the federal government created the Marine Hospital Service to provide medical services for sick and disabled seamen and to protect the nation's borders against the importation of diseases. Out of this movement, the United States Public Health Service emerged. Over the succeeding years, the federal government gradually undertook a somewhat broader public-health responsibility by establishing closer relationships with state and local health departments for the purpose of controlling communicable diseases and improving sanitation. Thereafter, it adopted programs to meet what it regarded as its obligations to provide medical services to specific beneficiaries who were otherwise not cared for, such as American Indians, members of the armed forces, and veterans.

The establishment of the National Cancer Institute in 1936 opened a new era for the federal role in health by offering direct federal support for biomedical research. Shortly thereafter, the National Institutes of Health were established, with authority both to conduct research and to support outside programs. At the same time the federal government became more active in regulation, especially food and drug inspections and control of the environment through programs designed to combat pollution of air and water. More recently, political and social pressures in the United States have resulted in the development of federal programs designed to meet the health problems of particular groups such as migrant workers, mothers and children among the poor, crippled children, alcoholics, drug addicts, and the mentally ill.

Because the role of the government in health has become increasingly complex in recent years and because the implications of its intervention in this field are so great as critically to influence people's lives, we should consider in somewhat greater detail the five broad areas in which the federal government now has responsibility.

1) It is directly providing health services to specific beneficiaries. It employs many thousands of physicians, dentists, and other health personnel and operates hundreds of health-care institutions for this purpose. The Department of Defense has a medical establishment that is now scattered throughout the world; the Veterans Administration operates one of the world's largest systems for the direct provision of health services to veterans; the United States Public Health Service dispenses care directly to merchant seamen, federal prisoners, members of the Coast Guard, and American Indians. Even at this time, the Public Health Service is experimenting with a National Health Service Corps which would render medical services to persons who live in geographically underserved areas when they have medical needs that private medicine will not meet.

2) The federal government provides health care indirectly through grants and contracts to private organizations and to state and local health departments. These units, in turn, provide health care directly to specific groups such as migrant farm workers, the urban poor, mothers and infants, and crippled children. Even though they operate systems of their own, the Veterans Administration and the Department of Defense are authorized to purchase private services to avoid unnecessary duplication.

3) The federal government has taken a major role in the development of health resources. The National Institutes of Health oversee the largest enterprise in the world in support of both basic and applied biomedical research. The Health Resources Administration supports the training of professionals and the construction of community hospitals through the federally financed Hill-Burton program.

4) The federal government has taken on increasing responsibility for quality control through the inspection and regulation of devices and consumable supplies that are used by medicine or affect public health more generally and are not adequately controlled by private industry. The Department of Agriculture, for instance, inspects and grades all meat and poultry products; the Food and Drug Administration reviews, tests, and regulates the flow of drugs, inspects the processing of foods, and assesses the safety of cosmetics. It also has responsibility for the regulation of hazardous substances and for radiological safety. The federal government also monitors the purity of water and air, a power derived from the Interstate Commerce clause of the Constitution.

5) During the last two decades the feeling has grown in the United States that convenient access to low-cost quality health care is a citizen's right that private medicine has not adequately met because it is intrinsically autonomous, self-serving, and interested in the individual patient, not in community health generally. In response to these pressures, the federal government has increasingly assumed the role of arbiter between the competing objectives of individual freedom and desirable social goals. It has so far chosen to use its considerable influence and resources to reform the traditional institutions for distributing health services rather than to assume complete control of the health industry. As a result, the past decade has seen a plethora of new federal programs designed to encourage modifications and reforms of our traditional American private institutions. Such programs as the Regional Medical Programs for cancer, heart, stroke, and kidney disease, comprehensive health planning, experimental community health-care delivery systems, emergency medical services programs,

the development of health-maintenance organizations, and the introduction of new methods for financing medical care, most notably by amending the Social Security Act to permit the introduction of Medicare and Medicaid to assist the aged and the poor, have been the result.

Unfortunately, the federal role in health is weakened by a lack of central guidance; like most government agencies, the health agencies expend much of their energies in reconciling opposing views. Thus, the assignment of priorities, the allocation of the nation's resources, and the development of centralized policies have often proved inordinately difficult and tend to encourage the attitude that our American society is a laissez-faire enterprise lacking in purpose and identifiable goals. Whether this is in fact a deficiency or a strength has yet to be determined.

There are those who believe that, to paraphrase an old saying, medicine is too important to leave to physicians. "Any sane nation," to quote Bernard Shaw's Preface for *The Doctor's Dilemma*, "having observed that you could provide for the supply of bread by giving bakers a pecuniary interest in baking for you, should go on to give a surgeon a pecuniary interest in cutting off your leg, is enough to make one despair of political humanity." The amount of unnecessary surgery in the United States lends credence to his view.

Not surprisingly, therefore, the consumers of health services are beginning to take part in the deliberations regarding health. Loosely organized, they are joining with labor-union interests and other consumer groups. The movement gained momentum following the Supreme Court decision on school desegregation in 1954, because its concerns also involved the civil rights and liberties of citizens more generally. Subsequently, the student movement, the consumer movement, and similar groups in the sixties began to challenge the "mystique" of medicine and the often self-serving decisions bearing on a subservient public who were otherwise in a poor position to render judgments on the quality of the medical care they were receiving. Around the same time, the Carnegie Foundation for Higher Education reviewed the production of health manpower, and the American Public Health Association began increasingly to devote attention to the underserved American citizen, particularly the impover-ished one. A "Committee of One Hundred," composed of citizens representing a broad spectrum of interests in the United States, was created to study the role of the federal government in the financing of health care, and its efforts culminated in the introduction into the Congress of the Health Security Act, which transferred dominance in the delivery of health services to government by manipulating the system of financing health care paid for under Social Security.

Meanwhile, several private foundations (the Robert Wood Johnson, in particular) directed an increasing portion of their resources to the study of health-care-delivery systems and to the development of pilot experiments designed to achieve reform in health-care delivery. The object was to modify the traditional medical monopoly of the private practitioner operating on a fee-for-service basis for a selected clientele. These contributions and others have already reduced the traditional sharp distinction between the public and private sectors in the health-care economy.

This movement derives from many sources. The American people watched impassively as their total health expenditures increased from approximately 6 per cent to over 8 per cent of the gross national product within a single decade. These expenditures now exceed $119 billion a year. As an outgrowth of this remarkable rise in expenditure for health, there has been a growing awareness of the need for public accountability both from voluntary and private institutions and from agencies that use public resources, operating in areas that have great impact on the public welfare. It is not unreasonable to expect that private agencies will consequently soon pursue a public objective along with their traditional private ones. The belief that differences in health indices are exclusively tied to the availability and use of the expertise and technologies of modern medicine has been eroded by a growing awareness that personal habits, lack of discipline, self-abuse, and ignorance are, in the long run, of equal if not greater importance.

These changing attitudes exposed several important contradictions. Technology was obviously expanding our capacity to treat disease, but its cost clearly limited its application. A universally high quality of education and training of health personnel was nullified by an inequitable distribution of its services. The remarkable increase in the investment of public resources in the health establishment further heightened public expectations, and although greater utilization of the health system by the poor was apparent, important inequities clearly remained and little improvement in the traditional health indices resulted.

The resolution of these paradoxes has been thwarted by an extraordinarily complex system. Locally, most county and state health departments are controlled by boards that have traditionally been dominated by members of the medical profession. Nationally, a non-integrated and uncoordinated system of congressional committees and subcommittees has proved incapable of generating an appropriate response to the needs of the American people, substituting instead the introduction and promulgation of single legislative steps to control specific diseases. The executive branch of government, while often espousing the cause of integration and rationalization of the health-care system, found that it could not do so without incurring one of two penalties: the inefficiency of reshaping the programs that emerged from the segmented congressional committees or, alternately, the commitment of large financial resources from the "controllable" portion of an already enormous federal budget at a time when other important claims were being made on these same resources.

This is not to say that the efforts of the consumer movement have gone unheeded. On the contrary, statements emerging from certain of the White House conferences such as those on aging and child health, and the marked increase in the sensitivity of Congress to the consumer, as evidenced by the number of public representatives who have been asked to appear before its committees in order to present their views on health matters, have had their effects. In 1966, for example, the "Partnership for Health" Act emerged as an instrument through which local health problems were supposed to be identified and priorities assigned them, so that they might be resolved through the establishment of comprehensive health-planning agencies dominated by consumers. Although of some symbolic significance, this legislation failed because it lacked the powers of veto and sanction. On the other hand, it created a new climate in local communities, when representatives from the health professions and consumers found themselves obliged to sit down and address local problems together. This small progress at least set the scene for the passage of the Health Planning and Resources Development Act of 1974 which provided both veto and sanction power to locally established Health Systems Agencies and which gave all the states certain regulatory functions, including the right to determine whether large capital expenditures were in fact necessary (so-called "certificate-of-need" legislation).

One can reasonably deduce from this sequence of events that the objective of providing all American citizens with access to the best that medicine can provide at a reasonable cost is a feasible social and political goal and that the chasm between the self-determining elements of health-care professionals and the needs of the public will narrow until responsibility for the implementation of this common objective is finally shared. Whether or not this will happen cannot be guaranteed, but it is evident that even those with vested or private interests are beginning to see this movement as a more acceptable alternative than complete federal domination of the health-care-delivery system in the United States. Reinforcing this viewpoint is the observation that we will soon no longer enjoy the unlimited resources that hitherto have allowed us to avoid having to make decisions that are truly difficult. If our population continues to expand and our resources to be overtaxed, the first test of our democratic form of government will shortly be upon us. A successful passage through this period of transition is more likely to be achieved by a cooperative effort than it is by defaulting to a single, centralized point of control.

The American health-care system has been described many times as being in a state of crisis. Since American resources for meeting its medical needs are at present strong and healthy, the crisis, if it exists at all, lies in choosing from among the options that are now to be faced. These options might be described as follows:

1) The social aspiration voiced in the nineteen-sixties and early -seventies to the effect that access to health care should be considered a right of all American citizens must be further defined. Does this right refer primarily to accessibility? Should it be all-encompassing? Should it be provided at no additional cost to the consumer? Who will provide it?

2) Traditionally the American "ethic" has dictated that we should do things simply because we have learned how to do them, regardless of cost. To continue to operate under such a philosophy virtually guarantees the early arrival of the law of diminishing returns, if for no other reason than that the nation's, indeed the world's, resources are limited. Thus we must make a choice between redistributing our resources so that less are expended for the rare and costly components of medical care and more are expended for meeting needs we all have in common. If we continue to insist on doing both, we shall have to increase the proportion of the gross national product that is allocated to health.

3) We must also choose between pursuing higher forms of technology designed to prevent disease and rehabilitating those citizens who are already afflicted with chronic disease. While it is possible to strike a balance between these alternatives, recent events suggest that it may become increasingly difficult to do so.

4) Most of the factors that bear on our health as individuals lie outside the control of traditional medicine. We must either educate health professionals to include the social, educational, economic, and environmental factors that bear on health among their responsibilities, or separate those factors more clearly from the medical domain.

5) Finally, we must determine whether or not to centralize (federally) the control and regulation of all health services and their distribution if we are to meet society's needs, or to extend the period of grace for the growth and development of methods that are designed to rationalize and integrate the contributions of the already existing private and public components of the American health-care system.

ERNEST W. SAWARD, M.D.

Institutional Organization, Incentives, and Change

In 1969, RICHARD NIXON PROCLAIMED A "HEALTH CRISIS," and he predicted "chaos" if a reorganization of the nation's health services were not soon undertaken. Although little has changed in the intervening years, the anticipation of "chaos" in health affairs seems to have abated. Even though the anticipated extraordinary cost increases that gave rise to the original alarm have proved accurate, that "crisis" has apparently been displaced in priority by newer ones. In his first speech as president, Gerald Ford proclaimed that national health-insurance legislation was to have top priority; but six months later he implied that this priority had been lost because the nation could not afford it. At the same time, political opposition looked at the same set of economic stresses and asserted that neither could we afford to go on as we were.

Americans have a tendency to adopt an Orwellian view when they look at the near future, and they consequently reach results far more suited to more distant times. To see this, one has only to look back a decade or so: 1966 is well within the memory of most and 1956 of many. Profound changes have been made in science and technology in that period; shifts in attitude and behavior have also been significant. But if one looks at health-care services, the movement has been glacial. Only a very small percentage of Americans now receive health services by a method that differs in organization in any basic way from what it was a decade—or even two decades—ago. What may at first glance look like progress becomes on closer scrutiny simply a tendency to mistake obvious advances in technology for changes in the institutions and organization of health-care delivery.

A century ago, little of what was called medicine would today be acknowledged as scientific in content: medical practice was still based more on art than on science. Only in the last half-century has there been any substantial progress, and even now, it is important to acknowledge what we do and do not know in medicine. The impression is often obtained from medical scientists and from the press that the scientific knowledge upon which medical practice is based is vast. If we look carefully, however, it appears more as an archipelago of knowledge in a sea of ignorance. And the efficaciousness in medical practice of much that we think we know has never in fact been substantiated. Nevertheless, a belief in medicine is a cultural myth we all share. Physicians have been honored, respected, and rewarded in almost all societies throughout history.

Human society has always displayed a willingness to devote a large share of its resources to the service of beliefs that are based solely on an unshakable faith. In

193

modern society, medical services would seem to fall into this category. Epidemiologists have demonstrated over and over again that factors other than the availability of professional health care largely determine the level of health in a population. Sanitation, nutrition, housing, education, occupation, and other habitual patterns of life statistically seem the major determinants. Nevertheless, whenever the subject of public health is raised, whether by health professionals or laymen, it rapidly comes to center on health-care delivery. Regardless of the statistical efficacy, let alone the value, of the data used, it is clear that we are dealing with an unshakable belief system having its roots in shamanism, the Judeo-Christian ethic, and faith in salvation through science and technology. Just as medieval society did not ask the price of a cathedral in order to achieve salvation, so ours in its search for health has not yet questioned the price of medical care. Instead of dispelling unrealistic beliefs, the expansion of education and access to information have tended to reinforce them. Procedures such as organ transplants have little to do with health, but the aura that surrounds their practitioners reinforces the belief system.

When we admit that one's state of health is only in small part related to medical care and that it is significantly linked to behavior, finding ways of influencing personal habits becomes critically important. Methods for doing this, however, are clearly as lacking as is evidence of accomplishment. The presumption has been that if people knew what was beneficial and what was harmful they would act accordingly (hence, for example, the ubiquitous admonitions regarding our health on television and radio). But the problem is clearly one of motivation, and the motivations of our culture are quite the contrary of the message. Can anyone who smokes not know that "smoking may be harmful to your health"? Can the physician's conspicuous lack of success in managing obesity in his patients be simply a problem of communication? The results he seeks can even be in harmony with a common social value—sexual attractiveness—and the regimen still fail. Smoking, obesity, alcoholism, and drug abuse are very rarely the result simply of ignorance on the part of the user regarding the likelihood of harm. The problem is obviously more complex.

Some insight might be gained by looking at the interplay in societies between individual freedom and the demands of social conformity. Maoist China, ruled by a potent belief system, displays a high degree of conformity and apparently low rates of alcoholism, drug abuse, venereal disease, and crime, and the foreign visitor to China is often shown records of efforts to control family size filed by each woman in the office of the manager of the apartment house! In such a society, individual freedom is hardly a concern. In American society, a similar phenomenon on a lesser scale can be seen among certain religious groups, where the interdiction of smoking and drinking has the incidental effect of preventing certain diseases. Perhaps the most successful method of achieving abstinence in clinical alcoholism has been Alcoholics Anonymous, which also has a formalized belief system. Hence, it would seem that for any significant beneficial change in habits to occur that would result in an improved level of public health, one has first to institute a major change in the value system of the society. How this is to occur in American society short of an apocalypse is unclear.

For at least a decade, health care has, at least by slogan, become an inherent "right" of all, a "right" that is often couched in terms of a demand for equal access to medical services. Since World War II, Western societies have attempted to implement this right by national legislation. But the extraordinary affluence of the United States and the attitudes of the medical profession have delayed our society from following suit. In no developed society has radical change in health services come in advance of general social change: the organization and financing of health services usually lag behind other changes in the society. Each society that has acted, has acted from stress. The stress may be as dramatic as that of the epidemics raging in Russia during its Revolution, or by the bombed and bankrupt institutions of the United Kingdom at the end of World War II, or, more characteristically, by the electorate's giving support to a government that is redistributing other forms of wealth, as in Scandinavia. Seldom, if ever, do organized practicing physicians assume leadership in making such changes: vigorous rear-guard action, with threats of non-compliance, or even, in some instances, strikes, has been the pattern.

The institutional providers of health services—the most powerful of which in our country have been the private, voluntary hospitals—have traditionally had their policies determined by their professional staffs. The financial consequences that would result from desertion by the leading members of the medical staff have usually, but not always, prevented the board of trustees or the administration of the voluntary hospitals from expressing attitudes that differ significantly from those held by that conservative profession. However, the American Hospital Association, the professional organization for this group, has not been under this constraint to the same degree: doctors can abstain from using a hospital; they cannot abstain from using hospitals. But there is no question that the rationalization of hospital function is largely controlled by the medical profession. To date, the planning done by these institutions is widely acknowledged to have been inadequate; hence the repeated attempts to legislate more effective remedies, both for the appropriateness of the array of services within a hospital and of the distribution of hospitals within a given area.

During the period immediately following World War II, general practitioners predominated in the medical profession. Consequently, both the profession and the public felt that quality of care would be improved by having more certified specialists. Although there was, and always has been, some maldistribution of physicians, no one claimed any significant general shortage. A shortage of hospitals was claimed, however, resulting in the passage of the Hill-Burton Act which was intended to provide hospital facilities throughout rural America. Hundreds of small hospitals (less than fifty beds) were built as a result of this legislation.

While medical care was comparatively inexpensive by current standards, it was still often burdensome and was a common cause of personal indebtedness. Less than 10 per cent of the population was covered by health insurance in 1940. During the Truman administration, a national health-insurance plan proposed in the Wagner-Murray-Dingell bill was bitterly debated in Congress. By 1948 it had been defeated, and the great and largely unregulated growth of voluntary health insurance was begun. In spite of its expansion, however, by 1974, according to the Social Security Administration, 42 million Americans still had no hospital insurance, 123 million still had no insurance for visits to the doctor's office, 168 million had no dental insurance, 127 million had no insurance for nursing-home care, and 67 million had no insurance against the cost of prescribed drugs.

None of these developments—more specialists, more hospitals, and free-enterprise, voluntary health insurance—was an accident; they all represent deliberate choices. If we appear now to be suffering from the consequences, we cannot blame it on chance. These choices were made either by passing or by failing to enact legislation. Failing to legislate—and hence to regulate—is a decision to delegate the

resolution of problems to competitive market forces. The largely unregulated voluntary health-insurance industry, basing its coverage on the group's cost to the
underwriter ("experience rating") rather than the health level of the community
("community rating"), effectively excluded many. Groups of employees in major
industries managed, often through collective bargaining, to obtain reasonable coverage, but special-interest groups in the health and insurance industries also exerted
their influence, and they continue to do so. Our elected representatives either decide
or default: demands for "innovative" primary care, certificate-of-need laws to control
the expansion of hospitals, and national health insurance reflect the failure of our past
choices. Only our unprecedented affluence in recent decades has protected us from an
earlier and more conspicuous disaster.

But change was coming. Voluntary health insurance had, by 1960, reached a
plateau. Most of the working population had, through their employment, gained
access to some form of health insurance: it was usually insurance for hospitalization
and professional procedures occurring in hospitals, however, and did not cover
ambulatory care, a practice that forced the inappropriate and expensive use of hospital
beds. The system also excluded many of the aged and the poor, and the self-employed
often remained uninsured. The turning point came in 1965 with the modifications of
the Social Security Act known as Medicare and Medicaid.

The intense and bitter debate over that program lasted five years, and resulted in a
compromise solution involving three different social policies. Part A of Title XVIII,
for hospital coverage, gave entitlement in principle to everyone over age 65 who had
contributed Social Security taxes during his working years; Part B, for professional
services, was voluntary, contributory, and involved coinsurance. Title XIX (Medicaid) was a combined state and federal program and involved a means test; its benefits
and eligibility varied from state to state, and it was to be funded from general
revenue.

A decade later the policy issues leading to that compromise are still unresolved,
still bitterly fought, and have served both to sharpen the debate over national health
insurance and to delay the transition to it. As the consequences of the free-enterprise
provision of services in mandated insurance reveal themselves ever more clearly in
forms of excessive costs, inequities of access, and constantly increasing regulation, the
appropriateness of the system itself becomes ever more questionable.

The following are some of the questions that must be answered before national
health-insurance legislation can be decided: (1) Should all residents of the United
States be covered, or only certain prescribed categories? (2) Should the coverage be
voluntary or compulsory? (3) Should the scope of benefits include all health services,
or should certain services be emphasized and others limited or omitted? (4) Should
payment be made through private insurance carriers or by a governmental agency?
Should their administration be private or public? (5) Should different categories of the
population pay in different ways? (6) Should payment involve a high or low degree of
income transference apart from the income tax? (7) Should the insurance principle of
"experience rating" (i.e., higher rates for higher risks) be used on all categories of the
population? (8) Should the funds be unified and centrally administered or left
fragmented? None of these questions seems ostensibly to bear on the delivery of
health services, but in fact each and every one does, and the answers offer a myriad of
options for the American people.

The Congress of the United States has not yet formally considered the question of establishing a national health service. It has so far only legislated the provision of direct services for certain categories of the population through the Indian Service, the Veterans Administration, the Public Health Service, and the Armed Forces. Federal funds, however, have been contributed to local jurisdictions for creating large-scale, direct health-service systems for the poor. For example, in New York City one-third of the population receives services funded from public monies; and in the Commonwealth of Puerto Rico 60 per cent of personal health services are directly provided to the public by the Health Ministry.

One possible course (but in my opinion an unlikely one for the United States) is to institute a national health service similar to those in the United Kingdom, Scandinavia, or the countries of Eastern Europe. Under such plans, the state owns and operates the institutionalized forms of health care—the hospitals and the various ambulatory-health-care centers—with some practitioners remaining in solo practice but paid by salary. This type of service could be organized along geographical lines, using both regional and local area councils as a form of control, and a central authority for regulation and general policy.

This may well be the system in this country sometime in the twenty-first century, but at present it does not seem compatible with either our social mythology or our economic system: it is a rationalization out of context with the way we handle our other affairs. It would take a very severe crisis to force the institution of such a system—a depression, for example, as deep and prolonged as that of the thirties, or involvement in a devastating or protracted war. The development of a national health service of this type, in short, is dependent upon the evolution of all aspects of our society moving in that general direction.

The issues of personal health services are usually discussed separately: commissions devote themselves to the numerology of "manpower" without regard to how services will be paid for; other agencies focus on "primary care" without regard to the organization of health services generally; the community hospital is offered as the center of ambulatory care despite the vested interest of the staff members in their own private facilities. Many proposals appear on closer scrutiny to involve only the poor in society who have little choice, implying the continuance of a two-class health system in America.

If the entitlement and the mechanism of payment for the poor under a national health insurance are different from that for the rest of the population, this surely will perpetuate a two-class system, which would ultimately be as untenable as a de jure two-class school system. The usual argument against comprehensive benefits for poor and rich alike is that "we can't afford it." But it must also be clearly acknowledged that we cannot afford to stay as we are. The devotion of over 8 per cent of our gross national product to health ought to have bought us a higher rung on the health-status ladder compared with other developed nations—and particularly more equity of access for the general population—than it is buying today. Comprehensive eligibility might be the mechanism for improving this record.

In personal health services today, competition and free enterprise still dominate. Consequently, it is economically essential for private medical facilities such as the voluntary hospital to maintain full occupancy in order to stay in business; to do so, they compete by having a full panoply of services whether it is appropriate to have them or not. For example, they may provide facilities for open-heart surgery, though they may perform so few procedures that proficiency cannot be maintained. Obstetrical units performing few deliveries have a higher morbidity and higher costs than those operating near capacity, but the procedures must be reimbursed regardless of outcome or costs. The continual and unsuccessful struggle to close unneeded obstetrical and pediatric units in competing urban facilities clearly illustrates the strength of the private competitive structure. Among individual physicians, unrestricted entrepreneurship with the sacrosanct fee-for-service payment continues to be regarded as a right not to be compromised.

In addition to direct public services and private free enterprise, there are still some other variants which, although in the minority, provide examples for almost every possible innovation in the organization of personal-health services. Some of these may well be the models on which future systems can build.

The last few years have taken this country through two devaluations of the currency, double-digit inflation, and an energy crisis; nevertheless we are still an affluent country, though no doubt less so than a decade ago, when to do everything at once seemed economically feasible. Now the nation is beginning to rank its priorities and allocate its resources more carefully. A few years ago, some, by projecting rates of increase in health expenditures, predicted a rise from the prevailing 8 per cent to 10, 12, or an even greater percentage of the gross national product. While it is now quite clear that health expenditures will indeed soon consume a somewhat larger percentage of the gross national product than at present, these extravagant figures seem unlikely. Americans will probably not reverse their dedication of substantial resources to health services, because the value placed on these services is too high, but expenditures will be limited by competition from other priorities in a no longer rapidly expanding economy.

In 1953, 23 per cent of health expenditures were from tax funds. By 1975, this had increased to 41 per cent. Every session of Congress amends the law to make the percentage even greater. Whatever the variety of national health insurance that is finally passed, some significant portion of its funding must come from additional tax money, for the poor of our society must be paid for. It is estimated that a decade from now, at a minimum, at least one-half of all funds for health services will be tax funds. Even today, more than half the support for hospitals in the United States comes from tax sources—federal, state, and local.

Another seemingly irreversible trend is the progressive control and regulation of private health insurance. In many jurisdictions, for example, Blue Cross and Blue Shield are mandated to have public hearings before making rate increases. (Blue Cross has a somewhat ambiguous public image. After considerable controversy as to whether it was serving hospitals or its subscribers, it dissolved its official ties to the American Hospital Association in 1972 and took that symbol from its insignia.) Medical-insurance-rate hearings are analogous to those for setting public utility rates: the public interest is presumed to be the paramount circumstance in their determinations. It is often regulation and control through an adversary process. If part of national health insurance is placed in private hands, there will of necessity be federal guidelines for this process—whether it is carried out by the federal government or by the states. The role of a regulated private insurer will become increasingly similar to the role of "fiscal intermediary" under the Medicare plan. What is politically perceived to be the "public interest" will be the determining factor.

The regulation of the institutional provider—particularly of the expensive short-term general hospital, but of the chronic-care institutions as well—is another, and to some extent a related, phenomenon. We have seen in the past decade, principally through the "Conditions of Participation" and "Methods of Reimbursement" of the Medicare-Medicaid programs, a series of constraints and regulations put upon the institutional provider that affects every aspect of hospital operation. Inasmuch as the support of such institutions is largely from taxes and funds of the regulated third-party payers, these institutions will continue to undergo control and regulation, reflecting a more general trend to make all our institutions publicly accountable.

Increasing regulation of the individual practitioner is also present, but it has been more subtle. A physician's hospital work has been subject to a—usually ineffective—utilization review for decades. His work outside the hospital has in part been regulated by "usual, customary, and prevailing" fee, but with no "quality" standard applied to it other than that of fraud. The rise in malpractice litigation is one aspect of the trend toward greater accountability. The enactment of the modifications of the Social Security law in 1972 to include mandated Professional Standards Review Organizations (PSRO) throughout the land provides another method of control. Whatever one's opinion regarding the methodology required by this act, the demands for control over competence and appropriateness of treatment can only increase.

The system required by PSRO legislation involves the organization of physicians in local areas to conduct "peer reviews" of the specific ways services were provided. Although at present only hospital review is mandated, it is clear that the intent is eventually to review all medical care. The act only applies to Medicare-Medicaid and maternal and child health programs, but it has already been voluntarily extended to Blue Cross-Blue Shield plans in certain jurisdictions. In other legislation (PL 93-222), the Congress has gone beyond the requirement of PSRO in seeking to measure the level of medical care. As a result, the profession is involved in a long search to find methods by which to determine accountability.

Still another form of control can be found in attempts in the past decade to regulate the specialties of the health professionals produced, in order to have them more accurately reflect public needs. The support of medical education by government is being proposed and would provide federal control over curriculum and choice of field. Either directly or indirectly, the government will try to influence the number of primary-care physicians and of those choosing each of the various specialty categories. The program will also affect the number of physician substitutes, nurse practitioners, and physician assistants that are trained to meet health-care needs.

One of the major complaints registered against present medical services is the lack of reasonably prompt personal attention for routine medical needs. The reasons behind the problem are many, in addition to geographic maldistribution and over-specialization in the profession. Yearning for the good old days of the general practitioner as a solution ignores the technological imperative that produced special-ization in the first place. The attitude is probably in some respects a part of the nostalgic mood that has caused a boom in the sales of such things as Franklin stoves and "natural" foods. A new family-practice specialty is emerging, nevertheless, and primary-care programs are developing across the nation; pediatrics and internal medicine are also developing aspects of primary care. These are useful and substantial modifications in the system that are long overdue and will help redress the imbalances in those being trained for medical practice.

However, access to appropriate medical service involves the organization of all its aspects, not simply the training of physicians. How medical care is financed, how the providers are paid, how organized responsibility for communities is assumed, and how it is administered in budgetary terms all shape the system. Factors seemingly as diverse as record keeping, transportation services, night and day care of equal quality, and consumer organizations are but a few of the governing aspects of a comprehensive system. The time-worn statement of physicians that "there can't be any real need in this community, for I will see anyone who comes to me whether they pay or not" epitomizes the blindness to responsibility for communities, as opposed to responsibility for individual patients. This attitude has contributed to increasing the numbers of underimmunized children and uncorrected handicaps that are revealed by surveys of school populations. Training for family practice will not correct this, unless the organization of health services generally is also appropriately changed.

In the past decade, emphasis has been placed on the training of physician substitutes as another way of filling the gaps in primary care. Physician's assistants and nurse-practitioners have demonstrated their usefulness and, in this sense, the programs are a success. Physician substitutes are particularly useful for serving the poor because of the dearth of physicians willing to do so. The result, however, is often as much additional services as physician substitution: for this reason, it can in fact end up by adding to the price of an already costly system. The established fee-for-service payment system also produces a dilemma over how the substitute's services should be remunerated. Physician substitutes are more apt to be used in the interests of economy, in salaried positions in a community practice responsible for a defined population and having a predetermined budget.

All these trends—in funding, regulation, and control—are growing ones; an attempt at coordinating them through more rigorous, comprehensive health-care planning has given rise to the concept of, and legislation for, "Health Systems Agencies" (PL 93-641). It is quite conceivable that this movement toward regionalization will strongly influence, through coordination of resources, the nature of the delivery of health services in the last years of this century. For many states—those small either in geographic size or in population—the unit may very well be the state itself. But for at least half the states, organization and control of health services must be subdivided so that familiarity with local problems can be combined with local responsibility.

Initially, regionalization concentrated on restricting capital expenditures, usually by avoiding duplication. In time, this regional authority will plan the use of all third-party operating funds devoted to the health-care system in order to assure equity of access and quality of services. How it will do this in the over two hundred jurisdictions will vary, but all of them will be subject to the same federal guidelines. The reason why strict allocation of funds must be maintained is clear, for the resource allocation to health will not be sufficient to make possible all the services that technology can provide. Only in rare instances will the regional health authority directly assume the responsibility for providing service. Ownership of capital facilities will remain predominantly in private hands. The regional authority will interest itself in evaluating the efficiency and effectiveness of the providers and either encourage or discourage their expansion on the basis of performance. It is hoped that an evaluative process will have been developed in time to use it in lieu of the tedious orthodoxies that now lie behind planning and decision-making.

When resources are limited and an ever-expanding, costly technology makes them insufficient, priorities must be set to determine what will and what will not be done, and for whom. Some of the reordering will be done simply on the basis of what is thought to be most urgent, but other issues will also be involved. For example, America allocates far less money to the age group 0-10 years than to the age group 65-75 years. As we become less affluent in a competitive world, will this decision be changed? Congress has legislated an "End-Stage Renal Disease" program alleged soon to cost one billion dollars a year. Will this continue to have priority? Will a serious study be made to demonstrate what medical procedures are genuinely efficacious? Will these then be used to the exclusion of the rest? These are dilemmas all organized health-care systems will have to face.

These considerations also suggest that we should reexamine the concept of the health-maintenance organization (HMO), i.e., an organized system in a geographical area responsible for medical care for all its members. The HMO provides a comprehensive set of basic benefits. It has a voluntary, multiple-choice enrollment for its members that provides a constant market test of consumer satisfaction, and it is financed by fixed, periodic payments. Two major types of organizations fall under this definition: prepaid group practice, where physicians function as a group and share income in a common facility, and the foundation for medical care, where physicians practice in individual or small-group offices, are paid as individuals on a fee-for-service basis, but also serve voluntarily enrolled populations for comprehensive services. The payment is fixed, regardless of the frequency with which the services are used. Either form of HMO must anticipate financial risks and be based on sound actuarial principles to fulfill the definition. The ease of access and the efficiency of decision-making inherent in the "one-stop shopping" concept of the prepaid group practice and neighborhood health center adds to its appeal. The name "health-maintenance organization" is an obvious political euphemism and undoubtedly will be changed, but the concept and the principles will remain relevant.

Interest in these organizations first arose in the legislative and executive branches of the federal government in response to the extraordinary cost increases of the Medicare and Medicaid programs. It has long been known that prepaid group-practice organizations have a cost saving ranging from 20 to 30 per cent and that most of this saving is clearly attributable to reduced hospitalization. Obviously a cheaper system is an option appealing to government if—as had been demonstrated—the quality of care is at least to equal that in private practice.

However, the appeal to the administration and to Congress goes beyond this obvious benefit. The HMO is also a competing, voluntary system in harmony with an economy based on choice and a free market, i.e., with the avowed free-enterprise policy of our nation. In addition, though less obviously, the idea of contracting for medical care for a voluntarily enrolled population had a similar appeal. Contracting with an organization provides a control almost totally lacking when dealing with a myriad of individual practitioners paid on a fee-for-service basis and having only fragmented responsibility for patients and none for populations. Government is on familiar ground when it can contemplate contracting with large organizations that will deliver a product of desired specification for a fixed price. The state of California has already initiated some prepaid health plans, although at first without adequate controls, in an effort to reduce the expenditures of the Medi-Cal program. Attempts are now under way in other states, notably New York and Maryland. A similar organization has recently planned responsibility for the care of all Medicaid and poor persons in Newark, New Jersey. Unfortunately, many of these efforts have not followed the widely recognized "genetic code" for prepaid group practice: such a program must be conducted in the interests of its membership; the membership must have comprehensive coverage and be voluntarily enrolled in the presence of a meaningful, alternative choice; the medical group serving the membership must be an organized, self-governing structure of predominately full-time members, pooling all income, and with an equitable prearranged method for its distribution. In some new programs, many other essentials have been ignored as well.

Nevertheless, the HMO is one of the viable choices for Americans, and it is a system unique to America. The alternatives—progressive control and regulation or direct provision of services to populations with no choice—have already produced the dismal vision of the impoverished city or county hospital. The principles of operation ascribed to the HMO are responsive to possible budgetary constraints, they are flexible in allowing competition, and they are a constructive alternative to the direct governmental provision of health services. Americans demand pluralism in health services, a demand that will probably be met at least for the balance of this century. The HMO is now a legally mandated voluntary choice.

Although the prepaid group practice and the foundations for medical care are perceived by the public to be quite different choices, each has in common the assumption of risk for enrolled memberships at a prospectively budgeted rate and a set of internal controls that make it adaptable to the period of constrained resources for health. It is probable that over the years the trend in medical practice will be toward one or the other of these two different cost-controlling mechanisms.

In summary, if we look ahead a decade, we see a period of transition in the organization of health services that will reflect the attitudes, culture, and customs of a society interacting with a prestigious and conservative profession. In the past, our society has prided itself on free enterprise, the independence of the individual, and competitive institutions; medical care has well reflected this. The system will continue to reflect it in the decades ahead, but it will adjust itself to the restraints that competition for funds will place on health care. Although it is rarely mentioned, the classic fee-for-service payment has shaped the present form of the medical profession and its institutions. And just as this method of payment has shaped the present system, so will the method chosen for any national health insurance affect the delivery system in the future. Publicly mandated, limited resource allocation will force a discussion of priorities and policy. Despite Orwellian projections, it seems unlikely that the choices the public makes will in any way violate cultural values that have been characteristic of our society thus far. There may or may not be many funding sources—this is not a central issue with the public, although for obvious reasons it is of paramount importance to the private insurance industry and to some members of the profession—but our value system seems to dictate that both pluralism and competition will remain in health-service delivery during the balance of this century.

SUGGESTED READING

René Dubos, *Mirage of Health* (Garden City, 1959).

Marc Lalonde, *A New Perspective on the Health of Canadians (A Working Document)*, (April, 1974).

Primary Care: Where Medicine Fails, ed. Spyros Andreapoulos (New York, 1974).

The Kaiser-Permanente Medical Care Program (A Symposium), ed., Anne R. Somers (The Commonwealth Fund, New York, 1971).

Robert Maxwell, *Health Care, The Growing Dilemma* (New York, 1974).

Committee for Economic Development, *Building a National Health-Care System* (New York, 1973).

ELI GINZBERG

Health Services, Power Centers, and Decision-Making Mechanisms

As a social scientist with over three decades of interest and involvement in health policy and programming, I will describe briefly what I find to be the critical questions regarding our health goals, power centers, and decision-making mechanisms as they exist today. Next, I shall look backward to the period following World War I, which some of my colleagues in this undertaking have defined as the golden age of modern medicine. It was then that physicians first gained access to a wide array of powerful drugs and therapeutic devices which permitted them to reverse or control major diseases. The primary objective of this backward look will be to extract from our half-century's experience with modern medicine some generalizations about the manner in which the health-care system has adapted to the new opportunities that emerged.

Once these generalizations are at hand, they should prove helpful in outlining the manner in which the present health-care system is likely to respond in the next quarter of this century to the pulls and counter-pulls which will be exerted upon it. These will come from the desire of the public to benefit fully from advances in modern medicine, the efforts of the interest groups to protect and enhance their power, and the capabilities and limitations of the critical decision-making mechanisms available in this country to reshape the component parts of the health-care system so that the American people can enjoy more of the benefits they seek at a cost they are able and willing to bear.

During the half-century following World War I, many changes were made in the structure and functioning of the American medical system in an effort to respond to new discoveries and challenges. A close study of these patterns of adaptation should provide some navigational aids for the decades ahead.

The ability of a society to respond to new opportunities depends upon its capacity to develop the necessary manpower and related resources, to have or create appropriate entrepreneurial organs which can marshal these resources effectively, and to have or put into place distribution mechanisms that can make them available to the public. We need only recall the structure of American medicine at the end of World War I to appreciate the flexibility demonstrated by the system in the intervening years. In the nineteen-twenties, scientifically based medical education was still attempting to establish its hegemony, and specialization was in its infancy. Hospitals provided room and board and nursing services, but only a small amount of effective therapeutic intervention. And philanthropy, with minor assistance from government, was able to cover the financial costs of the medical and hospital care for those who could not pay for their own. On the eve of World War II the average per diem cost in general hospitals in New York City was $6.70.

During the intervening decades, three innovations—the strikingly improved education and training of increasingly more specialized physicians, the greatly increased capability of the hospital to provide effective therapy, and the establishment and rapid growth of new systems of financing health care, initially through commercial and nonprofit insurance and later through the increased participation of government—radically transformed the system. In addition, the federal government, through rapidly expanding grants for biomedical research and later for medical education, took the lead in providing the financial resources which enabled the health-science centers at universities to blossom and expand. The magnitude of the change brought about by these mutually reinforcing developments is reflected in the proportion of the gross national product devoted to health services by the American people: in 1929, it was about 4 per cent; in 1975, it was up to 8.3 per cent.

This substantial transformation of modern medicine brought changes in interest groups and in their relative power. In the earlier period, the medical schools, organized medicine (represented by the American Medical Association, with which the medical schools were closely aligned), philanthropy (represented by private universities, hospital trustees, and a few foundations), and local and state governments (which had limited service responsibilities, primarily in the areas of public health and care of the chronically ill) dominated the system. Most major decisions came from the AMA and its state and local affiliates. Today, the power structure is very different. First of all, over the past decades, the American people have come to believe that medicine can contribute significantly to the betterment of their lives, and they have become determined to avail themselves of these benefits. Consequently, the electorate has become a major force in changing the medical establishment. The average citizen sees no way in which he, acting as an individual in the private market, can obtain better service. Accordingly, he presses for greater government involvement.

At the other end of the spectrum the physicians, no longer able to determine the structure and operations of health-care delivery (although no significant changes can be made without their acquiescence), have become more circumspect in their views. The influence of the medical establishment over its own membership and over the public is greatly reduced.

Much of the power that was formerly concentrated in the hands of the leaders of organized medicine is now divided up among the biomedical research and educational establishment, whose influence is derived from its large governmental subsidies and the critical contributions their results are making to modern medicine; the bureaucrats in strategic policy-formulating positions in government who can influence the system through appropriations and other actions; and, finally, academic, foundation, and other health specialists who help to determine the issues and public attitudes toward them on the nation's health agenda. In addition, the large sums which flow through commercial and nonprofit insurance channels, primarily into the nation's 7,000 hospitals, indicate the considerable leverage exercised by both the dispensers and recipients of these funds.

Since there are almost a million nurses currently employed, various nurses' groups are increasingly able to obtain hearings from legislators, hospital administrators, and the public. Furthermore, as trade unions organize paramedical employees, they are able to advance the demands of those heretofore largely voiceless groups.

This schematic classification of the multiple power centers in American medicine in 1976 points to the need for caution and restraint on the part of any analyst who attempts to forecast future transformations and their likely consequences. Only one conclusion can safely be ventured: the polemicist who believes he knows what will happen is likely to be wrong. There are simply too many interacting variables to permit even the most skillful analyst to anticipate all future developments. We can, however, consider the principal health-service goals on the nation's agenda and estimate the probabilities of accomplishing them in the decades ahead in light of the existing power centers and decision-making mechanisms. We know, of course, that neither these power centers nor these mechanisms are set in concrete. Since we also know that the desire of the public to enjoy more of the real (and some of the putative) benefits of modern medicine will not in itself assure large-scale reforms, we will address the question of how these expanded goals will be pursued in the face of competing power centers and weak or absent decision-making mechanisms.

No two students would agree in all respects about the principal health objectives to which the nation's efforts should be directed in the near and distant future. But the disagreements are more likely to involve emphasis, timing, and the methods of implementation than the objectives themselves. I feel confident that the following elements would be endorsed by most experts in the field.

First, the formulation that health care is a "right" is unacceptable in itself because the mere formulation leaves unspecified how this right is to be achieved and because such a right would conflict with other rights of other persons, e.g., enjoying more police protection or receiving higher welfare payments. However, there probably is a consensus that all individuals should have access to the health-care system and, irrespective of their financial circumstances, that they should be entitled to adequate care. The public is willing to tolerate large differentials in income and limited access to higher education—for example, persons who are qualified, but unable to pay, for a university education—but it is not willing to permit financial barriers to keep needed medical care from the poor and the near-poor.

Criticism in the media, malpractice suits, and recent legislation all point to the increased concern of the American people with the quality of health care. At a minimum, they expect the government to protect them from the unnecessary risks attendant on incompetence, inefficiency, or venality. There is no hard evidence of the extent to which people are suffering from deficiencies in the system, but there is ample evidence that many services are ineffective, some are harmful, and a few are lethal. The pressure is mounting on government to raise the standards of health care.

The outstanding successes of modern medicine, from therapeutic surgery through the stabilization of chronic illness to successful rehabilitation, have led the public to demand that all death-postponing, life-improving interventions be available to all citizens who can profit from them. Since the media are quick to report on new forms of medical interventions, frequently with premature conclusions about their effectiveness, the public has an exaggerated view of the rate of progress in scientific research and its potential benefits. There is a built-in mechanism in modern America that provides a ready receptiveness for anything new.

A major concomitant of the new prominence of health services on the nation's agenda is the growing belief that the system should be more responsive to the needs and desires of the public. This new emphasis on consumerism takes many forms, including the assumption that the voter should play an important role in health planning, that health providers, both hospitals and professionals, should be more alert to the needs and desires of those whom they treat, and that the quality of health services not only involve professional judgment but also require consumer approval.

Citizens, insurance carriers, and government are deeply concerned about the steep and continuing rise in health costs. With per diem costs to each patient in excess of $200 in major hospital centers, with the bill for a heart attack at about $5,000, and with total health expenditures amounting annually to $2,500 for a family of four, the concern over rising costs is natural. But so far efforts to contain them have been ineffective.

The American people appear generally to be seeking the following improvements in health-care delivery: improved access for the underserved, improved quality, additional services, more responsiveness to the consumer, and lower costs. To achieve these, public policy must take into account the power of critical interest groups and the possibilities for altering existing decision-making mechanisms and devising new ones. The conventional wisdom looks to national health insurance (NHI), supplemented by physician assignment and assisted by a shift in the training of residents from specialities to family practice, to provide broader access for those currently underserved. With regard to improved quality, the preferred solutions lie in making the legislated Professional Standards Review Organizations operational and in mandating that physicians and other health professionals participate in continuing education to refurbish their skills. In addition, there is some support for periodic relicensing. Some analysts believe that important gains can be made by shifting the licensing responsibility to institutions, primarily the hospital.

Relatively little attention has been directed to the ways of assuring that the American people can benefit from additional health services and medical care, but, if we project from the recent past, we can expect that government will foot most, if not all, of the bill (witness the recent inclusion of renal dialysis for kidney disease under Medicare). Some analysts believe that a shift to preventive and ambulatory care, which is expected to follow NHI, will free for new services a large part of the funds currently spent on the care of hospitalized patients.

The growing responsiveness of the health-care system to the public's needs and desires is to be obtained, it is suggested, by putting more consumers on decision-making bodies—the boards of hospitals, Blue Cross and Blue Shield, and the local, area, state, and federal planning and regulatory agencies. In addition, the studied attempts of health professionals to keep the inner workings of the system from public scrutiny are to be vitiated by public hearings and reports.

On the urgent necessity to control costs, the conventional wisdom holds that if NHI shifts the locus of care from the hospital to clinics and doctor's offices this will result in significant savings, that more stringent fee control is a likely concomitant of NHI, and that third parties, under the lead of the federal government, will move to eliminate excess beds and duplicated services, and will insist that prescriptions be written in generic rather than brand names. Most important, many believe that the government will simply limit the annual amounts that it will make available for the purchase of health services.

In sum, the principal elements of the reform program currently taking shape are predicated on: national health insurance, Professional Standards Review Organizations, expanded governmental financing for new services, placing more laymen into decision-making roles, and limiting annual governmental expenditures for health. Each of these proffered solutions, together with their supporting measures, warrants a closer inspection.

It is probable that Congress will pass some form of national health insurance in the near future because, among other reasons, the legislation contemplated will not threaten the interests of either the commercial and nonprofit insurance companies or the principal provider groups—physicians, hospitals, and other health professionals. For the same reasons, it is equally likely that the reach of the NHI that is passed will be modest. It will probably encompass catastrophic illness and little more, since more ambitious legislation is likely to be so expensive that the legislators would find it difficult to pay for out of Social Security taxes or general revenues.

New entitlements to care would presumably make it easier for the poor to gain access to the system, but only if additional services become available as a result of the new coverage. There is little reason to expect physicians and other health professionals, most of whom are earning a good living, to relocate in the small towns, the rural areas, or the urban ghettos where most of the underserved populations live. This explains the interest of Congress in inducing or compelling those medical students whose education is heavily subsidized by government to spend their early years practicing in these areas.

If compulsion is used, it may not withstand a legal challenge. If service is to be secured by inducements, the cost may be too high (the bonus for a physician serving in the military can exceed $13,000 annually). Most important, the direction of physicians into the ghetto may make little sense if they are to provide routine ambulatory care. Nurse practitioners and health aides drawn from the community are likely to do a better job, especially if they are effectively linked to hospitals.

The challenge of improving quality is more complex. First, the medical profession has given only grudging approval to professional standards review. And many who have followed its legislative and administrative implementation believe that the effort will contribute little to quality, although possibly it could contribute more to controlling costs. The record to date of deliberate avoidance by the profession of controlling its aberrant members warns us not to expect much from the new approach. And although it is relatively easy to legislate new regulations governing licensing and continuing education, it is more difficult for such changes to have a significant impact on quality. In sum, there are no external control mechanisms that can force professionals to behave responsibly other than their own individual and collective self-discipline and conscience.

The heart of the quality issue, as Walsh McDermott points out elsewhere in this issue, lies in widespread misconceptions about objectives, methods, and costs. Such basic issues as what is worthwhile measuring to assess quality, the state of the methodology, and the societal gains from alternative efforts at assuring quality have not been adequately probed, much less clarified. This being so, one cannot overcome the conviction that Congress would have been well advised not to have legislated on the subject to begin with.

The desire of the American people to benefit from the continued advances in therapeutic and rehabilitative medicine is as easy to appreciate as it is difficult to assure. Over time, most medical advances are incorporated into customary modes of practice and do become available to the citizenry. But at any given moment only a minority enjoys the costly breakthroughs. Under national health insurance, there will be great pressure on the system to treat all persons equitably, especially when it comes to life-extending procedures. But because of its cost, it is highly improbable that everything that is possible and desirable will be made available to all who require it. The arbitrary inclusion or exclusion of major new interventions, or their restriction to specified categories of patients, is far more likely. In either event the wealthy can probably obtain what they desire outside the national health insurance system, thereby assuring the continuance of more than one level of care.

So long as American medicine remains as loosely structured as it now is, with diverse power centers and multiple decision-making mechanisms, it will be difficult to make it more responsive to the consumer. Leverage on the system rests with those who control the critical resources—men, money, management. Consumers can, of course, play more of a role then they have in the past when they did not even have the opportunity to be heard. But it is difficult to see how they will be able to affect, except very selectively, the behavior of physicians, the managers of large insurance companies and hospitals, and government bureaucrats. There is little comfort in the record of consumer participation in less specialized sectors of the society such as education, urban planning, and environmental control.

There is little evidence that NHI and the changes it will bring will result in the kinds of improvements in the use of health resources that will lead to cost constraints. On the contrary, increasing entitlements will make necessary the enlarging of facilities that will require additional funds. There may be some economies in shifting the locus of treatment from hospital to ambulatory services, but only if the resulting superfluous facilities are closed. But no one acquainted with the "political" problems associated with the closing of installations and the dismissal of employees will expect many early gains from this form of rationalization.

In any case, the very notion of cost restraints may be beside the point. Conceivably the American people will be willing to increase the resources they invest in health care until they reach 10 or even 12 per cent of the gross national product. If that is so, cost will not be a pressing issue, at least for the time being.

But if it is more likely, as it appears to be, that we are approaching a socially acceptable limit for health expenditures, then the resolution must be an arbitrary ceiling on annual governmental contributions. In that event we will have a variant of the present allocation system.

The number of health services currently being performed is determined by the combined expenditures of the individual consumer, insurance, and government, with government accounting for 40 per cent of the total. Under NHI, the governmental share might reach 70 per cent or even more. But the range and quality of services will be determined by the resources available for their production. And if resources are limited by government, as they ultimately will be, services will be correspondingly curtailed. Services will always be short of demand whether produced under private or government auspices, or both.

In sum, problems of access may be moderated—but will surely not be solved—by NHI, even if the plan is supplemented by the reallocation of physicians to underserved areas. Nor will problems of quality be solved by new legislation. Solutions to both rest with the slow internal reform of the medical profession itself.

Most of the public is not even dimly aware that its immediate and full access to the many new life-extending and life-improving techniques will eventually run into budgetary constraints that will restrict the types of procedures and the numbers of those eligible for them. Consumers will unquestionably be more broadly represented on a great number of planning, operating, and controlling bodies, but they will have only marginal influence on restructuring the system in the face of the vigilant self-interest of the principal producer groups.

So far, the analysis has proceeded largely within the conventional parameters of the extant health-care system and the likely modifications that loom ahead. Another way to look at it is to regard the health-care system as a major service industry and then to consider what we know about the characteristics of service industries, particularly about their manpower. Many, though not all, of them are highly labor intensive. The health industry certainly is: labor costs account for about 60 per cent of hospital expenditures, and labor costs dominate the other principal sectors as well, with the exceptions of drugs and appliances. But the role of labor in health transcends the question of its share of total costs. In addition, its approximately 4.5 million employees make health the largest industry in the country in terms of workers and the third largest, next to construction and agriculture, in terms of income produced. When a labor-intensive industry accounts for 1 out of every 20 members of the labor force, its capacity for continued growth will be affected by its ability to attract and retain large numbers from competing sectors of the economy. During the post-World War II period, the health industry demonstrated this ability by more than doubling its numbers; it was helped in this by employing even larger numbers of women who needed work or were pressed into service during the war (the majority of health workers are women), and it was further assisted by new sources of funding to absorb substantial wage increases.

With regard to continuing large-scale growth of the health-services industry in the future, we have to postulate that it can be achieved, if at all, only at the price of substantially improving wage structures, and this will mean substantially increasing total costs. The likelihood of rapid increases in labor costs under conditions of continuing expansion is reinforced by the fact that the principal institutions within the industry—hospitals and nursing homes—have only recently been brought under the Fair Labor Standards Act, which has a tendency to push wage costs higher in two ways: by bringing the work force within the Social Security system and by making it easier for workers to organize themselves into trade unions. The consequences have already been suggested by the experience of a few cities where unions have succeeded in organizing hospital workers and raising the pay levels of unskilled staff by almost 200 per cent in a decade, albeit from a substandard wage level.

With or without unions, the work scene in the United States is being transformed in a manner that assures those currently employed considerable discretion over the scope and pace of their work. This trend helps to account for part, though not all, of the striking increases in the number of hospital employees per daily patient census, which increased from 1.78 in 1950 to 3.15 in 1973, or by about 80 per cent—at a time when patients were insisting that the attention they received from hospital workers was declining.

The increase in numbers and the splintering of responsibilities have had untoward consequences. The rapid expansion of health personnel during the past several decades has created many new professional and paraprofessional groups, and each one has attempted to broaden its responsibilities through certification, licensing, and similar devices at the expense of groups higher in the hierarchy, while protecting its domain from those seeking to enter or advance from below. This can be seen in the various factions among nursing personnel, which include nurse's aides who are trained on the job, practical nurses with a year's didactic instruction, registered nurses who may be graduates of a two- or three-year program, and baccalaureate nurses and nurses with graduate degrees. Although these distinctions with respect to general and specialized educational background are clear, they tell little about the experience, competence, or interest of the members of these several groups; they also tell little about their relative ability to perform a wide range of tasks independently or under supervision. We can deduce from such an overlapping structure—and this has been empirically validated by case studies—that labor costs in a hospital structure in which each group of employees operates as a quasi-independent guild are inflated.

The outsider, especially a management consultant, when he learns about this pattern, has a simple solution: increase the power of the hospital director to manage the entire work force. But in fact no administrator can effectively supervise large numbers of professionals and paraprofessionals. In the military, the formula has been one corporal for every two soldiers, if the detail is to be productive. The low productivity that is characteristic of white-collar employment in large offices, industrial research settings, college faculties, and the civil service reflects the same dilemma: it is difficult to ensure that service workers are seriously engaged in their work. Many prefer talking to working.

Another naive assumption held by economists who have little knowledge of the health industry is that the increased use of paraprofessionals will result in gains in productivity. The American health industry certainly has made major accommodations since the beginning of this century, when the ratio of physicians to all other health workers was 1:2. In 1975, the ratio approximates 1:15. But somewhere along this substitution course, the gains must come to an end when allowance is made for the difficulties of directing and supervising the ever larger numbers of paraprofessionals. It may be worth noting in passing that the Academy of Orthopedic Surgeons recently reversed itself and decided to phase out its support for training orthopedic physician's assistants after it became convinced, on the basis of controlled experimental studies, that these assistants were not being usefully absorbed in office practice.

A critical contribution to the tight professional control that has been exercised over the training and licensing of health professionals in the United States, at least since the implementation of the Flexner Report, has been the establishment of a common educational base and related training (internships and residencies) to assure a minimum level of competence for all independent practitioners, at least at the beginning of their professional careers. Since physicians, nurses, dentists, optometrists and opticians, druggists, and other individuals all provide health services, one could not assume that they are qualified to render particular services except upon evidence of their successful completion of a standardized course of study with subsequent granting of credentials or licenses.

Despite this system of credentials and licenses, which mandates some order of national qualifications at least for those at the top of the health hierarchy, we cannot enforce a single standard of health care in a nation of continental proportions with great variability in income levels, education, cultural attitudes, and population concentrations. A single standard might be possible but only within a completely controlled system in which health personnel, facilities, and equipment were centrally allocated. Even then, a single standard of care would not prevail, as we have seen in the marked differentials between England and Scotland, and between urban and rural areas in the Soviet Union. A sensible objective of public policy in a democracy should be the improvement in the use of available resources within each area and subdivision, with some contributions from the pool of national resources to strengthen the position of areas with particular weaknesses.

All services, including health services, are unevenly distributed. The educational opportunities in Boston are clearly superior to those in western Texas. Good theater is more readily available along the Eastern seaboard. Competent lawyers, accountants, architects, and most other professionals are heavily concentrated in metropolitan areas. With the possible exceptions of postal and telephone services, no critical services are as readily available in rural as in urban areas. So long as people are free to choose the locations where they work and so long as consumers are free to use their income as they desire, services will be unequally available to different population groups. At most, government can exert some leverage at the margin, but its power to alter the pattern of service delivery is limited indeed.

One final observation about manpower in the health-services industry: As the source of payment for health services shifts from consumers to government, we must anticipate that controversy over the distribution of the dollar will intensify as each organized group of health professionals recognizes that its current income and future prospects will increasingly be determined by the decisions of the bureaucracy which allocates the available governmental funds. If, as has been postulated earlier, the total amount of governmental money entering the system levels off, we must anticipate increasingly acrimonious struggles about decisions affecting relative shares. If foreign experience is any guide, the struggles within the medical profession are likely to be as intensive as those between physicians and those outside.

It would take us too far afield to explore all the ramifications of the approaching struggles over the distribution of the health dollar, but one is worth noting. If physicians feel that they are not properly remunerated, it is likely that they will trade income for leisure, as many now do when they join group practices, with the result that their hours of effective work per year may shrink by 20 per cent or more. There is some evidence that this is happening in general surgery. When the additional reduction in the hours of work that is almost certain to accompany the rapidly growing proportion of women physicians is taken into account, a further significant shrinking in work time must be anticipated. Here is one more important cost-increasing variable which health planners must take into account.

These, then, are some important clues to the future of health services that are suggested by considering the characteristics of other labor-intensive service industries:

1) The critical role of manpower in the provision of health-care services ensures that any improvements in access, quality, and range of services will be associated with additional substantial expenditures. Cost constraint is not a realistic goal.

2) There is little or no possibility that Congress can control the quality of services rendered by professionals. Consequently, to establish elaborate machinery for quality assurance is likely to prove disappointing. Quality improvement will hinge in the future, as in the past, primarily on the self-discipline and responsibility of the purveyors of services, especially physicians.

3) Even if the public were able and willing to allocate an ever larger share of its

total available resources to the health-care industry, there is no prospect whatever that all citizens would have access to the same range and quality of services, since the elements required to provide the services—people, facilities, traditions, money—differ substantially from one area to another and from one population group to another. Although those differences can be reduced, they cannot be eliminated.

4) All labor-intensive service industries find it difficult to structure an effective management and supervisory structure, and without such a structure the productivity of the work force is likely to be low. A point can be reached (and it may be near in general hospitals) where additional people provide almost no increment of useful work because of the difficulties of supervising and coordinating it.

5) Since governments are providing an ever larger part of the total flow of funds into health care, and since organization among health workers, professionals, and paraprofessionals is increasing, we must anticipate acrimonious struggles over the division of the medical dollar, particularly if budgetary exigencies retard the flow of additional monies.

Now that we have engaged in both a historical and an analytic exercise better to understand the elements that are likely to determine the reconstruction of the American health-care industry during the decades ahead, we should look more closely at the realities hidden in our title. What does this analysis imply for the critical issues of goals, power, and decision-making?

First, our national goals are too ambitious. No matter how enthusiastically the American people support enlarged expenditures for health, there is no reason to anticipate that the major current difficulties relating to access, quality control, additional services, and a broadened role for the consumer will be substantially attenuated in the years ahead. We can expect, of course, significant improvements in the health-care system. However, serious problems will remain in our attempts to realize each of the first four specific goals. And if cost containment, the fifth goal, is introduced into the equation, we can expect only failure.

With respect to the critically important dimension of power, the analysis points to its continued diffusion among a few centers with some shifting in the relative strengths of the parties. The members of the medical profession, both as individuals and as members of organized groups, will continue to play a determining role because (if for no other reason) in the absence of a dictatorship the work that professionals do must be elicited; it cannot be demanded according to specifications laid down by others. But, although physicians will continue to exercise a powerful voice over the direction and speed of structural changes, a much larger role will be assumed by government bureaucrats as the inevitable result of the larger funds flowing through public channels and the growing concern with control over quality. In addition, there will be some increase in the leverage exercised by organized professional groups (other than physicians), who will be in a better position to press their claims for higher salaries and benefits in the legislature than in the marketplace. So far as the consumer is concerned, he is likely to enjoy a more prominent role on planning and policy boards, but it is questionable whether he will be able to exercise much effective leverage on the system against organized professional and political interests.

With regard to decision-making mechanisms, it is important to note that although the federal government can alter the flow of funds into the system, select the targets to which they are directed, influence the production and allocation of health manpower, and promulgate rules for quality assurance, the effective transformation of the health-delivery system depends on the behavior of individuals and groups in specific locations. And, at present, there are few decision-making mechanisms in neighborhoods, cities, and other areas that are capable of engaging in the complex processes of structural and operational change. Moreover, even as the existing decision-making mechanisms are strengthened and new ones put into place, it is necessary to remember that the goals they pursue will reflect the relative power of the competing interest groups. These remarks have import for the future of health-maintenance organizations and professional standards legislation. If I had to estimate the future of these, I would argue that, as presently conceived, the health-maintenance organization has at best a dubious future, and that, if professional standards legislation survives, it is unlikely to contribute significantly to an improvement in quality.

It is almost "un-American" to look into the future and find disappointment and failure. Efforts at reform are supposed to produce successes that will improve life for the individual and the society. Nevertheless, while the health-care system is responsive to the most urgent needs of most of the population, there is no prospect whatever, no matter how much money we invest in it, for the system to serve as broad support for the host of ills that already beset modern man and that may well multiply in the years ahead. In consuming over 8 per cent of the gross national product, the health-care system is crowding the margins of family and public income, and we should consider carefully what we are likely to buy if we increase our expenditures to any significant degree.

Questions of investment aside, we must also consider whether we have, or are capable of designing, the social machinery needed to exercise tighter control over the uses to which health resources are put. The streets have not been made safe for pedestrians; the schools have not learned to teach many pupils how to read and write; and corruption permeates much of our public and business life. In light of these failings in the provision of services, a call for moderation in the setting of health goals and for realism in the assessment of power and decision do not represent a doctrine of despair and defeat so much as a plea for the role of reason in the search for a better society.

SUGGESTED READING
   Eli Ginzberg with Miriam Ostow, *Men, Money, Medicine* (New York, 1969).
   Stephen P. Strickland, *Politics, Science, and Dread Disease* (Cambridge, Mass., 1972).
   Rosemary Stevens, *American Medicine and the Public Interest* (New Haven, 1971).
   Eli Ginzberg, ed., *Regionalization and Health Policy* (U.S. Government Printing Office, Washington, D.C., 1977).

HERBERT E. KLARMAN

The Financing of Health Care

MEDICARE AND MEDICAID HAVE BEEN IN OPERATION since 1966. Since then, expenditures for health care in the United States have increased at an annual rate of 12 per cent. This is well above the rate of increase of 8 per cent in the preceding decade. Most years, the rate of increase in health-care expenditures has exceeded that of the gross national product (GNP)—the market value of all goods and services produced by the economy. Consequently, the proportion of the GNP devoted to health-care expenditures has also continued to rise: indeed, between 1940 and 1975, it doubled, rising from 4.1 to 8.3 per cent.

We shall begin our discussion with a description and analysis of past trends in health-care expenditures in this country, and then estimate future prospects, with emphasis on the potential effects of national health insurance. Finally we shall discuss alternative approaches toward containing future increases in health-care expenditures and consider certain distributional aspects of health-care financing.

The official data on health-care expenditures in this country, which are issued annually by the Social Security Administration, have become familiar to the student of the health-care industry since they assumed their present form in 1962. For each year, the expenditures by category, such as hospital care or physicians' services, are cross-classified by source, such as tax funds or voluntary health insurance. The most recent official figures on health-care financing in this country, those for fiscal year 1975-76, estimate total expenditures for that year at more than $133 billion. These figures come, however, from the Congressional Budget Office, a new source of data.[1] All other figures on health-care expenditures have been taken from the Social Security Administration, where they appear in one of the winter-month issues of the *Social Security Bulletin*.[2] Its estimate for fiscal year 1974-75 was $118.5 billion, giving an increase between fiscal 1975 and fiscal 1976 of more than 12 per cent. The increase between fiscal 1974 and fiscal 1975 was 14 per cent.

As Table 1 shows, the period 1966-75 had an average annual rate of increase in health-care expenditures of 12 per cent, compared with 8 per cent a year in the preceding decade, 1955-1965, or the longer period, 1950-65. During the approximately three-year period, 1972-74, of the Nixon administration's Economic Stabilization Program, when wage and price controls were applied, the annual rate of increase was 10.5 per cent, still higher than before 1965. In the other years of the Medicare-Medicaid era, the rate of increase in health-care expenditures averaged 13 per cent.

If attention is limited to expenditures for services that were most heavily affected by Medicare and Medicaid—the two major health-care-financing programs enacted

TABLE 1

INCREASE IN HEALTH-CARE EXPENDITURES, UNITED STATES,
SELECTED INTERVALS, 1929-75

Interval	No. of years	Increase during interval	Average annual rate of increase
1929-75	46	3201.8%	7.9%
1929-35	6	− 20.7	−3.8
1939-40	5	35.7	6.3
1940-50	10	211.4	12.0
1950-55	5	44.1	7.6
1955-60	5	49.2	8.3
1960-65	5	50.4	8.5
1965-70	5	77.9	12.2
1970-75	5	71.2	11.4
1950-60	10	115.0	8.0
1950-65	15	223.3	8.1
1955-65	10	224.4	8.4
1966-70	4	64.3	13.2
1966-75	9	181.4	12.2
1971-74	3	34.8	10.5

Source: Appendix Table A.

under the Great Society of President Johnson—the findings by time period are similar, but all rates of increase are higher.

Table 2 shows rates of increase in the sum of expenditures for short-term hospital care, physicians' services, and nursing homes. In the period 1950-65, these expenditures rose at an average annual rate of 9 per cent; for the period beginning in 1966 the annual rate of increase averaged 14 per cent. If the period of the Economic Stabilization Program is excluded, the annual rate of increase in the Medicare-Medicaid era averaged 16 per cent.

These rates of increase are important in themselves, given the awful power of compound interest. Thus, if the rate of increase compounded annually is 8 per cent, it takes 9 years for a given amount to double. The period for doubling drops to 6 years if the annual rate of increase is 12 per cent, and to 5 years if it is 14 per cent.

The increases in health-care expenditures can also be viewed in relation to the GNP. They have exceeded the increases in the GNP in most years. As the proportion of GNP devoted to health-care expenditures has steadily risen, there has been an outpouring of public concern and of efforts to curtail the rate of increase. As Appendix Table A shows, it took 20 years (from 1940 to 1960) for the proportion of the GNP spent on health care in this country to increase by one percentage point—from 4.1 to 5.2 per cent. Subsequently, increases of one percentage point took 7 years (from 1960 to 1967); 3 years (from 1967 to 1970); and 5 years (from 1970 to 1975), with 3 of those 5 years comprising the period of the Economic Stabilization Program, when the proportion of health-care expenditures to the GNP was constant at approximately 7.8 per cent.

TABLE 2

INCREASES IN SUM OF EXPENDITURES FOR SHORT-TERM HOSPITAL CARE, PHYSICIAN
SERVICES, AND NURSING-HOME CARE, UNITED STATES, SELECTED INTERVALS,
1929-75

Interval	No. of years	Increase during interval	Average Annual rate of increase
1929-75	46	4755.2%	8.8%
1929-35	6	− 15.7	−2.8
1935-40	5	31.7	5.7
1940-50	10	234.5	8.9
1950-55	5	44.8	7.7
1955-60	5	59.3	9.8
1960-65	5	60.6	9.9
1965-70	5	90.1	13.7
1970-75	5	85.7	13.2
1950-60	10	130.7	8.7
1950-65	15	270.5	9.1
1955-65	10	255.8	9.8
1966-70	4	79.7	15.8
1966-75	9	233.7	14.3
1971-74	3	38.0	11.3

Source: Appendix Table A.

The United States is far from unique in experiencing a marked rise in the proportion of health-care expenditures to GNP. Most developed nations for which data have been reported manifest the same tendency.[3] The noteworthy exceptions, those with a stable proportion, are attributable to special circumstances: In the United Kingdom, National Health Service expenditures are determined by the central government, and for many years after World War II other claims on the public treasury, such as housing and education, received a higher priority than did health care. In Israel, national security has been an overwhelming competitor for resources. In Japan, national income in current dollars (which reflects inflation in the economy as a whole) grew at such a high rate in the period 1965-70—18 per cent a year—that health-care expenditures rose less than commensurately in three of the five years.

Long lists of explanations have been presented to account for these persistently high rates of increase in health-care expenditures over the past decade in this country. They include such factors as the growth in total population, the aging of the population, advances in medical technology, heightened public expectations from medicine, and growth in third-party financing. But not all of these proffered explanations can withstand scrutiny. For example, with respect to the effects of an aging population, a difference prevailing at a given time—such as an above-average rate of utilization of services by persons 65 years and over—may not contribute to an increase in total utilization over an extended period, if the ratio of consumption of services by these people relative to the rest of the population remains the same. The reason is that the over-65 group is a small minority to begin with. Since the aging of a population is a slow process, it cannot by itself make a sizable contribution to total utilization in a period as brief as a decade.

As for other, competing explanations, such as advances in technology or the growth of prepayment, it is possible for the former to be the predominant factor in one period and for the latter to be predominant in another. One single explanation is not likely to hold true at all times.

Sometimes the explanatory forces at play are confounded, and it is difficult to distinguish between their respective influences. For example, in 1966 the amount of third-party funds to pay for health care increased substantially, but simultaneously new methods and formulas for reimbursing health-care providers were adopted. A further complication arises when a change is adopted widely and uniformly; the very lack of variation precludes the discovery of the effects of the change through standard statistical techniques, such as multiple regression analysis.

It is fair to say that there is still no consensus among economists, even when they look at the same data, on the reasons why health-care expenditures have continued to rise as much as they have since 1965. Some explanations that have been advanced, such as the catching up in earnings by hospital employees relative to earnings by comparable occupations in other industries, are fairly easy to examine and reject. Obviously an increase in expenditures from that source should cease when the hospital employees' salaries have caught up. By contrast, the question whether the inflow of additional third-party funds was more important in the continuing increase in hospital-care expenditures than was the decision by Congress to reimburse hospitals at their own individual costs remains unresolved. In these circumstances, it is not surprising that the policy proposals offered to remedy the escalation of expenditures differ a good deal.

Even so, the fact that economists are able to agree on the data and on the accounting framework within which the data are organized is no minor achievement. It is now possible to state that under the Medicare program expenditures for general hospital care rose by $7.4 billion from 1967 to 1975 and that of this amount, as calculated from data compiled by the Comptroller General of the United States, 78 per cent is attributable to the increase in patient-day cost, 16 per cent to the increase in enrollment, and only 6 per cent, to the increase in per-capita utilization.[4]

It will be recalled that the official data on health-care expenditures also show sources of payment. The major trends in sources of payment for the past genera-tion can be summarized as follows: out-of-pocket payments by patients at the time of illness have declined in relative importance and third-party payments have gained; although philanthropy is no longer identified separately in the published statistics, its relative importance has presumably also declined; and, while the major source of growth in the third-party payments before 1965 was voluntary health insurance, after that date it became public programs.

Closer examination of the several sources of payment shows that tax funds assumed increased importance with the enactment of Medicare and Medicaid in 1965. According to the Social Security Administration, as shown in Table 3, the public sector accounted for one-fourth of all health-care expenditures in 1950, 1955, and 1966. This fraction rose to one-third in 1967, and has continued to creep upward since then, exceeding two-fifths for the first time in 1975. Virtually the entire increase in public funds has occurred in the federal government's contribution, with the state

TABLE 3

PUBLIC AND PRIVATE EXPENDITURES FOR HEALTH CARE, UNITED STATES, SELECTED YEARS, 1929-75

Year	Proportion of total: private	Proportion of total: public	
		All	Federal
1929	86.7%	13.3%	na
1935	80.9	19.1	na
1940	79.8	20.2	na
1950	74.5	25.5	na
1955	74.5	25.5	na
1960	75.3	24.7	na
1965	75.5	24.5	11.9%
1966	74.3	25.7	12.8
1967	67.0	33.0	20.5
1968	62.7	37.3	24.3
1969	62.2	37.8	25.1
1970	63.5	36.5	24.0
1971	62.9	37.1	24.3
1972	61.6	38.4	25.5
1973	61.8	38.2	25.5
1974	60.7	39.3	26.4
1975	57.8	42.2	28.6

Sources: Reference cited in note 2 and Office of Research and Statistics, Social Security Administration, *Compendium of National Health Expenditures Data* (Washington, D.C., 1976), Table 5.

and local governments' share remaining almost constant at one-eighth of total health-care expenditures.

The figures so far presented reflect outlays, and do not take into account so-called "tax expenditures," which are steadily gaining in prominence. Today, tax expenditures appear as a regular feature of the federal budget, and show revenue losses to the federal treasury due to special provisions of the tax laws. Revenue losses from tax deductions or credits are meant to be seen as alternatives to subsidies through budgetary expenditures. In health care, tax expenditures are important because they constitute potential offsets to estimates of the cost of national health insurance to the federal treasury.

The most common estimate of the health-care tax expenditure in 1975 is $5.6 billion, as reported in the Budget of the United States.[5] This figure is the sum of two components under the individual income tax: $3.3 billion, the revenue loss due to the non-taxability to the employee of employer contributions to voluntary health-insurance premiums, and $2.3 billion, the revenue loss due to the itemized medical-expense deduction. Several additions to this amount have been suggested. The non-taxability of employer contributions to voluntary health-insurance premiums under the payroll tax for Social Security is estimated at another $2.4 billion.[6] The deduction of philanthropic contributions to health causes and agencies is estimated at another $0.9 billion.[7]

The Council on Wage and Price Stability has suggested that allowance be made for the real-estate-tax exemption enjoyed by voluntary, non-profit, and public hospitals;[8] this item serves to reduce private and federal health-care expenditures. Based on data for New York City, it is estimated that for the country's short-term hospitals the tax exemptions amount to between $1.7 billion and $2.0 billion.[9]

While the relative importance of federal expenditures has increased substantially in the past decade, that of voluntary health-insurance benefits has remained fairly stable. The history of the thousand and more health-insurance plans in this country is short, though longer than that of Medicare or Medicaid. Their formal beginning is generally traced back to the founding of the first Blue Cross plan in Texas in 1929. By 1935, several Blue Cross plans had been established in other parts of the country. The voluntary health-insurance movement did not, however, gain momentum until World War II, when wages were frozen while fringe benefits were negotiable. Employer contributions to voluntary health-insurance premiums then became an important item for collective bargaining between labor unions and management. It is noteworthy that while fringe benefits are deductible as business expenses under the corporation income tax—just as wages and salaries are—they are not taxable under the individual income tax. In effect, enrollment in group health insurance is federally subsidized.

The relative importance of voluntary health insurance in health-care financing is best illustrated by looking at the proportion of voluntary health-insurance benefits to personal health-care expenditures; the latter exclude certain non-personal health-care items, such as expenditures for construction, research, public-health departments, and administration of health-insurance plans. As Table 4 shows, this proportion rose steadily from one-eighth of the total in 1950 to one-quarter in 1965. The proportion declined somewhat for a short period, because of the immediate impact of Medicare. It returned to one-quarter by 1971 and has continued to increase slowly ever since.

In addition to providing insurance, many Blue Cross and Blue Shield plans and some commercial insurance companies serve as fiscal intermediaries or agents for government, especially in the administration of Medicare. The data shown in Table 4 pertain only to their role as underwriter for private health insurance.

Although most Blue Cross plans and some Blue Shield plans offer service benefits—as do Medicare and Medicaid—commercial insurance companies offer cash benefits to patients. As a result, the former have to maintain a direct relationship with participating providers for reimbursement, while the latter do not, except when they serve as fiscal intermediaries or agents for government programs.

From the outset, hospital care has been the most widely held and best covered benefit under voluntary health insurance in this country. Notwithstanding this, the exact proportion of the population below the age of 65 that has insurance coverage is not known: the current range of official estimates is between 80 and 85 per cent.[10] Nor is it really possible to calculate precisely how much hospital care is paid for by voluntary health insurance because some hospital care is defrayed by major-medical-insurance benefits, which encompass a wide range of services that are all subject to a common deductible. Nor can one state readily and on a current basis what proportion of general hospital care is covered by voluntary health insurance. While the official expenditure figures are for all hospitals, the bulk of voluntary health-insurance

TABLE 4

VOLUNTARY HEALTH INSURANCE BENEFITS AS PERCENTAGE OF PERSONAL HEALTH-
CARE EXPENDITURES, UNITED STATES, SELECTED YEARS, 1929-75

Year	Total expenditures (in millions of dollars)	Insurance benefits	
		Dollar amount (in millions of dollars)	Per cent of expenditures
1929	$ 3,165	na	na
1935	2,585	na	na
1940	3,414	na	na
1950	10,400	879	8.5%
1955	15,231	$ 2,358	15.5
1960	22,729	4,698	20.7
1965	33,498	8,280	24.7
1966	36,216	8,936	24.7
1967	41,343	9,344	22.6
1968	46,521	10,444	22.5
1969	52,690	12,206	23.2
1970	60,113	14,406	24.0
1971	67,228	16,728	24.9
1972	74,828	18,620	24.9
1973	82,490	20,955	25.4
1974	90,088	24,100	26.8
1975	103,200	23,340	26.5

Source: Table 6 of reference cited in note 2.

benefits are paid out for short-term hospital care. According to one study, the relative importance of voluntary health insurance declined between 1961 and 1971 from 60 to 48 per cent of all expenditures by non-governmental community hospitals. (By contrast, in all hospitals voluntary-health-insurance benefits declined only from 38 per cent to 36.5 per cent in the same period.[11])

With respect to enrollment, it is important to note that most voluntary-health-insurance enrollment in this country is job related. Members of an employed group pay lower premiums than do separately enrolled individuals because they pose a lower risk of adverse self-selection for illness and consequent health-care utilization. In addition, a given dollar premium often turns out to be cheaper for the employed person because, as previously noted, the employer contribution to the premium escapes taxation. Finally, the low-income employee finds it cheaper to enroll on the job, because then the premium paid either by him or on his behalf is computed as a percentage of his wages. Under individual insurance, the premium is a dollar amount, not graduated with earnings.

As the amount spent on health care in this country continues to increase, as the proportion it absorbs of the GNP also increases, and 'as the fraction of the total derived from taxes increases even more, the point—whether expressed as a statement or as a question—is frequently made that this nation cannot "afford" to devote more of its total resources to health care than it is now doing. If this statement is intended to mean that no single activity can absorb 100 per cent of the GNP, or close to it, then its validity is obvious and, were it not for the power of compound interest, even trivial. The point warrants examination, however, because even those who have projected a limit on health-care expenditures for this country of 11 or 12 per cent of the GNP have not really given convincing reasons why this figure should prove to be a maximum, if recent tendencies are allowed to persist.

What a nation can "afford" to spend on a given set of activities, such as health care, depends largely on the choices it makes in the face of alternative opportunities to spend and on the value assigned to the particular category of expenditure. The way in which such choices are manifested differs according to whether the spending is public or private, or whether it is incurred individually or as a group. Group and public decisions call for a more systematic analysis of alternatives than do individual and private decisions, which are made independently by consumers in the light of their own budgetary constraints and preferences. The expansion of third-party payments for health care, both through voluntary health insurance and through tax funds, has increased the demand for the role of systematic policy analysis in the health-care industry.

In this context, one question that has been raised in the past decade is the extent to which additional expenditures are likely to be dissipated in the form of higher incomes for health-care providers. In good part, any answer to this question will reflect one's opinion of the worthiness of the recipients of the higher income. If most of them are low-wage earners, such as nurse's aides, they may be perceived as deserving of salary improvement, at least up to the point where they will have caught up with their peers in other industries. Conversely, if the recipients of higher incomes are professionals already near the top of the income distribution, the additional income might be seen as justified only if it serves to attract to the industry manpower that is believed to be in short supply. Otherwise, the additional income will be viewed as an unnecessary transfer of income to the well-to-do, and therefore as inequitable.

It has been observed that, for certain types of services, appropriating more money may not elicit the desired response from providers. For example, despite financial inducements, physicians and hospitals in leadership roles in the mainstream of medicine have been unwilling or unable to sponsor health care for long-term patients. By contrast, making funds available has elicited a strong response from commercial investors, who are commonly regarded with suspicion in the health field. This negative attitude may have contributed to the recruitment of owners and operators of facilities who have proved uncommonly zealous in their pursuit of high profits.

For the most part, additional expenditures do result in some additional health-care services. The question then becomes one of determining whether these services are worthwhile. This question has been posed by two different disciplines, each in its own terms: the epidemiologist asks whether a given diagnosis or treatment is effective—that is, whether it yields a measurable improvement in the health of the population—while the economist asks whether a particular program yields the largest possible surplus of benefits over costs. The economist's notion is that, given the relative scarcity of total resources in any society, it is never possible to undertake every effective health-care program. Rather, every such program must compete for scarce resources not only with all other health-care programs but also with all other proposed avenues of expenditure.

Both the epidemiologist and the economist try to relate the outcomes of health-care programs, as measured by improvements in health status, to their inputs, as measured by program costs. Both disciplines share the difficult problems of measuring health outcome and of relating changes in health status to changes in program content. However, the economist faces the further difficulty of trying to put a value on a particular health outcome, a value that somehow must be expressed in money terms in order to make it commensurate with program costs. When the health outcomes in question are potential gains in life expectancy, the valuation of benefits is virtually impossible in the present state of the art. Properly put, the economist's question concerning the balance between benefits and costs should apply to changes—usually small ones—in the volume of services used. An answer to this question has nothing to do with the answer to another question that is sometimes posed, namely, whether an entire health-care system or one of its major components is worthwhile.

In light of these considerations, it is evident that answering either form of the question is not easy. The difficulties of measuring health outcome and of valuing it have already been noted. Unfortunately, there are further difficulties. Although improvement in the health status of a population is a major objective of the health-care system, it is not the only objective. The health-care system also serves to relieve pain, stabilize the patient's condition and arrest deterioration, offer assurance and support, and render sympathetic care in a considerate manner when nothing else can be done. Even with respect to health status, the health-care system may be seen as serving to counteract the unhealthful personal habits of people. The relative weights attached to the several objectives of the health-care system are a matter of value judgment. The expert can help by spelling out the implications of different weights, but he cannot substitute his judgment for that of organized society.

The problem of valuation is further complicated by the fact that different groups in the population receive different services and consequently different presumed benefits. For example, dental services for children are favored by their parents. Medicare is favored by the aged and by their middle-aged children, who also have responsibilities for their own families. Including benefits for patients with chronic kidney disease under Medicare is favored by the middle-aged patients, by their families, and by their co-workers.

When funds are made available and, as a result, services are utilized, something of value has been achieved—at least in the opinion of many. The trend observed since 1966 toward equality by income class in the use of hospital care and physician services, though perhaps overstated on technical grounds, is a reassuring sign that some programs do work, at least to some extent, in achieving their stated objectives.

If the preceding argument is valid, it follows that setting priorities among health-care programs and between health care and other avenues of expenditure is not a simple determination that can be made solely on the basis of data. A large component of value judgment, in the best sense, must always be involved.

Sometimes a proposed program necessitates substantial changes in the organization and operation of the health-care system. Then it is sensible to inquire into the magnitude of the anticipated improvements in health status and the probability of their occurrence. Allowance should be made for the fact that the ultimate consequences of such changes are unpredictable. On the cost side, implementation of substantial changes may be impeded by the opposition of providers who are comfortable with the existing arrangements to which they are accustomed. In that case, the cost of securing acquiescence is high, while the estimated benefits remain unchanged.

The issue whether to spend more or less on health care is simplified when a given set of agreed-upon health outcomes or health-care services can be produced more cheaply than before. Under most circumstances, in a world of relative scarcity of total resources, the more efficient health-care program is preferred. Thus, in caring for patients with chronic kidney disease, kidney transplantation costs less per life year gained than does continuing hemodialysis; furthermore, the patient with the trans-planted kidney usually leads a freer and better life. There may be one exception to society's general preference for efficient production: under conditions of high unemployment in a local area, the desirability of providing jobs may outweigh the usual objective of producing output at the lowest possible cost. But, subject to this occasional exception, it is always desirable that additional health-care expenditures be justified in terms of their efficiency in achieving the accepted purposes of the health-care system.

Multiplicity of objectives, difficulties in measuring health status and in placing a value on differences or changes in health status, and diversity of interests among various consumer groups and between providers and consumers all combine to make the total amount a nation spends on health care collectively a matter of negotiation and repeated renegotiation among the interested parties. Moreover, these consid-erations point to the impossibility of determining how much a nation can afford to spend on health care on the basis of data alone.

It is generally believed that enactment of national health insurance would lead to further increases in health-care expenditures. The reason is that the scope and depth of health insurance exert a major influence on the utilization of services and price per unit and therefore on the total amount spent. For the four major health-insurance bills pending in the Congress, the estimated increases for the year 1975 ranged between $3 billion and $13 billion. [12] In reality, the size of the increase will depend not only on the provisions of the law passed by Congress, but also on details of implementation as reflected in its regulations and on the future course of expansion of health-care facilities and manpower.

Why should national health insurance lead to additional expenditures? In part, the answer is that, to the extent that national health insurance does not merely replace existing voluntary health insurance, any prepayment plan for health care effects a transfer of funds from the well to the ill. Erratic and sporadic payments are converted into steady and reliable ones. More money is designated for health care under prepayment than in its absence; some persons who previously went without care because they were unable to pay for it will then be receiving it. In addition, providers will be less inclined to provide care free of charge or to reduce charges to some patients below their customary fees. For some health-care services, national health insurance would involve an expansion of enrollment or of benefits or both. Even for hospital care, 15 to 20 per cent of the population under 65 would be acquiring insurance protection, although some of the recipients would be shifted from Medicaid or from Veterans Administration hospitals. While shifting patients from other government programs to insured status leads to an increase in insurance costs, it need not lead to an increase in total government expenditures for health care.

As economists have increasingly emphasized, health insurance establishes, in effect, a two-price system. The provider charges one price—the gross price—and the consumer faces another—the lower net price—of his out-of-pocket expenses at the time of utilization. The result is that the consumer sees health care as cheaper than it really is, and his use of services is greater than it would be without insurance. In addition, when the presence of insurance is taken as a measure of a person's ability to pay for care, it may also lead to higher prices.

Historically, the wholesale financing of health care, as of other goods and services, by government has been accompanied by the large-scale production of services under government auspices or by purchase of services from existing providers. The tenor of the last decade or so, in this country as in Canada, is to leave intact the ownership or forms of organization by which health-care services are produced and to purchase services from existing providers. In the absence of simple measures of the quality of care that consumers can gauge, this has led to payment geared to the cost and charge patterns of individual providers. Reimbursement at the cost that was actually incurred is bound to be inefficient; the provider cannot earn more money without spending more, while he is virtually assured of getting back what he has spent. It is necessary to establish a rate of payment ahead of time independent of the expenditures that are actually incurred. How to do this is now a subject of intensive exploration and evaluation. Similarly, it is now apparent that the Medicare formula for reimbursing physicians was conducive to increases in stated fees and even more conducive to increases in actual fees charged and collected.

The purchase of services by government may yield a saving over production of services by government. The reason—apart from possible differences in efficiency of operation—is that owners of hospitals are inclined to "round out" their facilities in order to make the range of services more complete. By contrast, government as the purchaser of service has no interest in any one particular facility and can exert its power to block attempts at expansion.

Obviously the record of the past decade affords no grounds for complacency. We have had a high rate of increase in health-care expenditures in this country even without national health insurance. New steps will have to be taken even to maintain the same rate of increase if national health insurance were enacted, and stronger steps would be needed to reduce it. What measures are available? Several approaches toward moderating increases in health-care expenditures have been developed, ranging from changes in financing to limitations on the supply of resources and reorganization of the health-care-delivery system.

One approach favored by many economists is to return to greater reliance on the financial incentives that operated before the introduction and growth of prepayment. The idea behind "co-payment" or cost sharing is for consumers to pay a larger share of the total health-care bill out-of-pocket at the time of illness, so that they will be led to make more considered decisions on how many services to buy and at what price. Under co-payment, the price paid by the consumer will come closer to cost for a large fraction of care purchased, as it already does in the market for other goods and services. The expected result is that under conditions of substantial co-payment by consumers, per-capita utilization of services would be lower than under full insurance and the average price per unit of service would also be lower, because consumers would be induced to shop around for the lowest price.

There are, however, several practical difficulties with co-payment on a large scale. First, the notion of a knowledgeable consumer acting independently of a physician in a competitive health-care market is not a realistic one. The patient is usually unable to judge the quality of care and is guided by his physician with respect both to types and to quantity of services used. Indeed, in discharging his professional obligations, the physician is expected to act in the interests of the patient even as he pursues his own.

Introduction of a larger measure of co-payment would be opposed by many labor unions which have successfully negotiated first-dollar (full) coverage for their members. More members receive benefits under first-dollar coverage than do under sizable deductibles, and unions prefer that as many members as possible receive benefits. In light of this characteristic of unions, it is too simple to attribute the growth of health insurance with first-dollar coverage to the subsidy of fringe benefits under the federal tax laws.

In the real world, the operation of co-payment may also be thwarted by consumers who buy supplementary insurance to pay for the deductible and co-insurance provisions of their principal health-insurance plan. The aged in this country have already done this, by purchasing senior-citizen's health-insurance policies to supplement their Medicare benefits. It is unlikely that a law prohibiting such supplementation would be passed.

It is also worth examining the probable quantitative effects of co-payment. The best source of information on this is Scitovsky's study in the Palo Alto Clinic, which found that introduction of a co-insurance factor for physician services of 25 per cent resulted in an average decline in per-capita visits of 24 per cent in the first year.[13] It is not yet known what happened subsequently, and it is also not clear whether the group involved in this "natural experiment" represented a sufficient proportion of the clinic's patients to exert an influence on physician behavior in prescribing visits. The study indicates that the lowest of the three socioeconomic groups involved had the largest reduction in utilization. If desired, such an effect could be mitigated by relating out-of-pocket expense to income and by imposing a top limit on the total amount spent out-of-pocket. In that case, the presumed deterrent effect on utilization would not operate for low-income persons, and it would not operate for anybody after some sum had been spent. Beck's study in Saskatchewan covered a whole Canadian province; there the deterrent effect on utilization wore off after a few years.[14]

While it is well known that co-payment raises the visible costs of administering insurance plans, it is not equally appreciated that co-payment provisions impose certain costs of compliance on beneficiaries, such as record keeping, correspondence, and follow up; these are not easy to measure. An unintended loss of benefits may also take place. It is suggestive, according to an early report by Loewenstein on Medicare, that aged persons failed to obtain one-fourth of the benefits they were entitled to under Part B of the program.[15] Personal experience suggests that some aged persons are not capable of handling the intricacies of reimbursement when the physician declines to accept assignment of the bill.

Nevertheless, there is no denying that health insurance brings about greater utilization and higher prices than would obtain without it. The technical term, "moral hazard," that is sometimes employed to describe these effects of insurance is somewhat misleading, because the behavior in question is usually consistent with the changed incentives introduced by the insurance; it is not immoral. However, for the reasons given above, co-payment may involve greater costs than benefits and is not a good solution to the problem.

It will be recalled that health-insurance plans were established in this country in order to reduce the heavy financial burden that illness imposed on some individuals and families, by spreading it across the entire population. The movement gained support from providers who were eager to promote a reliable source of funding for their services, especially during the depression of the nineteen-thirties. The fact, which emerged fairly early in the literature, that individuals with insurance use more services than individuals without insurance was seen as a desirable attribute of insurance. More services were obviously better than fewer services, since, prior to health insurance, the well-to-do received more care than the poor. The association of "more" with "better" did not change until it emerged in the later nineteen-fifties that subscribers to prepaid group-practice plans had a lower rate of hospital use than subscribers to other health-insurance plans and did not suffer any adverse health effects from it. Indeed, its proponents felt that prepaid group practice provided better care, including preventive services, to its subscribers than the usual solo-practice, community-hospital, fee-for-service arrangement. At the same time the idea arose of a possible "availability effect," that is, under conditions of prepayment the physician's prescription and the patient's use of services are greatly influenced by the existing supply of facilities and manpower. This idea was formally expressed by Milton Roemer about 1960, but it did not gain widespread acceptance for another decade. While the availability effect suggests that per-capita utilization of health care will vary by geographic area in accordance with variation in the supply of resources, it also locates much of the power of decision-making in the provider, especially the physician. If this is the case, there is little point in applying strong pressure upon the relatively powerless patient.

Even if the deterrent effects of co-payment on utilization are neither desirable nor attainable, it can be argued in its favor that substantial out-of-pocket payments serve to reduce the burden that national health insurance would impose on the public treasury; otherwise, total reliance on public funding of national health insurance would reduce the amount of tax funds available for desired public programs that have no other source of funding. This point is valid. However, a strong case can be made for increasing the proportion of public funds in health-care expenditures. The arguments are as follows: Health insurance is necessary in order to spread the costs of expensive illness; for reasons already given, it may not be practical to remove less costly illness from the benefits package. Everybody should be insured because our society chooses not to deny health care for lack of ability to pay for it. The most direct way to make health insurance universal is to have it mandatory. The simplest way to make health-insurance enrollment both universal and mandatory is through the tax system. Moreover, a single source of financing reduces the danger that a dual standard of health care will be perpetuated.

If it is desired to hold down the amount of public funds devoted to health care, certain services can be kept out of the health-insurance-benefits package. Services not covered should not be potential substitutes for services that are covered. For example, hospital care and physician's services are partial substitutes for one another; dental care is not a substitute for either. There is, moreover, some leeway for private payments for amenities, such as an extra degree of privacy in the hospital or television in the patient's room.

If co-payment cannot be relied on and third-party payment increases in absolute and relative importance, it will be necessary to seek other approaches for curtailing the rise in health-care expenditures. Among the approaches that have been proposed are improved methods for reimbursing providers. When the purchase of services from providers who are paid by third parties becomes the predominant mode of financing health care, the method by which providers are paid assumes central importance. It is hard to believe that the method of provider reimbursement will make no difference with respect to the efficiency of operation of hospitals or physician charges and incomes. This seems obvious, despite the fact that little can be said today about the quantitative effects of different ways of paying providers. Students of hospital finances will probably all agree in principle that paying each hospital at its own patient-day cost, computed retrospectively after the expenditures have taken place, is an invitation to administrators to spend more. It is not clear, however, what method or formula is to be put in place of that system.

One reason that we do not yet know the precise effects of reimbursement is lack of experience with a single reimbursement mechanism and formula operating in a given local area. In the presence of several separate sources of payment, competent administrators are able to adapt to, indeed exploit, this diversity. Another reason has been the general lack of access to hospital data on costs and revenues; the replication of routine analyses on a regular basis is thereby precluded. A major problem faced by analysts is that regulators seldom adhere to a particular method of payment or formula long enough for its effects to be observed. They may change the elements of cost that are reimbursable, the formula for calculating permissible increases, the size of the overall limit on payment, or various internal limits on components of the hospital operation. Limits may be imposed on the rate of increase or on the size of permissible deviation from the average cost of the group in which a hospital is classified. Finally, even experiments at the state or local level especially designed to study prospective reimbursement have been confounded by the intrusion of other events, such as federal price and wage controls.

The reimbursement problem remains intractable principally because we do not yet understand why costs differ among hospitals to the extent that they do. If variations in cost could be accounted for by known and measurable differences in patient composition and in the quality of care, it would be possible to set uniform payments for the care of a patient with a given condition at a specified level of quality. As it is, reimbursement of hospitals on an individual basis must continue for the foreseeable future.

In paying for nursing-home care under Medicare and, even more, under Medicaid, proprietary ownership has posed the additional problem of how to reward capital investment and entrepreneurship. If the license to operate a nursing home of a given size constitutes a legal property right to care for that number of patients and to receive payment for them, as some courts have ruled, the sale and resale of the property can continually raise the capital value on which the rate of payment is calculated. When Congress voted to reimburse nursing homes in the same manner as hospitals, it disregarded differences in ownership. It is fair to add, however, that the problem is further complicated by the traditional distrust of proprietary ownership of health-care facilities. The usual response has been to impose a plethora of detailed controls on the proprietors.

In reimbursing physicians the new formula adopted by Medicare—paying at the usual, customary, and prevailing fee—has had a greater effect on fees and earnings than might have been expected from the relative size of the over-65 population. The customary fee was changed frequently; the usual fee served as an inducement to raise charges to younger patients; and, although the prevailing fee has been repeatedly set at a lower percentile in the local array of fees, such reduction has been offset by the tendency for the range of fees to become narrower. In 1965, there was no experience with such a formula. Nor was it anticipated that fees would be "fractionated," imposing additional charges for services, such as routine laboratory tests, formerly incorporated into the visit fee.

Reimbursement of providers is a crucial problem that needs urgently to be dealt with, whether national health insurance is enacted now or later. The incentives to economize at the state or local level are perhaps greater under the present system than they would be under national health insurance, when all funds are seen as flowing from a distant, central source.

Another crucial factor in health-care expenditures is the supply of health-care resources. If the availability effect is so important, it is imperative to try to curtail the expansion of health-care resources and, in the case of hospital beds, even to reduce them. Such curtailment of the overall supply does not imply interference with the practices of individual physicians in caring for individual patients.

By now many observers of the health-care industry accept the existence of an "availability effect." What this signifies is that variation in the use of hospital care or of physician services is heavily influenced by variation in the quantity of providers, much more so than by variation in other factors that influence utilization. Both consumers and providers learn to adapt and to accommodate to the existing supply of providers. No less important is the realization that an increased total supply of health manpower may not lead to a more equitable geographic distribution. Apparently physicians are absorbed and are able to earn a good living wherever they choose to settle. The assumption that physicians would relocate to poorly served areas is apparently invalid, though it has been a pillar in support of the expansion of medical education in this country. From the importance attached to the availability effect follows the corollary that close monitoring of the appropriateness of use of existing health-care resources is not likely to yield appreciable savings in expenditures— indeed, the monitoring activities entail costs of their own.

The available evidence indicates that the extent to which health-care resources are used "appropriately" depends a good deal on the pressures exerted on the several participants in a transaction. Physicians are more likely to adhere to a hospital's admission queue when the rate of occupancy is high. They are more likely to delegate tasks to assistants when their case loads are heavy. With the large increase in physician supply that is taking place in this country, there is no reason to expect extensive substitution of cheaper paramedical personnel for more costly physicians.

If the increase in third-party funds is considered the major factor behind the increase in health-care expenditures, the most likely deterrent to further increases is either substantial co-payment by patients or curtailment in the number of providers, depending on one's view as to where the locus of decision-making power in health care lies. The limitations of co-payment have been noted; in the light of experience, effecting a curtailment of supply may be difficult to accomplish. If the method by which providers are paid is held to be a major factor in the marked increase in health-care expenditures in the past decade, considerable effort must also be invested in changing reimbursement mechanisms and formulas. The implications of more effective regulation are very serious, posing a challenge to those who would want the process to be open and impartial, the meaning of regulations clear, their contents stable for some time, and the results reasonable and conducive to the sustenance of an adequate health-care system.

The health-maintenance organization (HMO) was put forth in 1971 by Paul Ellwood as a possible solution to the problem of how to halt the increase in health-care expenditures. The HMO is a political and legal amalgam of prepaid group practice, which for many years was opposed by the organized medical profession, and its arch rival for clientele in California, the community medical foundation. Prepaid-group-practice plans combine the group form of medical organization with financing by health-insurance premiums. The community medical foundation is usually established by the local medical society as a vehicle for organizing its members to render care to groups of employees or public dependents without changing the usual arrangements of solo practitioners charging fees for service. What the medical foundation does is assure the party financing the care for a group of consumers that premiums will be sufficient to pay for all the services rendered. It accomplishes this by monitoring the appropriateness of the services utilized and by prorating individual fees when necessary.

The evidence that has been adduced on behalf of the HMO derives almost exclusively from prepaid group practice and emphasizes its record of hospital use and expenditures for health care that are lower than under other health-insurance plans. The HMO was proposed as a fundamental change in the health-care industry by bringing competition into it between the HMO and the traditional health-care system as well as among HMOs. The contention is that the effective working of competition would obviate the need for government intervention by planning and regulation and would even reduce the need for certain types of public spending.

Since knowledgeable consumer behavior in health care is unlikely, it is not evident that free competitive behavior is desirable. The basis for lower hospital use by prepaid-group-practice subscribers has not been established, because prepaid-group-practice plans usually operate with a tight hospital-bed supply. Nor do HMOs provide more preventive services, designated or identifiable as such, than do other forms of health-care delivery. Whether HMOs incorporate preventive features in their regular medical care has not been studied.

For reasons that are not fully understood, the HMO movement failed to take off in the early nineteen-seventies, even after a federal law was passed to promote their growth. Therefore, the HMO cannot today be considered seriously as a major vehicle for curbing health-care expenditures in this country in the foreseeable future.

Programs and policies outside the health-care industry can also influence health-care expenditures. For example, mandating a reduction in the maximum speed of automobiles on highways in order to conserve gasoline has led to a reduction in the number of traffic-accident casualties. The growth rate of the economy is another external influence on the size of health-care expenditures. In a labor-intensive industry, such as education or health care, gains in labor productivity lag behind those in the economy at large. As wages rise in the several sectors of the economy in accordance with average productivity gains for the entire economy, unit costs in labor-intensive industries rise. If the overall growth rate of the economy were to decline, unit costs in health care would rise at a lower rate than formerly, as would expenditures.

The possibility that concentrated unemployment in an area may lead to efforts to maintain or create jobs in the health-care industry has been noted. The danger exists that once inefficiencies are introduced into the system, they may become impossible to eliminate.

Finally, a major issue in health-care financing, and in formulating a plan for national health insurance, is how it will be paid for. Whether a plan is financed through general revenues, payroll taxes, employer premiums, or employee premiums, a shift toward more third-party payments is usual. As previously indicated, the magnitude of the shift toward public funding will be overstated unless tax expenditures are taken into account. It can be argued, perhaps, that the extent of the shift toward compulsory insurance will also be overstated, since acquisition of health insurance today at an individual's place of work is not entirely a voluntary act. The favored tax treatment of the employer contribution to health insurance, as well as its seeming positive influence on take-home pay, is a potent persuader for employees to join.

Most discussions of health-insurance plans pay a good deal of attention to the specific sources of financing, on the grounds that these have direct implications for the distribution of the tax burden and for its equity. Although economists display a good deal of diffidence in measuring the incidence of taxes—in locating the ultimate burden—they seem to hold certain common views. The payroll tax is generally held to be regressive because it applies only to wages and salaries and the rate is proportional up to a point (the maximum earnings base) where the tax stops. General federal revenues are held to be progressive because they draw heavily on the individual income tax.

The distribution of the costs of national health insurance can be approached in two different ways. One is to ascertain the effects of a particular health-insurance plan, income class by income class. The other is to consider the distribution of all taxes, by income class and by the percentile distribution of taxpayers. The first approach is exemplified by a recent Rand Corporation study of the distributional effects of four major health-insurance bills pending in Congress.[16] The findings of this study may be summarized as follows:

1) The amount of redistribution by income class that is entailed by a particular plan is a function of the size of the program—universality of enrollment plus scope and depth of benefits—and the proportion of total expenditures devolving upon the public sector. (In this context public financing today means federal financing.)

2) When both revenues and benefits are considered, the four plans display different patterns of net burden (benefits less taxes) by income class. This is particularly true for incomes above $30,000.

3) When account is taken of the financing of existing programs of health care that would presumably be displaced by health insurance, however, the differences among the four bills in net burden by income class are appreciably diminished.

4) For families with low incomes, undesired effects can always be mitigated by subsidies.

The other approach, that of looking at the total tax burden, is exemplified by a Brookings Institution study.[17] For the year 1966, it found that for most of the range of the income distribution—between the 10th and 97th percentiles of family units arrayed by size of income—the effective burden of the totality of all taxes is proportional. This holds true for all eight sets of incidence assumptions used in the Brookings study. The reasons that the effective rate of all taxes combined is virtually constant at 25-26 per cent throughout the distribution of taxpayers are: the offsetting behavior of individual taxes, the availability of devices for avoiding taxes legally as income increases, and presentation of the effective rates of tax by population percentile rather than by income class. The specific choice of financing mechanism will, however, make a difference at both extremes of the income distribution.

Choosing to finance an insurance plan through general·revenues or a payroll tax may, however, lead to other consequences. In an international comparison of health-care expenditures, it was found that the single common feature of countries with the highest rates of increase was the presence of "earmarked" social-security funds.[18] With the incorporation of Social Security funds in the federal budget, the increase in payroll taxes, and the emergence of doubt as to the actuarial soundness of the funds, it is no longer certain that increased appropriations would be voted almost automatically in the future, as they have been in the past.

Whether earmarked taxes and separate funds for health care would lead people to regard themselves as more entitled to services than they would be if health care were financed by general revenues is not known. It is conceivable that individuals would learn to keep an eye on the earmarked tax and try to curb their use of services in an effort to keep down the size of the tax.

Maintaining a separate health-care fund can serve to promote stability of funding from year to year. Given the persistence of the patterns of incidence of disease and injury in a population and the habitual patterns surrounding the utilization of health-care services, stability of funding may have many advantages.

Finally, although earmarking of funds for health care may deserve consideration on its own merits, the distributional effects of the payroll tax would change if some of the proposals to reform it or to integrate it with the federal individual income tax were adopted.

The findings and arguments of the paper can now be summarized. Health-care expenditures in this country have moved steadily and markedly upward. Over the past decade, the rate of increase has accelerated. In relation to the GNP, the trend in the United States is similar to that in most developed countries.

It is reasonable to expect that in the normal course of events, national health insurance would lead to an increase in expenditures for health care. The size of the increase obviously depends on the enrollment provisions of the particular plan and on the breadth and depth of the benefits provided. In addition, the size of increase would depend on the regulations promulgated in order to implement the plan and, perhaps even more, on the future expansion of health-care resources—facilities and manpower. Steps are therefore in order to constrain further increases in health-care expenditures, whether national health insurance is enacted now or in the future.

The question, how much can a country afford to spend on health care, is not meaningful. Rather, the question should be, how much does it choose to spend. It is difficult to arrive at a single answer for several reasons: differences of opinion concerning the ultimate objectives of health care, problems in measuring the effectiveness or outcome of health care, difficulties in valuing improvements in health status, especially reductions in mortality, lack of consensus on how society is to deal with poor personal health habits, and lack of agreement on the standard of equity to be pursued—equality of access to health care or equality of utilization. There seems to be no objective, scientific way to determine how much a country is to spend on health care either in total or in its individual categories.

Among the prominent approaches that have been proposed to curb future increases in health-care expenditures are cost sharing by consumers, changes in the mechanisms and formulas for reimbursing health-care providers, curtailing the future expansion of health-care resources, and promoting the rapid growth of the HMO. But for a variety of reasons, substantial reliance on cost sharing is not desirable. The HMO likewise has its limitations, and its future prospects are, at best, uncertain.

One is led to stress improvement in reimbursement policies and practices and slowing down the rate of expansion of health-care resources. Each approach poses difficulties of its own. The former is pervaded by all the concerns that currently surround government regulation. The latter may not be possible to accomplish, if past experience is any guide. We cannot exercise too much vigilance with respect to regulation to insure its fairness as well as efficiency, or exert too much effort in the attempt to curb the growth of resources at the national, state, and local levels.

In considering alternative national health-insurance plans, sources of financing are always an issue. However, when the distribution of the total tax burden is kept in mind, the proportion of the burden imposed on most taxpayers is approximately equal. As Fuchs has observed, most families will pay the same share under any health-insurance plan.[19]

REFERENCES

[1]Congressional Budget Office, Congress of the United States, *Budget Options for Fiscal Year 1977: A Report to the Senate and House Committees on the Budget* (U.S. Government Printing Office, Washington, D.C., 1976), pp. 151-67.

[2]Marjorie Smith Mueller and Robert M. Gibson, "National Health Expenditures, Fiscal Year 1975," *Social Security Bulletin*, 39:2 (February, 1976), pp. 3-21.

[3]David Alan Ehrlich, *The Health-Care Cost Explosion: Which Way Now?* (Bern, 1975), pp. 12-16 and 22-23.

[4]Comptroller General of the United States, *History of the Rising Costs of the Medicare and Medicaid Programs and Attempts to Control These Costs: 1966–1975* (General Accounting Office, Washington, D.C., February 11, 1976), pp. 4-8.

[5]Budget of the United States Government, *Special Analyses, Fiscal Year 1977* (Analysis F, U.S. Government Printing Office, Washington, D.C., 1976), pp. 116-37.

[6]Council on Wage and Price Stability, *The Problem of Rising Health Care Costs* (Executive Office of the President, Washington, D.C., 1976), pp. 16-17.

[7]*Budget Options, 1977*, cited above, note 1.

[8]*Rising Health Care Costs*, cited above, note 6.

[9]Herbert E. Klarman, *Hospital Care in New York City* (New York, 1963), pp. 477-78.

[10]Marjorie Smith Mueller and Paula A. Piro, "Private Health Insurance in 1974: A Review of Coverage, Enrollment, and Financial Experience," *Social Security Bulletin*, 39:3 (March, 1976), pp. 3-20.

[11]Julian Pettengill, "Financial Position of Private Community Hospitals, 1961-71," *Social Security Bulletin*, 36:11 (November, 1973), pp. 3-19.

[12]Bridger M. Mitchell and William B. Schwartz, "The Financing of National Health Insurance," *Science*, 192 (May 14, 1976), pp. 621-29.

[13]Anne A. Scitovsky and Nelda M. Snyder, "Effect of Coinsurance on Use of Physician Services," *Social Security Bulletin*, 35:6 (June, 1972), pp. 3-19.

[14]R. G. Beck, "An Analysis of the Demand for Physicians' Services in Saskatchewan," Ph.D. Dissertation, University of Alberta, Edmonton, Alberta, 1971.

[15]Regina Loewenstein, "Early Effects of Medicare on the Health Care of the Aged," *Social Security Bulletin*, 34:4 (April, 1971), pp. 3-21.

[16]Mitchell and Schwartz, cited above, noted 12.

[17]Joseph A. Pechman and Benjamin A. Okner, *Who Bears the Tax Burden?* (Brookings Institution, Washington, D.C., 1974).

[18]Henry Aaron, "Social Security: International Comparisons," in Otto Eckstein, ed., *Studies in the Economics of Income Maintenance* (Brookings Institution, Washington, D.C., 1967), pp. 13-48.

[19]Victor R. Fuchs, *Who Shall Live?* (New York, 1974), p. 128.

Appendix Table A
SELECTED DATA ON HEALTH-CARE EXPENDITURES, UNITED STATES, SELECTED YEARS, 1929-75 (IN BILLIONS OF DOLLARS)

| Year | Total health-care expenditures | | Community hosps. expends. | Physician services | Nursing-home care | Sum of (3), (4), and (5) |
	Amount (1)	Per cent of GNP (2)	(3)	(4)	(5)	
1929	$ 3,589	3.6%	$ 380	$ 994	na	$ 1,374
1935	2,846	4.1	414	744	na	1,158
1940	3,863	4.1	551	946	$ 28	1,525
1950	12,028	4.6	2,234	2,689	178	5,101
1955	17,330	4.6	3,464	3,632	291	7,387
1960	25,856	5.2	5,706	5,580	480	11,766
1965	38,892	5.9	9,222	8,405	1,271	18,898
1966	42,109	5.9	9,721	8,865	1,407	19,993
1967	47,879	6.2	11,510	9,738	1,751	22,999
1968	53,765	6.5	13,967	10,734	2,360	27,061
1969	60,617	6.7	15,965	11,842	3,057	30,864
1970	69,202	7.2	18,669	13,443	3,818	35,930
1971	77,162	7.6	21,418	15,098	4,890	41,406
1972	86,687	7.9	23,925	16,527	5,860	46,312
1973	95,384	7.8	26,589	17,995	6,650	51,234
1974	104,032	7.7	30,115	19,571	7,450	57,136
1975	118,500	8.3	35,610	22,100	9,000	66,710

Sources: Tables 1 and 4 of reference cited in note 2, and Herbert E. Klarman, "Planning for Facilities," in Eli Ginzberg, ed., *Regionalization and Health Policy* (Washington, D.C., Government Printing Office, [forthcoming]), Table 1.

LEON EISENBERG, M.D.

The Search for Care

IT IS, AT FIRST GLANCE, CURIOUS that dissatisfaction with medicine in America is at its most vociferous just at a time when doctors have at their disposal the most powerful medical technology the world has yet seen. The "old fashioned" general practitioner, with few drugs that really worked and not much surgery to recommend, is for some reason looking good to many people—in retrospect, at least. In the past, if the patient had a serious infection, all the doctor could do was wait for its resolution; now he has powerful antibiotics. In the past, if the patient had cancer, the recommendable surgery was limited and uncertain in its effects; now, potent anti-metabolites, radiation, and many curative operations are available. Compared with the "good old days," modern treatment provides an effective range of drugs and procedures that are curative for a long list of diseases, and palliative for many more. How, then, can we explain the paradox that more effective medicine has resulted in nostalgia for a medically primitive past?

Some complaints concentrate on rising costs, and the new technology has certainly contributed to these, primarily because it requires more technicians. At the turn of the century, the ratio of supporting personnel to doctors was about 1 to 2; now it can be as high as 15 to 1. Because this shift occurred practically unnoticed, no effort was made to plan for the complexities it introduced. Other complaints concentrate on the difficulty of gaining access to care, and technology has indeed added to this also. Physicians tend to cluster around hospitals in big cities, partly to keep up to date with their specialties and partly to have available the technology, the supporting consultants, specialist nurses, machines, and technicians they may need. The maldistribution of available doctors between urban and rural areas is, if anything, even more pronounced in the developing countries, where the concentration of doctors in urban areas is almost complete. But there is small comfort in recognizing that this is a worldwide phenomenon. The patient who cannot find a doctor when he needs one will not be content with explanations about the sociology of medicine. Important as they are, problems of cost seem to have less to do with public dissatisfaction with medical care than access does, particularly in rural areas and in the central city.

Still, even patients with doctors to consult and the means to pay the bills are disenchanted. Neither cost nor access explains away the paradox that although we know the "old family doctor" had almost no decisive remedies to offer for serious disease, we nevertheless lament his disappearance. A part of this attitude is no doubt simply nostalgia for what only seems to have been a happier past, but is it not also possible that something the family doctor provided was lost or diminished in the transition to more scientific and more aggressive medical management?

Health practitioners of one sort or another are as old as human society.[1] As soon as some division of labor and specialization of function were required by the level of technology and accommodated by the culture, priest-doctors invariably made their appearance. Methods of diagnosis and ritualized regimes of treatment have been present in every society, however primitive its technology; so have the shaman, the witch doctor, and the faith healer. It was to these that ill members of the tribe or village turned for help. The potency of the witch-doctor's pharmacopoeia may not have matched ours, but many of his patients did get better, and even the ones that did not were likely at least to feel comforted. He gave a name to what had been mysterious, he offered an explanation for its cause, he prescribed a ritual for its exorcism, and he legitimized dying. At the least, the patient felt less alone; at best he was restored to his former health.

The folk wisdom that was transmitted by oral tradition guided those earliest "physicians"; trial and error added to their stock of remedies. But more powerful than their medicaments was the magical (psychological) influence of their rituals and ceremonies; they got—and still get—results. Whatever we may think of the rationale they offer for the mechanisms of disease and the superstition that surrounds their ministrations, we must admit their effectiveness.

Over succeeding millennia in the West, as science became more systematized, its metaphors were introduced into the formal training of physicians. The nature of "explanation" changed, but the empirical content of medical practice was not materially altered until the present century. As late as 1860, Oliver Wendell Holmes could still write that, except for opium and wine, "if the whole materia medica, as now used, could be sunk to the bottom of the sea, it would be all the better for mankind—and all the worse for the fishes!"

Why have human societies continued to support and to honor healers over so many thousands of years even in the face of their obviously limited effects on mortality and even on morbidity? Obviously they fulfill a vital function in responding to human distress, a function whose effectiveness cannot be measured simply by weighing the biological potency of their medicines. It is not merely that patients "get better" after they consult healers—they would have anyway, most of the time, because the common illnesses usually cure themselves (although that has never kept the doctor from assuming the credit nor the patient from granting it). But patients *feel* they have gotten better sooner for having consulted a practitioner certified as possessing special prerogatives in sanctioning illnesses and arcane skills in restoring health. A significant part of the discomfort and dysfunction that accompanies illness stems from apprehension, and apprehension is a relievable symptom by human interaction—all else being equal, less fear equals less pain.

Objective physiological functions themselves are equally altered by psychic factors. For example, an episode of asthma, though triggered by allergy or infection, is made worse by the agonizing feeling of not being able to get enough air. The arrival of a physician and the expectation that relief will be forthcoming may diminish the severity of the attack even before the medication has had time to reach an effective blood concentration. In a sense, the mere presence of the doctor is the medicine. When relief is produced, faith in the doctor is enhanced, and the power of the medical presence is even greater than before. What is true for respiration is true for any bodily function that is regulated by the brain through neural and hormonal pathways and therefore responds to psychosocial influences.

Thus far, we have emphasized the ritual qualities of the healing arts: the changes that are produced by belief, ceremony, and expectation. The capacity to evoke them resides in traditional practitioners and contemporary physicians equally. Both interact with sick persons in a cultural context that defines the possibilities for patient response; either, out of that context, is apt to be ineffective for the ordinary ailments of mankind, except insofar as the administration of specifically active drugs produces direct pharmacologic responses. Unfortunately, an excessively narrow view of what is "scientific" and an altogether unwarranted belief in the extent to which modern medicine is "specific" have caused disdain in some physicians toward these interpersonal aspects of medical care. They forget that psychophysiological responses to the physician are no less real than responses to drugs and, on the other hand, that solid evidence for the effectiveness of many contemporary medical procedures has yet to be provided. In a sense, both traditional and modern practitioners are unwitting captives of their own efficacy: they ascribe the benefit they produce to the things they give when—more often—it is how they behave toward the patient that is decisive.[2]

To disdain the "magic" in medicine is to cast aside a significant part of its effectiveness; to rely on it blindly is to use the lesser part of the considerable opportunity it represents. The changes produced by ritual have a significant toxicity. Responsibility for change rests with the physician; the patient remains passive. Benefit is almost independent of the rationality of the process: the patient remains dependent on the physician. Yet the apprehension that enhances the doctor's influence as magician also makes the patient more willing to confide his private concerns about family, job, and lifestyles to the doctor, which may provide significant cues to the source of distress. Three out of four people with minor illnesses treat themselves; the other quarter, who seek care, are therefore responding to something more than physical discomfort. Complaints of illness are unequally distributed in the population, recurring in disproportionately large numbers among people under stress.[3] Sympathetic exploration of personal circumstances in the course of the medical interview can show the patient options available to him for changing the conditions that have produced the stress in the first place and thus suggest how he can assume the responsibility for maintaining his own health.

These benefits apply with equal force when the physician has biological remedies to offer. Mere prescription does not assure consumption; drugs work only if they are taken. Studies of compliance with medical regimens reveal that one-quarter to one-half of the patients fail to take the drugs prescribed.[4] The very word "compliance" points to part of the problem; its connotation of subservience emphasizes the inequality in the relationship between doctor and patient. "Doctor" also used to mean "an educated man," and comes from the Latin *docere*, "to teach." The doctor's task ought still to be to educate the patient about the meaning of the illness and the methods for its remedy, after he has learned the patient's conception of its cause and how it might be treated. The process is one of exchange of information; the goal is the demystification of medical procedures, so that the patient is able to make his own decisions and thereby assume responsibility for acting.

The comfort that treatment brings—what has been termed "caring" as opposed to "curing"—is what accounts for the antiquity and the continuity of the physician's function in society. Present-day disenchantment with physicians, at a time when they can do more than ever in history to halt and repair the ravages of serious illness, probably reflects the perception by people that they are not being cared for. This is the result of much more than the way the physician behaves when the consultation occurs. It begins with difficulties in gaining access to care, including delays in obtaining appointments and frustrations with time spent in waiting rooms; it includes the attitudes and behavior of other health workers (the receptionist, the nurse, and the technician); it is influenced by the patient's own conceptions of what an "emergency" is, what complaints require attention, and whether it is "fair" to have to go to the emergency room or the physician's office rather than to have a home visit.

The very success of medicine, or at least the publicity about scientific advances and new cures, has had the effect of increasing demands for its services. Not so long ago, hospitals were viewed as places to die rather than as places where miracles could be worked. But this has in turn effected changes in health-care-delivery patterns: increased size breeds bureaucratization and impersonality. While these features of American society may be tolerated, however reluctantly, in certain other areas, they are particularly resented in so intimate and personal a matter as illness.

Encounter between physician and patient can also be marred by a mismatch between the consumer's and the provider's conceptions of what constitutes appropriate behavior. The patient wants time, sympathetic attention, and concern for himself as a person. The physical examination or laboratory test is acceptable insofar as it suggests thoroughness and indicates that the doctor is taking the complaint seriously, but the patient has few criteria by which to judge the appropriateness of the technical aspects of care. He will resent an apparent preoccupation with somatic matters if it supplants an interest in his individuality. Parents interviewed by Reader in a New York medical clinic, for example, mentioned interpersonal qualities as often as they did technical competence when discussing attributes they sought in a good physician.[5] Mothers interviewed at a Los Angeles pediatric clinic by Korsch reported lack of warmth or friendliness, failure to understand their worries, inadequate explanations of illness, and confusing medical terms as their principal causes of dissatisfaction.[6]

The physician, on the other hand, regards time as a precious commodity, given the number of patients he has to see and his interest in making what he thinks is a suitable income. Moreover, he regards accuracy of diagnosis as essential to effective management and is very naturally concerned with protecting himself against possible malpractice suits. He may regard a discussion of personal issues as quite superfluous to his primary medical responsibility, that is, identifying organic disease. Neither patient nor doctor is likely to be aware of what the public-health worker would regard as an equally serious lapse in their encounter—namely, the insufficient attention given to maintaining health rather than responding to individual episodes of illness. The patient, the practitioner, and the public-health worker view the doctor's role in very different terms.

The revolution in medical education produced by Abraham Flexner's remarkable study in the first decade of this century was extraordinarily successful in introducing a firm scientific foundation into the training of physicians. Shoddy proprietary schools were shut down; basic-science departments were immeasurably strengthened; the groundwork for systematic clinical investigation was established by assembling full-time clinical faculties. The cumulative triumphs of the new medicine led, however, to a spiraling, self-reinforcing trend toward specialization. The benefit was enormous: an increasing capacity for the successful management of severe and life-threatening illness. The cost was also enormous: an increasing disjunction between what the doctor was trained to do and what he or she was called upon to do in general medical practice. The public continued quite properly to want attention directed to its everyday problems, in addition to being assured of the full use of the new biomedical capabilities; the profession tended to lose sight of the former in grappling with the latter.

What are the nature and distribution of the complaints patients bring to a family physician's office? Fry has documented his experience in twenty years of general practice in London.[7] Two-thirds of the visits were for "minor conditions" described as illnesses of brief duration, usually self-curing and carrying small risk of consequential after-effects; about a quarter were for chronic illness, in which palliation and limitation of disability are the most that can be offered; and less than one in twenty were for major illnesses which carry a threat to life. The Cleveland Family Study conducted by Dingle and his colleagues at Western Reserve Medical School documents similar findings.[8] For example, 60 per cent of the illness episodes over a ten-year period in the study population were accounted for by "undifferentiated" respiratory illnesses, for which only general supportive measures are available; only 3 per cent were due to "specific" respiratory illnesses, responsive to drug treatment.

Paradoxically, in view of these figures, the medical student is trained, not in family practice, but in a university hospital and its clinics, where the proportions of minor and serious illness are reversed. When Hodgkin contrasted his clinical experience during his medical training with that in a year of general practice, he found that patients with cancer were seen 50 times as frequently in training as after it, while psychological problems were seen three times as often in practice as in training; lobar pneumonia was ten times as frequent in training as in practice, bronchitis, the reverse.[9] "Simple anxiety," rarely encountered (or better, rarely recognized) in training, was the most frequent disorder in practice; malignancy of the gastrointestinal tract, the most common entity in training, was rarely seen in practice. No doubt, learning how to manage severe illness also prepares the student for the management of lesser ones, but only if the emotional needs of the patient are not lost sight of in the midst of the technical complexities of care.

A sizable proportion (one-third to one-half) of the cases in general medical practice have a significant emotional or behavioral component.[10] Some emotional problems are obvious anxiety states or neuroses; many more appear in the form of bodily complaints that have no ascertainable organic basis and reflect response to psychosocial stresses; an important minority (one or two per cent) present themselves as severe psychiatric illnesses. Many medical and surgical disorders are the result of maladaptive behavior: cirrhosis from alcoholism, lung cancer and heart disease from smoking, obesity and its complications from over-eating. Accidents, suicides, and homicides account for three-quarters of the deaths in males from ages 15 to 24 and as many as a third from ages 35 to 44. Between 55 and 64, one-sixth of male deaths can be traced to cirrhosis and lung cancer. Estimates of the size of the problem derived from mortality data understate the magnitude of the associated morbidity: the number of individuals disabled by these causes at any given time far exceed those who die from them. Whether drinking, smoking, over-eating, or reckless driving are "medical" problems may be open to question, but their consequence for the health-care system is not. To recognize their prevalence and severity is not to have remedies for them; it does, however, identify aspects of social behavior that merit far greater efforts at modification, if there is to be any hope of improving the national health record. It serves also to reemphasize the importance of the educational function of health workers in helping patients to understand the relationship between personal behavior and illness.

Severe psychiatric disorders continue to constitute major public-health problems, despite progress in their management.[11] Resident state-mental-hospital populations have declined in the past twenty years from more than half a million to less than 200,000; now the average length of stay has been reduced from more than six months to less than six weeks. Not only does this mean a more rapid recovery, but shortening the hospital stay makes it less likely that the patient will settle into chronic patienthood. A major part of the statistical change can be attributed to the modification of the locked-asylum system and the introduction of powerful new drugs (the phenothiazines, the antidepressants, and lithium). However, reliance on state-hospital data alone exaggerates the gains that have occurred. For one thing, more psychiatric patients are now being treated in general hospitals and are not counted in state tabulations; for another, some patients have been transferred to nursing homes; worst of all, others have been administratively discharged to "welfare hotels" and rented rooms with dubious effect on their mental or physical well-being.

When figures from all institutions are combined the frequency of hospitalized cases of psychiatric disease in the general population has changed hardly at all during the past twenty years (remaining at a rate of about 800/100,000), although the length of each stay has been dramatically shortened. Over the same period, official counts of the number of out-patient episodes of care provided for by mental-health facilities have increased fivefold. Schizophrenia results in more than 900,000 episodes of care each year, a figure which undoubtedly understates actual prevalence because it includes only hospital and clinic reports; the figure for affective disorders, 650,000 episodes per year, is underestimated even more, and depression is frequently treated by family physicians who do not even report it. A conservative estimate would place the likely total at about 2 million acute psychotic episodes each year.[12]

Epidemiological studies of the prevalence of psychiatric disorder in the general population show wide variations by social class, residence, age, sex, marital status, and other demographic variables; impaired social function has been estimated to be as high as 15 per cent to 20 per cent and incapacitation, 2 per cent to 4 per cent. Yet, clinical training in psychiatric diagnosis and treatment is often an elective rather than a required course in the undergraduate medical curriculum. When it is offered, the time allotted to it is trivial compared to the frequency with which examples of these disorders will be met in primary care and to the period required for the acquisition of genuine skill in their management. Such training is rarely included in the residency training programs for internists and pediatricians, the groups that have supplanted the general practitioner. It should not surprise us that physicians will avoid problems they feel inadequate to manage by relying on the promiscuous prescription of tranquilizing drugs. The patient needs someone to listen, to sympathize, and to help him work out his problems, not to multiply maladaptive behavior by adding to it a dependency on drugs.

Another role of the doctor is to provide support for the patient and the family in the face of death.[13] Ours is a culture busily engaged in denying and avoiding the inevitability of dying, although even the most optimistic expectations for medical advance are for further postponement, but never the prevention, of death. At no time in his life is the patient so likely to need support, or be more afraid of abandonment than when he senses himself to be dying. When the medical staff itself perceives death as defeat, however, it may react by avoiding the patient or offering platitudinous responses to questions that deserve compassionate answers. Technical equipment may be injudiciously employed to prolong the agonies of dying by maintaining biological existence long after human life has ceased. An open admission of the universality of death may enable the staff to help the patient function as he or she has been until life ceases. The family, with its feelings of impending bereavement, its guilt for not having done more, or for wishing the end, and its anger at the unfairness of death, is also in need of support. Indeed, the psychological abandonment of the patient is often precipitated by the collapse of the family. Nor is the family immune to physiological stress. There is, for example, evidence that death rates are higher among widows and widowers than would be expected on the basis of age, while children are vulnerable to psychiatric disorders under comparable circumstances. Here again, we confront an essential function of physicians for which little or no time is afforded during training. The training should involve not so much what to *do* as what to *be*. Required is an opportunity for the open and honest sharing of feelings and for thoughtful reflection. The physician who ministers to the patient and the family during death not only performs a crucial function, but may be received more gladly and gratefully than in those far more dramatic cases where he has succeeded in reversing the biology of a disease.

It is evident that there is a large gap between the "need for support" and the capacity of the health-care system, as presently constituted, to provide it. The demands will almost certainly increase. By the year 2000, the number of persons over 65 will have risen by 50 per cent if there is no upward change in present life expectancy, and more if there is. More old people means more disability, less capacity for self-sufficient functioning, and more dependence on social and health supports. Medical advance itself is likely to add to the burden of chronic handicap by diminishing the mortality from acute illness. There is nothing on the horizon to suggest any diminution of life stresses; therefore psychological and psychiatric disturbances will continue to be a major source of demand for care. In the absence of a radical transformation in our culture and a revamping of its social institutions, it will be to the health-care system that Americans will turn for relief from distress. We may question whether this is wise, but there is little doubt that it will continue.

In what ways can the health-care system be modified to respond to these requirements? Elsewhere in this issue, David Rogers has outlined the possibilities with regard to professional roles and training for primary care. We will limit ourselves to a few additional points.

First of all, without a far more rapid expansion in the training of nurse practitioners and other paramedical personnel than seems likely to occur in the foreseeable future, physicians will remain the principal providers of primary care. Therefore, it will be essential to revise medical training by placing greater emphasis on the art and science of primary care. We do not propose that the epidemiology of illness in general practice alone dictate the allocation of training time in medical school. Not only the frequency but the consequences of an illness matter: the availability of means to prevent, to detect, and to treat it, and the relative complexity of the task of learning to understand it. Patients do not come to doctors with their problems all sorted out; distinguishing major from minor ailments requires a great deal of knowledge. Supporting the dying patient is no substitute for saving his life, whenever a meaningful life is possible.

But there is something wrong when training in therapy focuses on disorders so uncommon in general practice and so complex in their management that they would almost always be referred to a specialized center in any case. It is a rare generalist, indeed, who can maintain skills that are not frequently practiced. Providing human comfort and reassurance, and being ready to discuss problems are skills in frequent demand; such skills are slighted in training. It is this aspect of patient care that the "old family doctor" is thought to have managed so capably. New doctors must be taught to develop the compassion and skill that the practitioner of yesteryear acquired over decades in the course of the continuous and comprehensive care he provided;[14] training in the behavioral sciences and psychiatry should help to impart these skills more quickly. But unless the medical faculty is able to convey to students the importance of primary care, indeed, the intellectual challenge and satisfactions that primary care can provide, its practice will continue to be regarded as trivial, boring, and beneath the dignity of a professional physician.

Even if nurse practitioners and physician "extenders" are viewed as being most suited by temperament, role, and training for the increasing responsibilities of primary care, it nonetheless will remain vital that the physician be thoroughly familiar with this type of care. To the extent that physicians are to supervise primary care, they must understand it; if they consider it of no interest, it will have no interest for their surrogates and will be slighted whenever resources are allocated. Given the dominance of the physician within the health-care system, research, training, and service in primary care will almost certainly decline unless they remain among his central concerns. We are not recommending such Draconian measures as those employed in mainland China, where academic physicians are required to live and practice in the countryside, but more realistic priorities would surely result if academic physicians were better to acquaint themselves with community health problems.

A thorough understanding of the supportive aspects of medical care is as essential for the specialist as it is for the general physician, who practices or supervises primary care. The patient with a complex biological disorder is likely to be highly distraught by the time specialized care is required. Apprehensions multiply as illness evades correction by simple measures; dependency is increased in the face of a diminished capacity for self-sufficiency. The patient and family require understanding and explanation. Concern for the complexity of tertiary care need not require that the humanistic aspects of care be overlooked.

When there is need for continuing care, prescription of such care in a medical center does not guarantee its delivery. Designing programs of treatment requires an intimate knowledge of the social systems of the community. Moreover, it demands an ability to communicate effectively with the patient and those taking care of him. Specialized care differs from primary care in the biological problems with which it deals, the specific skills its practitioners acquire in the management of such problems, and the technologies they use. But both kinds of care share a common obligation to respond to patients as human beings.

To list the ingredients of a medical-practice pattern responsive to patient needs and to recommend changes in medical education are simple enough; to propose the means to bring them into being is far more difficult. Major institutional barriers stand in the way. Within academia, the premium is on diagnostic sophistication rather than on supportive care. There are few Brownie points given for compassion. Specialists dominate the scene. Change will require a revolution in the power structure.

More decisive are the conditions of medical practice. Third-party reimbursement schemes make procedures (drugs, tests, injections, surgery) profitable and penalize the doctor who takes the time to listen and to explain. The office fee is the same for a short encounter as for a longer one. The conscientious doctor will earn less than his counterpart who runs an injection mill. Escalating malpractice suits make it safer to rule out every remote diagnostic possibility than to treat the patient humanely on a pragmatic basis. For example, the clinical signs and symptoms after a head injury almost always distinguish minor from serious problems. Today, most doctors order skull x-rays "to be on the safe side" lest they be sued if an insignificant linear fracture should subsequently be detected. It costs more to order films and it exposes the patient to radiation. But it takes a courageous physician *not* to do it. Finally, the financing and organization of the health system concentrate money and power in hospitals and medical centers. Community services for ambulatory patients are on the sidelines, under-financed and secondary.

This analysis suggests the need for structural changes to make educational recommendations more than pious platitudes. More emphasis should be placed on commitment to human service in the selection of medical students than on good academic credentials alone. One suggestion would be a requirement for one to two years of service (the equivalent of a domestic Peace Corps) in an urban ghetto or remote rural area; the student's sensitivity to human needs would be evaluated not only by his/her job supervisor but by a consumer panel. Within the medical school, primary-care clinicians should be members of the curriculum committee in order to assure a proper balance between generalist and specialist orientation in the student's education. Accreditation standards for residency training programs must redress the balance between inpatient and outpatient experience.

The evidence we have, however, suggests that it is the organization of medical practice rather than undergraduate education that has the most decisive influence on a physician's professional behavior. More comprehensive insurance coverage for out-patient care will diminish the thrust for unnecessary hospitalization. Reimbursement schedules should bear a closer relationship to the time the physician spends with a patient and less to his specialty and to the procedures he carries out. There is a need for a major revision of malpractice insurance. Those patients who suffer from unpreventable misfortune deserve compensation in the same way as victims of industrial or automobile accidents. It is absurd to require proof of physician culpability, since the suffering of the patient is the same whether or not the doctor is at fault. When the doctor is at fault through negligence, the remedy is not an insurance settlement which has no effect on physician behavior since premiums are passed through to the patient. What is called for is disciplinary action against the offender. Doctors have to be judged on the basis of whether they act prudently on the basis of current medical knowledge; to hold them responsible for the patient's disease and the imperfections of medical science is absurd. It leads to increased costs and self-protective behavior on the part of doctors. Finally, professional audit, with the results of peer evaluation fed back to the practitioner, is essential if physician performance is to be improved. The goal of professional audit (in contrast to fiscal audit which aims at detecting fraud) is on upgrading the skills of doctors in practice by providing them with essential information on how well they are doing. In a teaching hospital, the public review of all medical decisions in the course of resident training keeps the staff on its toes. Peer pressure in a medical group exerts a powerful influence for professional excellence. Similar schemes in practice settings will have similar effects.

Over the long run, a medical care system is both inadequate and inappropriate as a mechanism for responding to the range of human needs that has been thrust upon it.[15] It is expected today to provide services formerly supplied by the extended family, the church, and the schools. Palliative responses to social dislocation are inevitably self-defeating; victims multiply faster than personnel can be trained to resuscitate them. If the twin goals of improving the public's health and reducing the demand for medical care are to be attained, three kinds of efforts are required: (1) research in educational methods must be undertaken to encourage health-promoting behavior; (2) biological research must be fostered for disease prevention, and (3) social innovation must be attempted on a new scale if a more humane society is to be created.

Diseases linked to bad habits in their pathogenesis are among the major producers of morbidity and mortality; destructive patterns of smoking, drinking, and eating have irreversible biological consequences. Better trauma surgery will be trivial in its impact on health compared with the institution of safe driving habits. Improved methods for treating lung cancer are poor substitutes for reduced smoking. Although accepting self-destructive behavior as a "fact of life" makes little sense, the success achieved in campaigns to alter disease-related behavior has so far been modest.[16] But so also have been the resources allocated to their design and testing. It is precisely the limitations of current methods that warrent a sizable investment in research to advance theory and practice in mass education. That change in long-standing patterns of behavior can be produced on a massive scale has already been proved by the Chinese. The only question we must ask when we look at their example is whether any modification of habitual behavior on a large scale will necessarily threaten the value we place on individual self-determination. We must assess the cost before we seek the benefit.

Medical intervention after the onset of illness has little influence on longevity, as is attested by the negligible change in adult life expectancy in the United States over the past twenty years despite the remarkable technical virtuosity of modern medical measures. However, when fundamental biological knowledge of disease is acquired and applied as a preventive measure, striking changes do result: consider the annual saving of 2,000 lives, 3,000 cases of severe paralysis, and $1 billion in costs which have derived from the total outlay of $40 million invested in basic research on the poliomyelitis virus.[17] Since the behavior-linked diseases we are concerned with here do not entirely fit the infectious-disease model, a more appropriate paradigm might be the inherited metabolic disorders such as phenylketonuria and galactosemia. Untreated, these conditions lead to severe mental deficiency and uncontrollable seizures; with routine screening of the newborn, however, cases can be detected early; the provision of special diets for infants and children with these abnormalities enables them to develop normally, or nearly so.

Some disorders associated with smoking, obesity, and alcoholism also have an important genetic link. The statistical relationship between smoking and lung cancer is unequivocal, but not all heavy smokers develop cancer. Genetic vulnerability, an additional key variable, intervenes.[18] Accurate identification by screening tests of those who are most vulnerable would permit the design of specifically targeted anti-smoking campaigns, less costly because they would have a smaller audience and probably more effective because the consequences of smoking for such individuals can be demonstrated with certainty.[19] There is, of course, another scenario possible. If research enables us to learn what it is that makes such individuals susceptible to carcinogenesis, measures to protect them even if they persist in smoking might be devised.

Similar approaches are possible for disorders arising from obesity and alcoholism. We are now able to detect some individuals with inherited disorders of fat metabolism that create high risk for coronary disease; modifications of diet and use of prophylactic medication can diminish that risk. Studies of alcoholics have demonstrated familial aggregations and links with other psychiatric disorders, so that alcoholism, too, would appear to be the result of social exposure combined with individual vulnerability. What we lack today is a way of determining when that vulnerability is present. If we could discover this, social programs for prevention could be directed to the 5 to 10 per cent at risk rather than diluting them among the entire population. Again, we may be able to devise methods to reduce vulnerability without requiring abstinence. Thus, additional knowledge derived from fundamental biological research can interact with new methods in behavioral sciences to permit the development of effective education for health maintenance.

Doctors and other health workers are even less able to assure happiness than they are to assure health. If work is unsatisfying to many in modern society, psycho-pharmacology is a toxic and inappropriate remedy for correcting the resulting tension and alienation. If unemployed workers are depressed, mental-health counseling may be a temporary source of comfort, but the only genuine solution is full employment. If children fail to thrive, child-guidance workers may diminish their misery, but they cannot guarantee their flowering in the midst of social disaster. As physicians, our daily practice with human ailments makes us aware of the extent to which problems of ill health flow from failures in our political, economic, and social institutions. The redesign of these institutions is the central challenge for the coming century, and gives the greatest promise for improving public health.

REFERENCES

[1] A. M. Kleinman, "Toward a Comparative Study of Medical Systems," *Science, Medicine, and Man*, 1 (1973), pp. 55-65.

[2] L. Eisenberg, "The Ethics of Intervention: Acting Amidst Ambiguity," *Journal of Child Psychology and Psychiatry*, 16 (1975), pp. 93-104.

[3] D. Mechanic, "Social Psychologic Factors Affecting the Presentation of Bodily Complaints," *New England Journal of Medicine*, 288 (1972), pp. 1132-39.

[4] R. J. Haggerty and K. J. Roghmann, "Non-Compliance and Self Medication," *Pediatric Clinics of North America*, 19 (1972), 101-15.

[5] G. Reader, L. Pratt, and M. Mudd, "What Patients Expect From Their Doctors," *Modern Hospital*, 89 (1957), pp. 88-94.

[6] B. Korsch, E. Gozzi, and U. Francis, "Gaps in Doctor-Patient Communication: Doctor-Patient Interaction and Patient Satisfaction," *Pediatrics*, 42 (1968), pp. 855-71.

[7] J. Fry, *Profiles of Disease: A Study in the Natural History of Common Diseases* (London, 1966).

[8] J. H. Dingle, "The Ills of Man," *Scientific American*, 229 (1973), pp. 76-89.

[9] K. Hodgkin, *Towards Earlier Diagnosis: A Guide to General Practice* (3rd ed., London, 1973).

[10]K. L. White, "Life and Death and Medicine," *Scientific American*, 229 (1973). pp. 22-33.

[11]L. Eisenberg, "Psychiatric Intervention," *Scientific American*, 229 (1973), pp. 116-27.

[12]Eisenberg, "Primary Prevention and Early Detection in Mental Illness," *Bulletin of the New York Academy of Medicine*, 51 (1975), pp. 118-29.

[13]A. D. Weisman, *On Dying and Denying: A Psychiatric Study of Terminality* (New York, 1972).

[14]J. B. Richmond, "Patient Reaction to the Teaching and Research Situation," *Journal of Medical Education*, 36 (1961), pp. 347-52.

[15]M. Lalonde, *A New Perspective on the Health of Canadians* (Ottawa, 1974).

[16]N. Maccoby and J. W. Farquhar, "Communication for Health," *Journal of Communications*, 25 (1975), pp. 114-26.

[17]H. H. Fudenberg, "Fiscal Returns of Biomedical Research," *Journal of Investigative Dermatology*, 61, (1973), pp. 321-29.

[18]National Research Council, *Genetic Screening: Programs, Principles, and Research* (Washington, D.C., 1975).

[19]B. Childs, "Prospects for Genetic Screening," *Journal of Pediatrics*, 87 (1975), pp. 1125-32.

JULIUS B. RICHMOND, M.D.

The Needs of Children

ANY EVALUATION OF THE HEALTH of a society's children includes an evaluation of the entire social fabric to which they belong. Relatively few issues involving public health are limited strictly to children, in part because the welfare and education of the family are so intimately interwoven with the well-being of each child. While there have been obvious achievements in the field of child health and welfare, there are also striking deficiencies, and both need to be considered for what they tell us about health care in the United States today. Some of the developments that have become apparent over the past ten years are discussed below.

1) *Reduction in infant mortality:* In the decade from 1964 to 1974, a decline from 24.8 to 16.5 deaths per 1,000 live births reflected the substantial improvement in the general welfare of families as well as in the delivery of health services. Although the 1974 rate ranked the United States below fifteen other countries, it nonetheless represented a consistent downward trend. As Wegman[1] has pointed out, the lowest infant-mortality rates achieved today (less than 10 per 1,000 live births in Sweden, for example) are better than any pediatrician would have thought possible twenty-five years ago, and the improvement is expected to continue. The reason this country is lagging behind fifteen others is entirely attributable to the relatively higher death rates among non-whites and the poor. According to Bronfenbrenner:[2]

. . . infant mortality for non-whites in the United States is almost twice that for whites, the maternal death rate is four times as high, and there are a number of Southern states, and Northern metropolitan areas, in which the ratios are considerably higher. . . . One illuminating way of describing the differences in infant mortality by race is from a time perspective. Babies born of non-white mothers are today dying at a rate which white babies have not experienced for almost a quarter of a century.

It was not until 1973 that non-whites achieved the rate of 26.8 per thousand that had been achieved for whites in 1950.

The introduction of an effective federally funded maternal- and infant-care program in low-income areas led to a further reduction in infant-mortality rates, and this suggests that it is possible markedly to reduce ethnic and racial differentials still further. Thus in Denver, for example, there was a dramatic drop in infant mortality—from 34.2 per 1,000 live births in 1964 to 21.5 per 1,000 in 1969—in twenty-five census tracts in a target area where the program was adopted. In Birmingham, Alabama, the rate decreased from 25.4 in 1965 to 14.3 in 1969, and in Omaha from

247

33.4 in 1964 to 13.4 in 1970. Significant reductions also occurred in rates of prematurity, in repeated pregnancies among teenagers, and in conceptions among women over 35 and families with more than four children.

The impact of the maternal- and infant-care programs cannot be attributed wholly to medical intervention. The programs brought with them improved nutrition and better social services, and these necessarily had some effect on health as well. Here again, however, the effectiveness of these services was different for various ethnic groups. The Kessner[3] study of infant mortality in New York City revealed:

> . . . for mothers at socioeconomic risk, adequate medical care substantially reduced infant mortality rates for all races, but the figures for black and Puerto Rican families were still substantially greater than those for whites. In other words, other factors besides inadequate medical care contribute to producing the higher infant mortality for these non-white groups. Again these factors have to do with the social and economic conditions in which these families have to live. Thus, the results of the New York City study and other investigations point to the following characteristics as predictive of higher infant mortality: employment status of the breadwinner, mother unwed at infant's birth, married but no father in the home, number of children per room, mother under 20 or over 35, and parents' educational level.

2) *Changes in the causes of morbidity and mortality in children:* Progress in the natural sciences at the turn of the century led to an expansion of our knowledge of disease, particularly those of infectious and nutritional origin. These advances have, over the decades, resulted in striking declines in the infectious diseases, the nutritional deficiencies, and the gastrointestinal disorders that were the major causes of morbidity and mortality in the early decades of this century (Tables 1 and 2). These mortality rates are now less than one-tenth of what they were in 1920. This is not to say that infectious diseases and nutritional problems are no longer present, but that, when they are, they result largely from a failure to apply our knowledge rather than from

TABLE 1

LEADING CAUSES OF DEATH IN CHILDREN, BOTH SEXES,
1–4 YEARS OF AGE, 1920 AND 1970*

	1920			1970	
Rank	Cause	No./100,000	Rank	Cause	No./100,000
1	Influenza and pneumonia	283.7	1	Accidents	31.5
2	Diarrhea, enteritis, etc.	141.3	2	Congenital anomalies	9.7
2	Diphtheria	90.5	3	Influenza and pneumonia	7.6
4	Accidents	80.2	4	Malignant neoplasms	7.5
5	Whooping cough	57.7	5	Homicide	1.9
6	Measles	56.4	6	Meningitis	1.9
7	Tuberculosis, all forms	45.4	7	Diseases of the heart	1.7
8	Scarlet fever	23.2	8	Enteritis and diarrhea	1.4
9	Dysentery	12.8	9	Acute bronchitis and bronchiolitis	1.0
10	Diseases of the ear, nose, and throat	12.3	10	Meningococcal infections	1.0
	All causes	987.2		All causes	84.5

*Adapted from *Facts of Life And Death* (DHEW, National Center for Health Statistics, 1974), pp. 33-34.

TABLE 2
LEADING CAUSES OF DEATH IN CHILDREN, BOTH SEXES,
5–14 YEARS OF AGE, 1920 AND 1970*

	1920			1970	
Rank	Cause	No./100,000	Rank	Cause	No./100,000
1	Influenza and pneumonia	45.1	1	Accidents	20.1
2	Accidents	44.3	2	Malignant neoplasms	6.0
3	Diphtheria	28.0	3	Congenital anomalies	2.2
4	Tuberculosis	22.4	4	Influenza and pneumonia	1.6
5	Diseases of the heart	21.8	5	Homicide	0.9
6	Typhoid fever	7.1	6	Diseases of the heart	0.8
7	Diarrhea, enteritis	4.1	7	Cerebrovascular diseases	0.7
8	Chronic and unspecified nephritis	3.5	8	All other neoplasms	0.4
9	Diabetes mellitus	3.5	9	Suicide	0.3
			10	Bronchitis, emphysema, and asthma	0.3
	All causes	263.9		All causes	41.3

*Adapted from *Facts of Life and Death* (DHEW, National Center for Health Statistics, 1974), pp. 33-34.

ignorance about them. Partly as a result of these scientific advances, accidents have now become the leading cause of death among children in the first to fifteenth year. The rates are 31.5/100,000 for the 1-4-year group and 20.1/100,000 for the 5-14-year group. Oddly enough, accidents occur at a higher rate in the younger group when the child is presumably under the close supervision of adults. Death rates from accidents are approximately 150 per cent higher for non-white children than for whites.

Congenital anomalies are the second major cause of death in the 1-4-year group and rank third in the 5-14-year group (malignancy ranks second). Among the non-fatal illnesses, the National Center for Health Statistics reports (Table 3) indicate that the majority of acute illnesses in childhood are various forms of acute respiratory conditions.

Another approach for determining morbidity patterns is to examine the conditions that lead to the hospitalization of children. Although hereditary factors cannot always be clearly distinguished, it is estimated that from 30 to 35 per cent of hospital admissions are related to genetic factors.

3) *Decline in birth rate:* A remarkable decline in the birth rate has been yet another notable trend over the past decade. This decline is illustrated in the following table:

	BIRTHS	BIRTH RATE
1955	4,047,295	24.6
1960	4,257,850	23.7
1965	3,760,358	19.4
1970	3,731,386	18.4
1971	3,555,970	17.2
1972	3,256,000	15.6
1973	3,141,000	15.0
1974	3,166,000	15.0

TABLE 3
ACUTE CONDITIONS IN CHILDREN,
BOTH SEXES, UNITED STATES, 1971–1972*

Rank	Condition	Incidence, cases/100 persons per year
		0-6 years old
1	Respiratory conditions	214.4
2	Infective and parasitic diseases	52.3
3	All other acute conditions	46.5
4	Injuries	40.5
5	Digestive-system conditions	12.5
	All acute conditions	366.2
		6-16 years old
1	Respiratory conditions	159.3
2	Injuries	39.0
3	Infective and parasitic diseases	34.0
4	All other acute conditions	30.7
5	Digestive-system conditions	17.4
	All acute conditions	280.4

*Adapted from National Center for Health Statistics, *Acute Conditions: Incidence and Associated Disability, United States, July, 1971-June, 1972*, series 10, no. 88, January, 1974. Excluded from these statistics are all conditions not involving restricted activity or medical attention.

Sociologists have speculated that the largest factor in this decline may be a temporary trend by the young to postpone having children, rather than a permanent trend toward smaller families. The availability of family-planning information, the legalization of abortions, and public concern over population growth all influence birth rates, but it is impossible to predict the long-range effects of these factors.

The implications of a permanently lowered birth rate for child health, welfare, and educational services are more readily apparent. If the rate remains low, we will, by the year 2000, be caring for about 25 per cent fewer children than we were caring for in 1960. Unless there is a substantial decrease in the productivity of the nation's child-health personnel, this ought markedly to increase the availability of professional resources for child-health programs.

4) *Reduction in incidence of dental caries:* Dental caries remain the most common health problem of children, although, through the fluoridation of water supplies, this very common disorder could easily be brought under control. There is still great resistance to fluoridation in many communities, but the practice will no doubt eventually become universal and, as it does so, it ought to diminish—if not eliminate—the current major shortage in dental personnel. Half of all children in the United States under 15 have never been to a dentist,[4] and 75 per cent in families with annual incomes under $2,000 have never visited one.[5]

In any review of the recent changes in the status of the health of children, it is also important to review social and educational factors that influence family life and therefore the well-being of children. Though not directly involved in the medical system, these factors nonetheless have striking effects on health. Some of them are:

5) *Improved educational level of our population:* According to Charles Lewis the single most important factor associated with increased life expectancy is literacy, a fact that has enormous bearing on the rearing of children, for many problems once managed by the health-care system can now be met directly by parents. Infant and child nutrition, for example, which used to be supervised by pediatric personnel a few decades ago, can now generally be managed by literate, comparatively well-educated parents. A literate mother pushing her food cart through a supermarket is able to feed her infant better than her predecessor would have done with the prescribed pediatric dietary regimes of the twenties and thirties.

As a consequence, there is now considerable resistance to the professionalization of child care, a new reliance on older, traditional methods (such as breast feeding) which in the past were part of the folklore and wisdom of the community, and a trend toward demedicalizing obstetrical and other child-care practices. Professionals should welcome these trends; they reinforce the movement toward greater confidence and competence on the part of the parents, and they free the professional to direct more of his attention to the complex clinical problems of pediatrics that require specialized training.

6) *Improved hygiene, housing, and nutrition:* The overall trend toward improved housing has had a generally favorable effect on child hygiene and health. Much obviously remains to be done for families of low income; we also need innovative planning for safe play space and after-school services for children and families. The introduction of safe water and food supplies has also had a major impact on the growth and development of our children. Wegman has pointed out that the major decline in infant mortality actually took place before 1940—that is, before the advent of antibiotics and the technologies of modern medicine. Through the reduction of the numbers of poor people and improvements in the handling and storing of food, there has been an overall improvement in nutrition of children and families in the United States. Nevertheless, significant numbers of children can still be found who go hungry. Thirty per cent of infants living in poor families have iron-deficiency anemia; one-fourth of the children in the United States live in families with incomes below the minimum considered necessary for adequate nutrition. Misleading advertising and over-processing practices by the food industry have deleterious effects on good nutrition as well—and for rich and poor alike. We have yet to learn what the results of the consequent early nutritional practices will be on such adult diseases as obesity, hypertension, and coronary disease.

7) *Changes in the structure of the American family:* There have also been dramatic changes in the structure of the family that are influencing the health of children. Half of all women with children from 6 to 17 years old are engaged in, or seeking, work, twice the rate of twenty-five years ago. One-third of all women with children under 6 were in the labor force in 1974; this is three times the proportion that existed in 1948. The great majority, two-thirds of these women, were working full time. At the same time, the number of adults in the household has dropped steadily to a current "average" of two. The extended family (grandparents and other relatives living with

the nuclear family) is becoming increasingly rare. Parents no longer can rely on relatives in times of stress, and children have far more limited experience with other adults as they are growing up. Over the past twenty-five years, the percentage of children under age 18 living with a single parent rose from 10 per cent to 16 per cent; for children under 6 the percentage has doubled, from 7 per cent to 15 per cent; among children under 3, one out of eight now lives in a single-parent family; half of those single parents are mothers who are working full time.

The "illegitimacy ratio" (illegitimate births per 1,000 live babies born) has risen from 35 to 130 in the last quarter-century. The number of teenagers in our population is growing, and the teenage population is the only group among whom the birth rate is also going up. According to a recent study, the number of children born to girls under the age of 15 has doubled since 1960.[6] Married teen-agers have the highest birth rate of all—twice that of married women in the 20-24 bracket.

While the highest pregnancy risk is among teenagers, the infants that result are more than twice as likely to be of low birth weight (less than five and a half pounds) than those born to older mothers, and comprise about 62 per cent of all infant deaths: 8.7 per cent of all babies born are of low birth weight; 18.2 per cent born to mothers under 15 years and 10.7 per cent born to mothers 15-19 years fall into this category. If these infants survive, they are also the most likely to develop major disorders.

The study quoted above also reports that 85 per cent of the infants born to mothers under 15 years of age were illegitimate, and 34 per cent of those born to mothers 15-19 years of age were illegitimate. Inadequate prenatal care, common among young unmarried mothers, may more than double neonatal mortality (deaths under one month of age). Neonatal-mortality rates were 58.7 per 1,000 live births for mothers under 15; 32.8 per 1,000 for mothers 15-19; 22.4 per 1,000 for mothers 25-29 years old.[7] The risk of low-birth-weight infants is not only much higher in very young mothers, it is also higher in illegitimate births.

8) *The shift from rural to urban poverty:* In 1959, the majority of poor people—56 per cent of the total of 39 million—lived in rural America; today, 60 per cent of the 23 million poor have moved to cities. Along with this population shift, however, was another—of professionals moving away from the central cities to the outlying districts. In 1945, the physician-patient ratio in the cities was 1:450; in the suburbs, it was 1:2000. Now it is the reverse—1:2000 in the cities and 1:5000 in the suburbs. These social changes, collated by Bronfenbrenner, have particularly disturbing implications for the health of children when we combine them with the fact that the unwed mother and the abandoned mother are the most apt to be poor: the struggles of raising children alone are compounded by the problems of poverty and of limited medical care.

Directions for the Future

These selected health, social, and demographic trends suggest the need to redesign efforts on behalf of the health care of children, particularly in the direction of improving resources and services to the urban poor, who constitute the majority of those who are now being neglected. If we examine the health record for the children of the more affluent families in the United States (the upper 75 per cent), they compare favorably with those of any country in the world, although this should not be construed as implying that further improvement is unnecessary.

Improvement in child-health care generally depends upon improvement in several areas including preventive medicine, the delivery of medical care for both acute and chronic illness, the quality of the environment, social problems (including child abuse and the perils associated with living in a modern industrial society), and, finally, the search for new knowledge, our ability to apply what we have learned, and to deliver it to the community in some effective way. Particular aspects of some of these problems will be outlined below.

The Application of What Is Known

Child-health workers (pediatricians, public health nurses, etc.) have been concentrating on preventive services, and they should continue to do so. In infectious diseases, for example, it is now possible to control measles, tetanus, diphtheria, pertussis, and poliomyelitis. Recurrent outbreaks of these diseases represent the failure of the profession to deliver those services adequately. Recent surveys by the Center for Disease Control of the Public Health Service have indicated that half the children in low-income areas are unprotected against one or more of these diseases.[8] Educational efforts are desperately needed; more concern should be shown for developing effective delivery systems. A cost-benefit model designed by Schoenbaum and his colleagues[9] is already available for use as a foundation for effective strategies. By the year 2000, these diseases ought to have completely disappeared. As was recently the case with smallpox, for which mandatory immunization has now been discontinued, the question will then be whether or not these immunizations can safely be eliminated.

Attention to nutritional status ought to be part of continuing child-health services, even though higher literacy rates and more universal public education will permit parents to assume greater responsibility in this area. Nutritional programs ought to be begun in the prenatal period and continued throughout childhood. Undernutrition is usually the result of poverty, though poor dietary habits in any class can lead to malnutrition. In that connection, serious efforts are needed to assure truth in the messages about nutrition purveyed to children through advertising.[10]

We clearly possess the information needed to reduce infant mortality significantly. Sweden's success in bringing infant mortality down to less than 10 per 1,000 live births provides a goal to which Americans ought to aspire, and which we can equal if low-income groups are adequately cared for. Accessible, high-quality prenatal- and infant-care programs must include family-planning information and services for those who wish it, improved nutrition, effective obstetrical, nursery, and social services, and efforts at reducing high-risk pregnancies—especially among adolescents.

Continuous and comprehensive pediatric care for families of infants and young children should also include preventive mental-health services; these are central to early detection of developmental deviations and emotional problems. Though we have relatively little data concerning what specific child-rearing practices will ensure mental health, clinical experience does provide data on which to base advice to families dealing with developmental problems.

The introduction of preventive methods has resulted in a steep decline in the numbers of acute illnesses in childhood. Pediatric supervision during acute illness is designed to minimize complications and in many communities is a function now performed by physician's assistants and/or nurse practitioners as well as pediatricians. Although the numbers of pediatric and other child-health workers are adequate to perform these functions, their distribution, as in many health services, is skewed, being particularly low in rural and in densely populated inner-city areas. The National Health Service Corps is a federal effort intended to attract physicians to underserved areas. If voluntary methods of redistribution of professional resources do not work, mandatory services for under-served areas may have to be instituted. New kinds of incentives and major institutional changes will have to be considered to ensure more equitable distribution.

Improving the quality of some aspects of general pediatric services also merits attention. A critical review of surgical procedures such as tonsillectomy and adenoidectomy, for example, is certainly in order. This surgical procedure accounts for nearly a million hospitalizations each year; almost half of all operations on children are for this purpose, and a few of them result in death; they account for 25 per cent of hospital admissions and 10 per cent of hospital days for children.[11] The costs run into several hundred million dollars each year. Yet the true indications for this procedure are few. In the next decade, tonsillectomies should become a rarity; whether or not they do depends in part on how effectively the Professional Standards Review Organizations do their work.

The Care of the Chronically Ill

Controlling some of the many acute infectious disorders has made professional time and energy available to deal with chronic ailments. A 1973 study[12] of children under 15 years old has estimated that 22.4 per cent of children in the United States have at least one chronic condition, and, for 8 per cent of those, its severity places some limitation on their activity. The most common of these conditions is asthma-hay fever, which affects 20 per cent of children who are limited in activity (Table 4).

In 1974, there was a total of 3 million mentally retarded or emotionally disturbed children under 17 years of age in the United States.[13] Another 700,000 suffered from learning disabilities. These estimates are unreliable, in part because of errors in classification, in part because of incomplete reporting. There is every reason to believe that the figures cited are in fact very conservative.

TABLE 4

LEADING CAUSES OF ACTIVITY LIMITATION FOR
CHILDREN UNDER SEVENTEEN YEARS*

Cause of Activity Limitation	Per cent
Asthma—hay fever	20.0
Impairments of lower extremities and hips	8.3
Paralysis, complete or partial	7.4
Chronic bronchitis and sinusitis	5.5
Mental and nervous conditions	3.8
Heart conditions	3.7

*Adapted from "Children and Youth—Selected Health Characteristics," *Vital and Health Statistics*, series 10, no. 62 (United States, 1958 and 1968), p. 18.

Haggerty, in the conclusion of a study of child health in Monroe County, New York, wrote:[14]

> The current major health problems of children, as seen by the community, are those that would have barely been mentioned a generation ago. Learning difficulties and school problems, behavioral disturbances, allergies, speech difficulties, visual problems and the problems of adolescents in coping and adjusting are today the most common concerns about children.

To indicate that this is not a phenomenon peculiar to the United States, the final volume of the family survey of Newcastle-upon-Tyne offers British evidence on a cohort of children born in 1947:[15]

> The health of the children in our city was never better than in the years of our study. Yet at fifteen not less than one in five had either handicap, recurrent illness, intellectual limitation, poor education performance or severe difficulties of emotional or social adaptation. This residual disability is the true measure of our failure to deal effectively with the physical and educational disorders of children, and we do not yet know how much of the effects of physical illness or emotional disturbance will only become apparent later in life.

While state programs for crippled children have been the most involved in the care of the handicapped, the responsibility for physical and mental health and for special education is increasingly shifting to departments of education and to local school systems,[16] reflecting the current trend toward focusing on the functional capacity of the child rather than on some common diagnostic label. It also expresses the desirability of keeping the child in his community and in his local school if that is possible. Static, traditional school health programs (with relatively few results considering the funds expended) are giving way to a more dynamic integration of the health-care system with education. This is a long overdue recognition of the need to apply knowledge of many kinds in the most effective way.

There is movement also toward integrating services among the local child-care and educational systems with the secondary and tertiary health institutions. Regional diagnostic centers are often used for consultation and for highly specialized services—particularly for children with mental retardation, seizures, learning disorders, cerebral palsy, and orthopedic and sensory handicaps. Because the consultation center is often too remote to implement the integration of service delivery, that must be done at the local level, and this in turn suggests a crucial role for the community pediatrician. Such integration may well become the province of pediatricians within the school systems, with schools in every community being held responsible for the total local child population. This would require schools to extend their services down to younger age groups, a proposition that may prove very attractive in an era of shrinking school populations, of unfilled school houses, and of unemployed teachers. Programs to identify handicapped children and provide remedial care prior to first grade ought to enhance the effectiveness of subsequent educational interventions.

The care of children with serious and potentially fatal illness increasingly rests with the tertiary medical-care system. This system includes the approximately 120 children's hospital medical centers as well as the university medical centers of this country; it is the best organized of all the child-health services in the United States. The system covers practically every geographic area rather well. Within the centers, medical care is delivered, young health workers are taught, post-graduate education is offered, and biomedical research on neoplasms, hypersensitivity, cystic fibrosis, and disorders such as congenital heart disease, renal disease, and disfunctions of the new-born are pursued.

Improvements in child health have diminished both the length and the frequency of in-hospital treatment. New reimbursement schemes ought consequently to be worked out (and this is also true of general hospitals) to sustain the fiscal solvency of these medical centers, for the current pattern of hospital financing through per diem bed costs encourages unnecessary hospitalization by placing a premium on keeping the beds filled.

The Environment

For the next several decades, the major problems in child-health care will be to cope with the negative effects of the environment. Many of the major problems of child health today are shaped by social forces that exist outside the health-care system. A discussion of some of them follows:

Accidents: Accidents are the leading cause of death in childhood. Repairing the results of accidents are medical and surgical problems; their prevention, however, is a problem for social and community action. Improved emergency medical services for the care of accident victims are clearly needed, but only preventive measures can reduce morbidity and mortality appreciably. All too little attention has been given to the design of cities, highways, motor vehicles, and household products for the safety of children.

Child abuse: Many cases of physical and psychological child abuse, as well as child-neglect syndromes such as "failure to thrive," are encountered in health-service institutions. The striking increase in cases reported may in part reflect legislative efforts throughout the United States to improve the accuracy of such reporting, but in part it may well also reflect a real increase resulting from some of the social changes already described.

Although the number of reported cases of child abuse is something like 200,000 a year, data acquired from a nationwide survey of a representative sample population of a standard metropolitan statistical area indicate that the numbers may in fact be as high as 2.5 to 4.8 million cases a year.[17] These data, combined with the day-to-day experiences of child-welfare agencies (and the limited resources of most of them), suggest a problem of great magnitude for those concerned with the protection and care of the young. Perhaps no problem is more dependent for its solution on an integrated system of health, social, and educational services. We are only now beginning to learn how to organize comprehensive and effective programs of care and protection.

Toxic substances and pollution: Another risk for the contemporary young lies in the ubiquity of toxic substances. Lead poisoning, for example, is an insidious health problem found almost exclusively in urban slums because of the common presence in antiquated housing of leaded paint. It is estimated that approximately 400,000 children are affected by it annually: of these, 16,000 require treatment, 3,200 incur moderate to severe brain damage; and 800 suffer brain damage severe enough to require care for the rest of their lives.[18] Treatment is complex and difficult; prevention would involve the renovation of the some 7 million housing units still harboring lead-based paint.[19] Industrial wastes and other pollutants pose similar hazards for children; prevention will involve even far more expensive and complex solutions.

Developmental attrition among the poor: Many children living in poverty fail to develop the verbal and social skills that are prerequisite to academic and vocational achievement. We do not know how to measure very precisely the degree of "developmental attrition" among our population; it is not recorded under the traditional health indicators of morbidity and mortality. There is reason to believe, however, that it results in a great loss of human potential in our society. Since 10 to 20 per cent of children live in poverty (the percentage depends on the definition of poverty), the provision of family-support systems is basic to the prevention of these intolerable losses in human potential. Family support systems (day care, home visitors, homemaker services, preschool programs, and the like) must be flexible if they are to meet the needs of such families.

It may seem odd to include a recommendation for adequate income in a presentation on health. However, as has repeatedly been pointed out, our major child-health problems—failure to immunize, infant mortality, undernutrition, developmental attrition, and developmental disorders—are all compounded by poverty. Just as basic to significant improvement in the health and welfare of infants and preschool children is an effective set of social and health indicators that will enable us to identify the children who are at greatest developmental risk. Such a system must go beyond the usual morbidity and mortality classifications and focus on the functional capacity of the child, taking into account discomfort and disability, on the one hand, and social and psychological competence, on the other.[20]

The Search for New Knowledge

Further reduction in childhood morbidity and mortality can only come through research in such fields as reproductive biology, genetics and genetic counseling, inborn errors of metabolism, fetal biology, and congenital malformations and fetal and neonatal insults that can result in handicapping conditions. Research in the behavioral sciences is almost equally crucial, however, particularly in such fields as accident prevention, the causes of emotional disorders and developmental disabilities, and the physiological and emotional bases for suicide and homicide. Problems such as child abuse and juvenile delinquency are poorly understood, as are the problems that lie behind our apparent inability to reintegrate our neighborhoods and regain our sense of community.

Community Services

In the United States, we know where children are when they are born (through birth registration) and we identify them again when they go to school, but between those two events, we have no adequate system for locating them. We should develop a system for finding children and families in need of services, but one designed not to transgress the privacy and integrity of each family.

Communities must ensure that families are aware of their entitlements to health and social services—particularly prior to school age when children (especially from low-income families) lack care. If an effective set of social and health indicators were available, local child-development councils reporting to health departments could carry the responsibility for knowing where the needy children are and for helping families to utilize appropriate resources for their care. Where government resources are not available, the child-development council could be made responsible for providing the services itself or for purchasing them from private agencies.

Just as significantly, a local child-development council could serve as an integrating force in bringing fragmented child-health, educational, and welfare services together to concentrate on the needs of the child rather than on the requirements of professionals and institutions. One of the greatest challenges for the next decades resides in the integration at the local level of our now much fragmented service systems.

Because the schools serve the universe of children after the age of five, they are also potentially good candidates for forming the community's child-development councils. Some enterprising school systems are already exploring this avenue, and these will help us identify the likeliest alternatives.

Toward a Presidential Council of Advisers on Children

There was a time when the affairs of children were concentrated in one federal agency—the United States Children's Bureau. The years have brought greater complexity, and now there are many agencies—even many agencies within the Department of Health, Education, and Welfare alone—which deal with the affairs of children and families. Virtually every department of government, including, among others, Agriculture, Housing and Urban Development, Transportation, Interior, Commerce, and Treasury carry on programs which influence the lives of children. Clearly, because of the importance of the welfare of children for the nation's future, a national policy for children is in order. Programs are now piecemeal and fragmented, with relatively little continuity and comprehensiveness. It would seem appropriate that they all be joined together on a supradepartmental level. Some have suggested a Presidential Council of Advisors, analogous to the Council of Economic Advisors (which has stability and continuity by which to provide analysis and planning, but which has no direct operational responsibility for any one agency). This, or some other integrating force, is needed to remedy fragmentation of federal programs and to provide a focal point for them within the federal government for serving the best interests of children and their families.

REFERENCES

[1] M. E. Wegman, "Annual Summary of Vital Statistics, 1974," *Pediatrics*, 56 (1975), pp. 960-66.

[2] U. Bronfenbrenner, "The State of American Families and Children," in *Toward a National Policy for Children and Families. Report of the Advisory Committee on Child Development, Assembly of Behavioral and Social Sciences, National Research Council, National Academy of Sciences* (Washington, D.C., 1976).

[3] D. M. Kessner, *Infant Death: An Analysis by Maternal Risk and Health Care* (Institute of Medicine, National Academy of Sciences, Washington, D.C., 1973).

[4] *National Center for Health Statistics: Decayed, Missing, and Filled Teeth Among Youths 12–17 Years: United States*, series 11, no. 144 (U.S. Government Printing Office, Washington, D.C., 1974).

[5] A. F. North, "Project Head Start and the Pediatrician," *Clinical Pediatrics* 6, pp. 191-94.

[6] *National Center for Health Statistics: Monthly Vital Statistics Report, Summary Report Final Natality Statistics*, vol. 23, no. 115.

[7] *National Center for Health Statistics: A Study of Infant Mortality from Linked Records by Age of Mother, Total-Birth Order, and Other Variables.*, series 20, no. 14 (U.S. Government Printing Office, Washington, D.C., 1973).

[8]*Center for Disease Control: Morbidity and Mortality Weekly Report*, 48 (1975), p. 405.

[9]S. C. Schoenbaum, J. N. Hyde, L. Bartoshesky, and K. Crampton, "Benefit-Cost Analysis of Rubella Vaccination Policy," *New England Journal of Medicine*, 294 (1976), pp. 306-10.

[10]R. B. Choate, Oral argument in children's television proceeding, Testimony before the Federal Communications Commission, Washington, D.C. January 9, 1973.

[11]A. F. North, Jr., *Medical Dimensions*, 1 (May, 1976), pp. 26-27.

[12]Alice D. Chenoweth, "Health Problems of Infants and Children" in *Maternal and Child Health Practices*, ed. H. Wallace, E. Gold, and E. Lis (Springfield, Illinois, 1973), pp. 641-42.

[13]*America's Children, 1976. A Bicentennial Assessment*, National Council of Organizations for Children and Youth (Washington, D.C., 1976).

[14]R. J. Haggerty, K. J. Roghmann, I. B. Pless, *Child Health and the Community* (New York, 1975).

[15]F. J. W. Miller, S. D. M. Court, E. G. Knox, and S. Brandon, *The School Years in Newcastle-upon-Tyne, 1952-62* (London, 1974).

[16]J. B. Richmond, "The Health Needs of the Handicapped Child," *Proceedings of the First National Conference of State Directors for Crippled Children* (Baltimore, 1974), pp. 7-14.

[17]D. G. Gil, *Violence Against Children* (Cambridge, Mass., 1970); E. H. Newberger and J. H. Daniel, "Knowledge and Epidemiology of Child Abuse, A Critical Review of Concepts," *Pediatric Annals*, 5 (1976), pp. 15-26.

[18]L. A. Blanksma, H. K. Sachs, E. F. Murray, and M. J. O'Connell, "Incidence of High Blood Levels in Chicago Children," *Pediatrics*, 44 (1969), p. 661.

[19]H. L. Needleman, "Lead-Paint Poisoning Prevention: An Opportunity Forfeited," *New England Journal of Medicine*, 292 (1975), pp. 588-89.

[20]O. G. Brim, "Macro-Structural Influences on Child Development and the Need for Childhood Social Indicators," *American Journal of Orthopsychiatry*, 45 (1975), pp. 516-24.

SUGGESTED READING

Doctors and Dollars Are Not Enough. How to Improve Health Services for Children and Their Families (Children's Defense Fund of the Washington Research Project, Inc., Washington, D.C., 1976).

T. W. Lash and H. Sigal, *State of the Child: New York City* (New York, 1976).

C. A. Miller, "A Bicentennial Generation of Healthy Children," an address for the Bicentennial Conference on Children, National Council of Organizations for Children and Youth, Washington, D.C., February 2, 1976.

E. H. Newberger, C. M. Newberger, and J. B. Richmond, *Child Health in America: Toward a Rational Public Policy* (in press).

Report of the Committee on Maternal and Child Health Research, National Research Council, National Academy of Sciences (Washington, D.C., 1976).

J. B. Richmond and H. L. Weinberger, "Session II: Program Implications of New Knowledge Regarding the Physical, Intellectual, and Emotional Growth and Development and the Unmet Needs of Children and Youth, prepared for the Invitational Conference on Health Services for Children and Youth sponsored by the American Public Health Association," *Journal of Public Health*, 60 (1970), pp. 23-73.

K. J. Snapper, H. H. Barriga, F. H. Baumgarner, and C. S. Wagner, *The Status of Children 1975* (Social Research Group, The George Washington University, Washington, D.C., 1975).

Toward a National Policy for Children and Families. Report of the Advisory Committee on Child Development, Assembly of Behavioral and Social Sciences, National Research Council, National Academy of Sciences (Washington, D.C., 1976).

PHILIP BERGER, M.D., BEATRIX HAMBURG, M.D.,
AND DAVID HAMBURG, M.D.

Mental Health: Progress and Problems

In the quarter-century since the inception of modern psychopharmacology, there has been a revolution in the care of the mentally ill. Drug treatments for psychiatric disorders have sharply decreased the numbers of severely ill patients in state and county mental hospitals. The advent of drug therapy has also led to more accurate methods for diagnosis, assessment of severity, and criteria of improvement of mental disorders. The optimism generated by the success of early pharmacological treatments created a climate favorable to innovation; psychological and socioenvironmental therapies for the mentally ill could then be introduced and evaluated.

But widespread adoption of psychopharmacology in the treatment of psychiatric disorders has had, at the same time, some negative effects. Psychopharmacological agents (like most other highly potent medicines) occasionally produce side effects which are dangerous or irreversible. Some drug-abuse problems of recent years have involved new psychopharmacological agents, often drugs of the same classes as those that, when properly administered, reduce suffering in patients with mental illness.

Pharmacological treatments for mental illness involve psychiatry in the powerful currents of modern biological science, an important part of which has been the investigation of possible biochemical mechanisms underlying the three main categories of mental disorder: schizophrenia, manic psychosis, and depression. It might be useful to describe each of these categories briefly before continuing with our discussion.

The symptoms of schizophrenia, a profound disorder of behavior, mood, thinking, and perception, usually begin in young adulthood. At present approximately 200,000 patients are hospitalized in the United States as diagnosed schizophrenics, while another approximately 400,000 are either patients in outpatient clinics or not being treated at all. About half of the available hospital beds for mentally ill and mentally retarded patients (and one-quarter of all available hospital beds) are occupied by schizophrenics. The number of patients who develop schizophrenia each year is approximately 300 per 100,000 population. The chances that a person will be hospitalized for schizophrenia in his lifetime have been estimated at one in one hundred. Although it is widely believed that the incidence of severe mental disorder has been increased by the complexity of industrial societies, the incidence of schizophrenia has in fact been nearly constant for the last hundred years in the United States, and recent international collaborative studies report that the situation is similar in all nations and cultures that have thus far been studied.[1]

The symptoms of schizophrenia include altered motor behavior, ranging from total immobilization to frenetic and purposeless activity, sometimes accompanied by peculiar mannerisms. Perceptual distortions, often including auditory hallucinations, also occur, as do disturbances in thinking that can lead to distorted concept formation, bizarre speech, and illogical thinking. This last is often expressed in paranoid delusions ranging from pervasive suspiciousness to fully developed beliefs in complex but improbable plots against the patient. Expressions of emotion are either completely absent or inappropriate to the speech and actions of the individual. Many victims seem incapable of experiencing genuine satisfaction.

Numerous attempts have been made to divide schizophrenic patients into subgroups, based upon one or another of these symptoms. Paranoid schizophrenia is the diagnosis given to patients whose major symptoms are highly organized delusions. Patients who are withdrawn and remain in fixed positions for long periods of time are called catatonic schizophrenics. Patients with less dramatic schizophrenic symptoms are more difficult to classify, but one important distinction is based on the clinical history of the symptoms: those who experience time-limited episodes of schizophrenic symptoms separated by periods of near-normal functioning are often called acute schizophrenics; those who, if untreated, continue to suffer from schizophrenic symptoms and insidious but progressive deterioration of social and mental functioning are called chronic or "process" schizophrenics.

Manic psychosis or mania, like schizophrenia, is disabling and usually reveals itself in an excited, pseudo-elated, and unstable mood, rapid speech, and increased motor activity. In mild mania, a patient talks easily and constantly, seems to have boundless energy, and often develops and tries to act out grandiose schemes for getting money, helping others (sometimes as a savior of all mankind), or making earth-shaking discoveries. The manic patient is easily distracted, easily irritated, impatient, and rarely able to complete a task. In its most severe form, mania leads the patient to move and speak so rapidly as to be incoherent, and to involve himself constantly in apparently purposeless activity. Hallucinations and delusions are also often present. There is obviously some overlap between the symptoms of severe mania and those of acute schizophrenia. In general, however, manic patients are easily distinguished from schizophrenic patients by their intense pseudo-elated mood and the ease with which they involve themselves with others.

The general term "depression" can refer to a normal mood, a psychiatric symptom, or several psychiatric syndromes. We have all experienced depressed moods—the ubiquitous sadness of everyday life. Whether depression is categorized as a mood or as a psychiatric symptom is in part simply a question of degree. However, "psychotic depression" is a distinct entity with a distinct collection of symptoms, of which only one is profound sadness or depression. The severely depressed patient often loses appetite and weight, has disturbed sleep patterns, has little interest in doing things, and suffers from feelings of guilt and worthlessness. Many depressed patients feel that their thinking has slowed down and that their movements are sluggish; it is difficult to concentrate. Others are extremely anxious and painfully agitated, and are often unable to sit still. Commonly they are preoccupied by thoughts of death and suicide—indeed, severe depression is the principal precursor of suicide. Some have delusions—for example, they may feel they are guilty of unspeakable crimes—or suffer self-deprecating hallucinations.

A number of efforts have been made to divide severely depressed patients into subgroups based on symptoms. The most important of these distinctions is probably between unipolar and bipolar depression. "Bipolar" is simply another term for the manic-depressive disorder. A bipolar depressed patient has a history of at least one episode of mania in addition to some depressive episodes. A patient with "unipolar" depression may have had several episodes of illness, but all of them show only depressive symptoms. Increasingly, evidence suggests that bipolar patients are a subgroup of depressed patients who can be distinguished not only by their history of mania, but also by specific metabolic abnormalities and specific responses to psycho-pharmacological agents. The prevalent view among research workers is that depressive disorders are heterogeneous.

The incidence of severe depressive illness has not been accurately determined. However, the incidence of bipolar depression (manic-depressive disorder) has been estimated at about 300 per 100,000 population, or about the same as the incidence of schizophrenia. The incidence of severe unipolar depression is probably considerably higher. The National Institutes of Mental Health have estimated that 1,500,000 people are being treated for depression at any given time. The approximately 24,000 reported suicides each year and the many unreported ones (suicide is the tenth major cause of death in the United States) are another indication of the numbers of severely depressed. Suicide can be associated with other illnesses, including schizophrenia, but most suicides occur among this class of the mentally ill.[2]

In order to understand the revolution that occurred in the treatment of the mentally ill after the introduction of pharmacotherapies, it is important to recall what conditions were like before these therapies were introduced. Many psychiatrists practicing today were also active in the pre-drug era, so firsthand descriptions are easy to come by.

Before drug therapies were introduced, few outpatient clinics for psychiatric patients existed, nor did the majority of general medical hospitals admit severely ill psychiatric patients. Those hospitals that did admit them often kept them only briefly; they usually ended up in state mental hospitals, which were more likely to be custodial institutions than medical facilities.

Pessimism toward severe mental illness was common because each year the number of patients admitted to hospitals increased, while very few were ever discharged. The patients' living areas were crowded and poorly furnished; schizophrenic patients with paranoid delusions crouched in corners in constant fear; catatonic patients were allowed to maintain the same rigid posture to the point of developing swollen legs and pressure sores; hallucinating patients paced the floor talking to their "voices" and unaware of what was going on around them. People sat year after year on benches or on the floor doing nothing, while their physical health deteriorated as well. Violent patients attacked staff members or other patients for reasons known only to themselves. Manic patients laughed, joked, and moved constantly for days at a time until they collapsed, exhausted. Combative patients were kept in rooms without furniture or strapped to beds that were bolted to the floor to prevent injury to themselves and others. Agitated patients were often placed in warm baths or tied in wet sheets in an effort to calm their frenzy.

The psychiatrists charged with the care and treatment of these patients were baffled by these disorders. Both cause and therapy were quite unknown and untaught in medical schools. Before World War II patients were in the care of physicians trained mainly in neurology, but by the postwar period many had studied psycho-analytic psychotherapy as well. But neither neurological diagnosis nor psychoanalytic psychotherapy had any substantial effect in the treatment of chronic schizophrenia or severe mania. Regardless of their training, psychiatrists functioned mainly as adminis-trators and custodians.[3]

While conditions such as these were widespread, for the most part they were not produced by inhumane individuals; many decent, well-meaning people worked in public mental hospitals. The situation was exacerbated by public apathy, by the social stigma attached to mental illness, by lack of funds for patient care, and especially by the lack of effective treatment.

A new era in the treatment of the severely mentally ill began in the mid-fifties. Before then, the number of patients in state and county mental hospitals had been increasing at an average annual rate of over 2 per cent, until it reached a peak of 559,000 in 1955. In 1956, however, for the first time in history, the number of patients in mental hospitals declined, and this decrease has continued, despite increases in national population and a steady increase in the admission rate to the present day. By 1967, the patient population had fallen to 426,000 and, by 1973, to 249,000. Without the advent of psychopharmacologic drugs, if the earlier trend had continued the number of patients in public mental hospitals by 1973 would probably have been at least 800,000. The patients who are now leaving these facilities are by no means free of all psychiatric symptoms; many continue to receive treatment in outpatient clinics and transitional facilities. However, most are able to return to work, to reestablish family ties, and to participate in community life.

But conditions are also changing for patients who remain in hospitals. Most hospital wards are now unlocked, and many are organized on the principle of "milieu therapy," resulting in what is often called the "therapeutic community." In a therapeutic community, patients and staff have regular group meetings, where patients are given a considerable voice in determining the conditions of their lives in the hospital. They are treated with respect and given an opportunity to make decisions for themselves. Many have also been moved from maximum security units to open wards.

In addition to the increase in patient government on individual wards, entire hospitals have been transformed by recreational facilities similar to those found in many small towns. Concerts, movies, plays, and equipment for games and arts and crafts are commonly available to patients. Some hospitals have small industries that contract to do "piecework" for local companies, allowing patients who have not improved sufficiently for community life to become economically productive while still hospitalized. These activities serve to ease the eventual return of the patient to normal functioning at home and in the community.

Although these dramatic changes were brought about through many interrelated factors, including the introduction of milieu therapy in the fifties, they gained most of their momentum when several pharmacological treatments for severe psychiatric disorders were discovered through research both in the United States and in other countries. These drugs, called phenothiazines or antipsychotics, were first tested in France and were introduced in the United States around 1955. They reduced the symptoms of schizophrenia and manic psychosis. Monoamine oxidase inhibitors, developed in the United States, and tricyclic antidepressants, tested in Switzerland, were used with reasonable success in relieving the distress of severely depressed patients beginning around 1956-57. Finally, lithium carbonate was developed in Australia in the late nineteen-forties and tested extensively in Europe in the fifties. It proved to be a remarkably effective treatment for manic-depressive illness, but, curiously, it was not introduced into the United States until 1970.

Pharmacological agents were not responsible all by themselves for the dramatic changes in the treatment of severely mentally ill patients, but they did add to the climate of optimism and innovation that encouraged other new forms of therapy. Gradually a set of useful therapies emerged: crisis intervention, brief psychotherapy, group therapy, family therapy, the therapeutic community, and behavior modification therapies. The last of these applied to the hospitalized patient the principles of learning theory that had been elucidated in psychology laboratories.

All these new hopes for the treatment of the mentally ill combined with a spirit of social reform that was prevalent in the nineteen-sixties led to the Federal Community Mental Health Centers Act of 1963, which was supposed to provide prompt, comprehensive, and continuous mental health services to all segments of society by creating community mental health centers. In contrast to state mental hospitals, which were often in remote locations, these centers were to be located within the geographical area they were meant to serve. They were supposed to supply the essential elements: emergency services, inpatient hospital facilities, and services for education and consultation throughout the community, and they also were to make available new treatments for mental illness at reasonable cost to anyone who needed help. These goals have not yet all been realized—and they may prove too ambitious—but significant progress has certainly been made in some areas.

As with all dramatic social changes, however, there have been some negative aspects to the revolution as well. In some cases, the attempt to move patients out of the large state and county mental hospitals proceeded too rapidly. Reich,[4] for example, reports that many chronically ill patients discharged from New York state mental hospitals are living in cheap hotels and deteriorated single-room-occupancy dwellings, where they are robbed and abused by people who have taken advantage of their helplessness. Arnhoff[5] has suggested that the community mental health movement tends to ignore important developments in biological psychiatry and the behavioral sciences, and is deficient in studying the effects of community treatment on family, siblings, and offspring, as well as on the mental patients themselves. He finds no convincing evidence that community or home treatment is superior to hospital treatment in either its short- or long-term effects.

In our view, the location of the treatment is much less important than its quality, although this comment is not meant to negate the positive effects of the Federal Community Mental Health Centers Act. A great deal of progress has been made toward the goal of prompt, comprehensive mental health services for all segments of society. Nevertheless it is clear that more research is required and more careful attention must be given to the administrative and operational aspects of community treatment.

The clinical research that has been stimulated by the need to confirm the effectiveness of medications as treatments for mental illness has also led to efforts to define mental disorders and their subtypes more precisely and to develop more rigorous methods for evaluating the vacillations of psychiatric symptoms. An important concept in this research has been the random-assignment, double-blind design.

Patients are assigned on a random basis to an experimental drug or to a capsule identical in appearance, which may either be a drug of known effectiveness or a placebo, if there is no treatment of established value. The capsules are coded so that neither the patient nor the treating staff knows which substance is being used. The staff then evaluates the patient's symptoms and records its observations on standardized rating scales. After a specified period of time, the code is broken and the data analyzed statistically.

This research method goes a long way toward eliminating the bias of the "placebo effect" of spontaneous recovery from symptoms and of the staff opinion either for or against the new medication, which might influence staff ratings. It was used in the initial evaluations of drug treatment for psychiatric disorders in studies conducted at numerous hospitals across the United States. This enormous effort was coordinated by the National Institutes of Mental Health, which also led the way in establishing high standards for research methodology.[6]

Some of these studies involved research on brain function and were undertaken principally as attempts to explain how and why these new drugs were working. To understand this important research, it would be well first to review a few hypotheses about how the human brain functions.

The brain is composed of some ten billion nerve cells or neurons whose long processes, or axons, conduct electrical activity. These axons connect to other neurons in complicated electrical circuitry, which is essential to the functioning of the brain; cessation of this activity is one criterion for death. However, not all brain activity is electrical. One axon or long-cell process does not quite touch the next neuron: there is a microscopic gap called the synaptic cleft that separates the two. This gap is chemically bridged by a small molecule appropriately called a neurotransmitter. A neuron releases a neurotransmitter or neuroregulator, which diffuses across the gap, attaches to a receptor on the second neuron, and activates a mechanism which may stimulate, inhibit, or modify the firing of the second neuron. Several neurons, some stimulating, some inhibiting, may be connected to one neuron by these neurotransmitters.

The chemicals that serve as neurotransmitters or neuroregulators include dopamine, norepinephrine, and serotonin (often called biogenic amines) and acetylcholine. Psychoactive drugs, both the drugs used to treat mental illness and those abused for their "mind-altering" effects, probably act by changing functional activity of one or more neurotransmitters. Research on the neurotransmitters was stimulated, and has since been aided, by the introduction of these psychopharmacological agents.

Two hypotheses of special interest relate neurotransmitter dysfunction to severe mental illness. Both had their origin in clinical observations on the actions of psychopharmacological drugs; both involve biogenic amine neurotransmitters. The first hypothesis states that vulnerability to depression is enhanced by a functional deficit of two neurotransmitters, norepinephrine and/or serotonin, while vulnerability to mania is increased by a functional excess of these same neurotransmitters. The second hypothesis states that excess activity of the neurons that use the neurotransmitter dopamine predisposes the individual to schizophrenia.

The biogenic amine hypothesis of depression had its origin in observations on the effects of two psychoactive drugs, reserpine and iproniazid. In the early fifties, reserpine was found to be the active principle in a herbal medication from India. It was soon found to be useful in treating hypertension, schizophrenia, and manic psychosis. There was a problem, however: some patients chronically treated for hypertension developed a syndrome remarkably similar to psychological depression. The medication iproniazid, also developed in the early fifties, was used to treat tuberculosis. Some patients given iproniazid for tuberculosis developed euphoria and hyperactive behavior. In 1956, this led two groups of medical researchers to treat depressed patients with iproniazid, and both reported encouraging results. Thus, reserpine caused depression in some individuals and helped patients with mania, while iproniazid was the first effective chemical antidepressant, suggesting that chemical changes in the brain could alter mood in predictable ways.

This suggestion was partially responsible for two parallel and important research directions. One strategy was to look for new agents that might alter the mood of severely depressed patients; the second was to study the chemical mechanisms by which these substances might alter mood. Reserpine was soon found to deplete the biogenic amines serotonin and norepinephrine from the brain. Iproniazid was found to be an inhibitor of an important brain enzyme, monoamine oxidase (MAO), an enzyme partly responsible for the metabolism or inactivation of the biogenic amines. When the MAO enzyme activity is blocked by iproniazid, the quantity of biogenic amines is increased in the brain. Thus reserpine causes depression and decreases brain biogenic amines (neurotransmitters), while iproniazid helps depression and increases biogenic amines. Numerous other drugs were subsequently developed which similarly inhibited the enzyme monoamine oxidase and, like iproniazid, decreased depressive symptoms.

In 1948, another drug with profound effects on mood disorders was developed in Australia. Lithium carbonate was found to be an effective treatment for manic psychosis, diminishing the number and frequency of manic episodes in patients who had suffered frequent recurrences. About the same time, the tricyclics, a new class of antidepressants, were found to be even more effective and considerably safer than the inhibitors of monoamine oxidase in the treatment of depression. In both cases, their action on brain chemistry is consistent with the biogenic-amine hypothesis which ascribes depression to decreased, and mania to excess, biogenic-amine activity. Lithium decreases the release of biogenic amines from neurons and speeds the removal of biogenic amines from the synaptic cleft, thus decreasing their functional activity. Tricyclic antidepressants, on the other hand, have been shown to slow the removal of biogenic amines, presumably increasing their functional activity.

The biogenic-amine hypothesis thus finds support in the action of all four of these pharmacological agents. Nevertheless, it poses several problems. Pharmacological agents exist that have effects similar to tricyclic antidepressants on biogenic amines and they still do not seem to be effective antidepressants. On the other hand, at least one tricyclic antidepressant exists that is effective in depression but that does not seem to block the inactivation of biogenic amines.

The so-called "precursor load" strategy has also failed to confirm the biogenic-amine hypothesis. The idea behind it was simple and elegant: if depression was caused by decreased functional activity of biogenic amines, why not feed patients large amounts of dietary substances that are converted to biogenic amines in the brain—that is, feed them the precursors of the biogenic amines? Three precursors have been tried and have so far produced disappointing results in depressed patients. They may have had some effect on mood, but they are clearly not effective treatments for depression. Direct attempts to find altered biogenic-amine levels in patients with mania and depression have likewise produced suggestive but inconclusive results. Thus, the biogenic-amine hypothesis of depression and mania has not been proven, and it may turn out to be an oversimplification. Nevertheless, the hypothesis has stimulated a broad range of research that has given significant new insights into brain function.[7]

The same can be said for another major theory of brain physiology and behavior, the dopamine hypothesis of schizophrenia, which states that excess functional activity of the brain neurotransmitter, dopamine, predisposes the individual to schizophrenic symptoms. Like the biogenic-amine hypothesis of depression and mania, this hypothesis found its origin in both biochemical and clinical studies with psychoactive drugs. Antipsychotic drugs seem to work by blocking the receptor for dopamine on brain neurons. This receptor is a complex system that includes an enzyme called adenylate cyclase. Dopamine, after diffusing across the synaptic cleft, activates that enzyme; antipsychotic drugs seem to prevent or inhibit the activation and displace dopamine from its receptor site. They have numerous other actions as well, but since they are a chemically diverse group of medications they do not all share the same biochemical actions—in fact, dopamine-receptor blockade seems to be the only biochemical effect these drugs have in common. Their antipsychotic potency also correlates fairly closely with their potency in blocking the dopamine receptor.

If dopamine blockade and the consequent decrease in dopamine neurotransmission are helpful in reducing schizophrenic symptoms, does increased dopamine activity cause or worsen schizophrenia? There is some evidence that it may. Some chronic users of the psychoactive drug amphetamine or cocaine develop a a syndrome that is remarkably like paranoid schizophrenia even though they may have no previous history of mental illness. The process is not completely understood, but the syndrome may be the result of increasing dopamine neurotransmission, while antipsychotic agents may act by blocking the dopamine receptor, decreasing neurotransmission in the dopaminergic nerves.

The dopamine hypothesis cannot be considered established fact: direct attempts to find increased dopamine activity in patients with schizophrenia have been disappointing. However, like the biogenic-amine hypothesis of depression and mania, the dopamine hypothesis has been an important stimulus to clinical and neurophysiological research and has led to the discovery of several pharmacological agents which have decreased the suffering caused by schizophrenia. It continues to stimulate the search for an explanation of the biochemical basis for that suffering.

The development of psychopharmacological agents has also been associated with some difficult clinical and social problems. We have already mentioned that caused by the massive discharge of patients from public mental hospitals. Other problems include the side effects of psychopharmacological agents, the tendency of people to abuse them, and the value conflicts associated with pharmacological treatments of mental illness.

Although the antipsychotic medications have generally proved to be remarkably safe, a few patients who use them for prolonged periods develop a syndrome, called tardive dyskinesia, of involuntary muscle twitches of the jaw, cheeks, and tongue. The syndrome sometimes gradually subsides, but it can be permanent.

The antidepressant drugs have thus far revealed no long-term side effects, but, unlike the antipsychotic medications, the tricyclic antidepressants readily lend themselves to suicidal attempts because fatal overdoses are easy to ingest. This is a particularly knotty problem because the tricyclic antidepressants are otherwise particularly useful for that large proportion of depressed patients who tend to be suicidal to begin with.

Another problem has been the abuse of psychopharmacological agents in their ingestion for effects on mood, thinking, and behavior. This is certainly not a new phenomenon; substance abuse is older than written history and found in most human cultures. Indeed, a remarkable amount of energy has been spent by mankind in producing and consuming substances with psychopharmacological actions.

These substances can be divided into four types: the hallucinogens, the stimulants, the narcotic-analgesics, and the sedative hypnotics. The syndromes produced by each of them are distinct, but members of each class produce similar alterations of mood, thinking, and behavior. Each pharmacological class also includes both substances derived from plants and those newer ones totally synthesized in the laboratory.

The hallucinogens produce symptoms which include perceptual distortions, illusions, and labile mood that can include euphoria and profound fear. They can result in some novel feelings and thoughts and some unusual experiences. The user often claims he has a better understanding of ultimate questions and purposes and has had feelings comparable to mystical or religious experiences. These reactions can be produced by ingesting part of the peyote cactus or psilocybe mushroom or by taking the chemical substance lysergic acid diethylamide (LSD-25).

The stimulants include amphetamines, which were synthesized in the nineteen-thirties, and cocaine, which is derived from coca leaves. These compounds produce seeming alertness and euphoria, decrease appetite, and diminish feelings of fatigue. Their continued use can produce a syndrome remarkably like paranoid schizophrenia.

The opiates are sedatives, decreasing pain sensation and producing a sense of well-being. The user tends to withdraw into himself for quiet reflection; sometimes he sleeps. The opiates include derivatives of opium, heroin, and morphine, and newer compounds synthesized in laboratories that produce similar biological reactions. One pattern of opiate use involves the daily intravenous injection of heroin. When this daily injection is stopped, the user experiences a characteristic three- to four-day withdrawal syndrome which resembles a severe case of viral influenza.

The sedative hypnotics include alcohol, perhaps the oldest and certainly the most widespread drug of abuse, and newer tranquilizers and sleeping pills, such as the barbiturates. These substances produce talkativeness, relaxation, and a sense of well-being. In higher doses, sedative hypnotics produce slurred speech, a staggering gait, and a markedly reduced ability to perform complex motor skills. As there are heroin addicts, so there are people who use alcohol or barbiturates every day. When this daily use is stopped, a dangerous convulsive withdrawal syndrome appears that requires hospital treatment. The chronic use of alcohol causes damage to cells, particularly in the liver, and can also damage cells in the brain.

The abuse of psychopharmacological agents is a significant public health and legal problem. Hallucinogen-drug users occasionally harm themselves or others, because of distorted perceptions or beliefs. Aggressive acts are probably more common with abusers of amphetamines and cocaine; their paranoia sometimes leads them to violence. Partly because their drug of abuse is expensive and illegal, heroin addicts are also frequently involved in burglary, robbery, and other criminal activities to sustain their habit.

Despite the widespread problems caused by other drugs of abuse, alcohol abuse continues to cause more problems for society than all other drugs of abuse combined. The damaging physical and mental effects of chronic alcohol abuse have been well documented. In 1964, 22 per cent of the first-admission males to state mental hospitals were diagnosed as alcoholics. Alcohol abuse is also the largest law-enforcement problem in the United States. In 1965, 40 per cent of all arrests were made for public drunkenness or drunken driving. Homicide and suicide are often associated with alcoholic intoxication. In a case study done in Ohio in 1954, 43 per cent of those who committed murder had done so under the influence of alcohol. A 1951 Maryland study reported that 69 per cent of the murder victims had also been drinking. In a study of 588 Philadelphia homicides, alcohol was present in both the killer and victim in 44 per cent of the cases. A 1962 study in the state of Washington reported that 31 per cent of suicides were committed by patients known to be alcoholics. The relationship between alcohol intoxication and automobile accidents is also significant. In one study, 50 per cent of fatally injured drivers had a blood alcohol level of 0.15 per cent or more, indicating serious intoxication, at the time of death.[8]

Although there are many causes for drug abuse, one hypothesis, pointing to the existence of psychoactive substances in nearly every culture, suggests that the gratifications of altered states of consciousness are apparently common among all peoples.[9] The sense of well-being produced by drugs of abuse is evidently a powerful reinforcer for repeated drug use. Psychoactive drugs may reinforce their own use by enabling the user to withdraw from a painful environment, or may represent an attempt at self-cure. The sense of well-being produced by amphetamines, for example, can bring transient relief from psychological depression, as can that produced by alcohol. Social factors, more distantly related to the pharmacological actions of the drugs of abuse, also play a role. Intoxication begins in a social setting; heroin, hallucinogen, and amphetamine users often share a specific subculture in which drug use is an important social behavior linked inextricably to membership in it.

The development of new psychopharmacological agents has posed in new form the question of involuntary treatment, part of a larger philosophical issue which is the subject of constant debate both within and outside the psychiatric profession. The basic issue is whether patients should ever be given psychopharmacological agents without their consent. While the exact legal mechanism varies from state to state, it is common to do so in the case of highly disturbed psychiatric patients who refuse medications. In California, for example, patients must be found to be a danger to themselves or to others or gravely disabled, and each of these problems must be regarded as resulting from a mental illness.[10] In practice, the patients who fall into these categories are suicidal or so schizophrenic that they are unable to care for their bodily needs.

There are those who argue that this involuntary treatment, however well intentioned, is an effort to alter an individual's conduct by external means, and that an individual should have a right to refuse it.[11] Szasz, representing the extreme of this view, feels that the government and psychiatry have joined together, as did the state and the church before them, to force individuals to conform to certain patterns of behavior and belief. Szasz feels that an individual has a right to determine his own behavior, his own beliefs, and his own future, and that he should retain these rights even if he is considered potentially dangerous, suicidal, or unable to care for himself.

The other side of the coin, however, is that if the individual commits a crime, he can also be tried, regardless of whether or not he is found to be sane.[12]

Szasz's viewpoint may have attractions for civil libertarians. Some of its logical consequences, however, would be difficult for many people to accept: Should a depressed patient be allowed to commit suicide? Should a paranoid schizophrenic who believes his food is poisoned be allowed to starve to death?

The prevailing consensus has been that it is more humane to treat some patients involuntarily. Many suicide-attempters often regret it later, respond to treatment, never try again, and are grateful for the help. Involuntarily treated schizophrenics are also usually thankful when they are able to resume their former lives and relationships. Thus, involuntary psychiatric treatments, if truly effective and humane, can be regarded as liberating rather than restricting. So long as the treatment is adequate and allows patients to return to society, to be free from disturbing thoughts or self-destructive impulses, this view is likely to prevail in the future.

The decisions are often not so straightforward. Consider the "spaceman" of San Diego, California. He lives in a rooming house in north San Diego and pays his rent with money he earns cleaning a small variety store. He wears a suit which appears to be made in part of aluminum foil and carries a device which looks like a radio transmitter. The spaceman will tell anyone who asks, and some who don't, that he is from a distant planet and has been sent to save the earth from destruction. This project is set to begin when the signal is received from his home planet. To most people who live in the area, the spaceman is part of the community. Some make fun of him, strangers are often frightened, but most tolerate this man and his eccentric beliefs. Psychiatrists would probably call him a chronic paranoid schizophrenic. But the decision to hospitalize him would not be easy. Antipsychotic drugs might diminish his belief in his origin and his mission, but why should they be given against his will?

Clearly there is no simple solution to the philosophical dilemma. Organ transplants and the mechanical means for keeping comatose patients alive are other medical advances posing similar ethical questions for society. Ethical inquiry will have to become a more important part of health care than it has been in the past. In this and other contexts, the biomedical sciences must more effectively integrate with the social sciences in tackling these difficult problems.

Despite the impressive progress that has been made in the drug treatment of psychiatric disorders, much remains to be done. The drug treatments for schizophrenia reduce symptoms but do not cure the disease, and sometimes have adverse side effects. Drug treatments for depression and mania do not seem to have major long-term side effects, but are not always effective either. The drug treatments for depression can also be fatal if taken in sufficiently large doses. The margin between the helpful and harmful dosage should ideally be much greater. Psychiatric treatments for substance abuse, violent behavior, and senility are still either only partially effective or non-existent.

Some new chemical substances with a potential for alleviating mental illness can be developed by systematic modification of existing medications, as many of the newer medications in use today were developed. Other pharmacological agents may arise from basic research that will tell us more about the biochemical factors that predispose people to psychiatric symptoms. The dopamine hypothesis of schizophrenia led to the trial in schizophrenic patients of alpha-methyl-paratyrosine (AMPT), which decreases dopamine synthesis. Preliminary reports suggest that AMPT may allow physicians to use lower doses of current antipsychotic medications to achieve the same reduction in schizophrenic symptoms. [13]

New chemical substances are tested in animals before they are given to human patients to screen them for toxic effects and help predict the pharmacological actions of drugs in humans. Animal pharmacologists have already developed a number of tests in rodents which predict antidepressant and antipsychotic activity of new medications in man. Animal paradigms may or may not have any direct relationship to human mental illness, but they are nevertheless always useful in predicting some drug actions in humans. They have often been criticized because they lead to a kind of circular process. Since the animal-test paradigms were based on drugs already used in human patients, new drugs which have similar action in these tests will probably act through similar mechanisms. A drug that might prove to be extremely effective in reducing the symptoms of mental illness, but that acts through a different biochemical mechanism, could easily be inadvertently eliminated by these animal screening tests.

A promising new approach to animal testing of new pharmacological agents is the attempt to develop animal models which more closely approximate human mental illness. Several non-human-primate models of behavior disorders not only test individual animals but also look at non-human primates in social groups. Mother-infant separation may produce in monkeys a parallel to human depression; the chronic administration of amphetamine or cocaine to non-human primates in social groups may lead to a non-human parallel for human schizophrenia. Basic research into the mechanisms of pharmacological actions should also yield information on the mechanism of the production of side effects. Current psychoactive drugs could then be tested in animal models in order to predict human side effects and systematically modified to reduce those side effects.

One possible approach to avoiding unwanted side effects is the placement of the drug near its site of action. Small plastic membranes placed in the conjunctival sac of the eye are currently used to release medication for the treatment of glaucoma. Intrauterine devices which release hormones locally are now in use for contraception. The advantage of this local placement is that the medication does not enter the general circulation and consequently cannot produce unwanted effects in other areas of the body. [14] But local placement of psychoactive medication would require placement in specific areas of the brain. Because the practical and philosophical problems of such a technique are formidable, here, as elsewhere, it is worth anticipating developments and analyzing their probable social implications.

Better treatment for the alcoholic and other substance abusers is another important public health need. Pharmacological treatments for the heroin addict have already improved the prognosis for some of these patients. Methadone is an opiate like heroin, but with three important differences. It can be taken orally; its effects last 24 hours (versus 6 to 8 hours for heroin), and it can be taken legally. Many opiate addicts have voluntarily given up heroin for methadone. One dose a day produces minimal sedation and allows a former addict to be economically productive and to remain on the right side of the law.

Maintenance with pharmacological agents which antagonize the effects of opiates is another pharmacological approach to heroin addiction. Naltrexone inhibits the effects of injected heroin and can help a former heroin addict to avoid opiates. [15] The disulfiram (Antabuse) treatment of alcoholics is based on a related concept. A former alcoholic who takes disulfiram daily will develop extremely unpleasant symptoms if he drinks alcohol. Alcoholic patients therefore voluntarily take Antabuse daily to help get through periods of stress, when they are especially tempted to drink.

A similar but highly speculative new approach to substance abuse based on biochemical research is now being experimented with. Spector has developed anti-bodies that bind steroid hormones and opiates to use in tests which assay the quantities of steroids or opiates in blood or urine.[16] The steroid antibody seems to modify the pharmacological actions of administered steroids. It is possible that antibodies to opiates could similarly prevent the pharmacological actions of heroin, helping a former addict to abstain from the drug.

More practical and less speculative is the continuing research by pharmacologists and psychiatrists into the mechanism of action of psychoactive drugs such as alcohol and opiates and into the psychological causes of substance abuse, and it is likely that new treatments for substance abusers will result. Because this form of abuse is prevalent—and increasing—among the young, substance abuse is an important public health problem and research on it deserves high priority.

The pharmacological treatment of violent behavior is still in its infancy. One reasonable drug treatment for assaultive behavior is available: antipsychotic medications can reduce paranoid delusions and hence the potential for violent behavior in cases of paranoid schizophrenia or amphetamine paranoid psychosis. Pharmacological modification of certain types of violent behavior in animals is an active area of research which may help, but the causes of human violence are extremely complex, and pharmacological treatment of violent patients is likely to involve only a small portion of future attempts to understand human aggression. The ethical issues of possible pharmacological treatments for violence are also particularly complicated. Despite these problems, this is an important area for psychiatric and interdisciplinary research: indeed, it is remarkable that human hatred and violence have so far attracted so little scientific investigation.

Clinical research has shown that many elderly people become senile and in-competent for social rather than medical reasons. If they are provided with social support, occupations, and, consequently, self-esteem, they can function effectively at advanced ages. Some, however, do have brain disease associated with the senile symptoms, and this is another area of active research in psychopharmacology. The memory loss and personality changes which occur in these organically damaged old people are poorly understood, but at least two areas currently show some promise for pharmacological treatments. Drugs which dilate blood vessels may be useful where symptoms are due to decreased blood flow to the brain. Such medication for this condition is already in clinical use, but further clinical trials are needed to determine how effective they are and which senile patients will benefit from them. Depression is common among the aged. Some patients with the personality changes and the thinking and memory defects of senility seem to be markedly improved by treatment with the same medications used for depression in younger patients, though typically at lower dosage. In retrospect, these elderly patients are said to have suffered from "pseudosenile depression." There is, to date, no reliable way to predict which patients are most likely to benefit from antidepressants. The aged have been neglected in respect both to current services and to future-oriented research. The recent creation of a National Institute on Aging should help to remedy these omissions.

A speculative approach to the treatment of senile brain disease involves the use of a medication which seemed at least in animal tests to improve learning and memory. This medication, called ACTH (4-10), is a fragment of a naturally occurring pituitary hormone in man. It is currently being tested in patients with memory deficiencies, including senile patients.[17]

In the course of this essay, we have noted several heavy burdens of distress and disability that have largely been neglected by science until the last quarter-century. One phase of the life cycle that is still being neglected in the field of mental health is the onset of adolescence, a time of lifelong importance in the formation of crucial behavior patterns involving habits that influence future health, such as cigarette smoking, alcohol and other drug use, automobile driving, nutrition and exercise, and human relationships. These extensive changes in behavior are associated with drastic physiological and biochemical changes in the body.[18] Messages from the brain influence the pituitary gland to release hormones which in turn control the output of sex hormones. These sex hormones have far-reaching biochemical influences throughout the organism, including effects on cells and circuits in the brain. Although it is plausible to suppose that there are specific links between certain hormonal changes and concomitant changes in fundamental components of sexual, aggressive, and emotional behavior, virtually no well substantiated information exists to confirm this supposition, despite its clinical significance.

Research on monkeys and apes, however, indicates that major behavioral changes occur in many species during adolescence. In non-human primate societies in their natural habitats, adolescent males are the most active, exploratory, and aggressive class of individuals. In most species, sex differences in behavior are apparent from early life, with males being more aggressive. Building on these differences at adolescence, the males play more roughly and threaten the adults. The adult males typically respond to these challenges by threatening in turn, then attacking, eventually driving the adolescent males back into peripheral positions. In rhesus monkeys and baboons, males commonly transfer to a different troop during these periods of turbulence. Although this behavior takes many forms, the upsurge of aggression and the struggle for enhancement of status in adolescent males is constant.

This research suggests that an evolutionary heritage is involved in the hormonal changes of puberty and concomitant changes in behavior. The biological changes of puberty now occur in a social environment very different from that of our ancestors. The interaction of these biological and social factors in adolescent development is ripe for study.

As sophistication has grown in the entire field of life-cycle studies,[19] it has become clear that research based on broad categories such as "adolescence" and "adulthood" have been disappointing, their findings confusing and often contradictory. Future progress probably depends on distinguishing appropriate sub-sets within those broad categories; there are many more phases in the life cycle than are conventionally described.

One of them is early adolescence, the neglect of which is deserved neither in terms of its intrinsic interest nor in the visible and increasing incidence of problems and distress it often brings. Attempts to deal with the alarmingly high rates of pregnancy, venereal disease, alcohol and drug abuse, vandalism and personal violence, dropping out of school, depression, and suicide in adolescents have been largely unsuccessful, probably because there have been no useful data on which to base action and no framework in terms of the developmental tasks and the range of coping strategies appropriate to the sex and sociocultural context of these children.

Early adolescence includes the phase in which status changes from child to adolescent, often marked by a major shift in school from elementary to junior-high or high school. The age range is ten to fifteen years old, on average. It is a time of sharp discontinuity with the past. Because of the profound biological and psychosocial changes occurring in early adolescence, it is a critical period of development. Relevant endocrine studies of puberty can now be carried out with precision. Careful simultaneous studies of the endocrine and bodily changes of puberty and the concomitant emotional and behavioral changes therefore can and ought to be done.

How early adolescents make decisions is important, not only for determining their immediate behavior, but also for establishing the attitudes and patterns of behavior which will shape the negotiation of later stages of adolescence. It seems likely that adult behavior may be strongly linked to the decisions of early adolescence. Determining this is but one example of why the cognitive, psychological, and psychosocial development of early adolescence is important for learning about the mental health of people in all stages of life.

In mental health, perhaps more than elsewhere in medicine, the life of the individual is increasingly being studied in terms of its various stages. We have called attention to early adolescence and the problems of the aged, but we might equally well have considered the formative influences of early childhood or the stresses of mid-life. Viewing the organism in its trajectory through the life course, as genetic endowment interacts with environmental vicissitudes, is of singular importance in the understanding of behavior and its disorders. There are important behavioral factors in cancer and heart disease (e.g., heavy cigarette smoking), in accidental injury (e.g., risky and drunken driving), and in other casualties which are clinically dealt with, but which for too long have been neglected in the scientific study of behavior. The burden of illness and the opportunities for relief of that burden surely call for an awakening of interest in behavioral aspects of health. Indeed, we predict that the next decade will see a closer integration of mental health with medicine in general—including services, research, and education. The understanding of human behavior in sickness and in health is surely one of the critical problems of our time.

REFERENCES

[1] A. M. Friedman, H. I. Kaplan, and B. J. Sadock, eds., *Modern Synopsis of Comprehensive Textbook of Psychiatry* (1972).

[2] *Ibid.*

[3] F. J. Ayd, Jr., "The Impact of Biological Psychiatry" in F. J. Ayd and B. Blackwell, eds., *Discoveries in Biological Psychiatry* (Philadelphia-Toronto, 1970), pp. 230-43.

[4] R. Reich, "The Chronically Mentally Ill: Their Fate in New York City." *Bulletin of the New York State District Branches, American Psychiatric Association*, 15 (November, 1972), p. 6.

[5] F. N. Arnhoff, "Social Consequences of Policy Toward Mental Illness," *Science*, 188 (June 27, 1975), pp. 1277-81.

[6] D. A. Hamburg, ed., *Psychiatry as a Behavioral Science* (Englewood Cliffs, New Jersey, 1970).

[7] P. A. Berger, "Brain Neurotransmitters and the Affective Disorders," presented at the Houston Neurological Symposium on Basic and Clinical Aspects of Neurotransmitter Function (in press).

[8] *Task Force Report on Drunkenness, President's Commission on Law Enforcement and Administration of Justice* (U.S. Government Printing Office, Washington, D.C., 1967). The data reported were collected by F. A. Thomas, Plaut, and Judge John M. Murtagh. Studies by L. M. Shupe, H. A. Bullock, R. S. Fisher, and M. E. Wolfgang were cited by R. H. Blum.

[9]A. H. Weil, *The Natural Mind: A New Way of Looking at Drugs and the Higher Consciousness* (New York, 1972).

[10]The California Community Mental Health Services Act, Lantermann-Petris-Short Act, Division 5, Part 1, Chapters 1, 2, and 3.

[11]T. A. Gonda and M. B. Waitzkin, "The Right to Refuse Treatment," *Current Concepts in Psychiatry* (1976), pp. 5-10.

[12]T. Szasz, *Law, Liberty, Psychiatry* (New York, 1963).

[13]J. D. Barchas, G. Elliott, and P. A. Berger, "Biogenic Amine Metabolism in Relation to Schizophrenia," presented at the Second Rochester International Conference on Schizophrenia, University of Rochester (in press).

[14]H. K. H. Brodie and R. L. Sack, "Promising Directions in Clinical Psychopharmacology," in D. Hamburg and H. K. H. Brodie, eds., *American Handbook of Psychiatry*, VI (2nd ed., 1975), pp. 533-51.

[15]P. A. Berger, "The Addict in the Emergency Room," in P. Rosenbaum and J. Beebe, eds., *An Introduction to Treatment in Psychiatry: Crisis Clinic and Consultation* (New York, 1975), pp. 161-71.

[16]S. J. Spector, "Quantitative Determination of Morphine in Serum by Radioimmunoassay," *Journal of Pharmacological and Experimental Therapeutics*, 178 (1971), pp. 253-58.

[17]C. A. Sandman, J. M. George, J. D. Nolan, H. Riezen, and A. J. Kastin, "Enhancement of Attention in Man with ACTH/MSH 4-10," *Physiology and Behavior*, 15 (1975), pp. 427-31.

[18]D. A. Hamburg, B. A. Hamburg, and J. D. Barchas, "Anger and Depression in Perspective of Behavioral Biology," in L. Levi, ed., *Emotions—Their Parameters and Measurement* (New York, 1975), pp. 235-78.

[19]B. A. Hamburg, "Early Adolescence: A Specific and Stressful Stage of the Life Cycle," in G. V. Coelho, D. A. Hamburg, and J. E. Adams, eds., *Coping and Adaptation* (New York, 1974), pp. 101-24.

Notes on Contributors

IVAN L. BENNETT, JR., M.D., born in 1922 in Washington, D.C., is executive vice-president for health affairs, provost of the Medical Center, and dean of the School of Medicine at New York University. He has written numerous articles for scientific and technical journals and is the editor of *Internal Medicine* (1977).

PHILIP A. BERGER, M.D., born in 1943 in Newark, New Jersey, is assistant professor of psychiatry and behavioral sciences at the Stanford University School of Medicine and director of the Psychiatric Clinical Research Center of the Veterans Administration Hospital in Palo Alto, California. His published works focus on the biochemical aspects of psychiatric disorders.

DANIEL CALLAHAN, born in 1930 in Washington, D.C., is founder and director of the Institute of Society, Ethics and the Life Sciences at Hastings-on-Hudson, New York. He is the author of *Abortion: Law, Choice, and Morality* (1970), *Ethics and Population Limitation* (1971), and *The Tyranny of Survival* (1974).

MERLIN K. DUVAL, M.D., born in 1922 in Montclair, New Jersey, is vice-president for health sciences at the University of Arizona, Tucson, and the author of numerous articles on medical subjects.

ROBERT H. EBERT, M.D., born in 1914 in Minneapolis, is dean of the faculty of medicine at the Harvard Medical School. His publications include studies on tuberculosis and inflammation, and essays on the problems of medical education and medical care.

LEON EISENBERG, M.D., born in 1922 in Philadelphia, is Maude and Lillian Pressley Professor of Psychiatry at the Harvard Medical School and Senior Associate in Psychiatry at the Children's Hospital, Boston. He is the author of *Conceptual Models of Physical and Mental Disorders in Research and Medical Practices* (1976), and articles in the field of psychiatry.

RENÉE C. FOX, born in 1928 in New York City, is professor of sociology, psychiatry, and medicine at the University of Pennsylvania, and chairman of the Department of Sociology. Her published works include *Experiment Perilous* (1959), (with Willy de Craemer) *The Emerging Physician* (1968), and (with Judith P. Swazey) *The Courage to Fail* (1974).

DONALD S. FREDRICKSON, M.D., born in 1924 in Canon City, Colorado, is director of the National Institutes of Health. He is the author of many articles in biomedical research and an editor of *The Metabolic Basis of Inherited Disease*.

ELI GINZBERG, born in 1911 in New York City, is A. Barton Hepburn Professor of Economics and director, Conservation of Human Resources, Columbia University. He is the author of *Occupational Choice* (1951), *The Ineffective Soldier* (1959), *The Pluralistic Economy* (1965), and *The Human Economy* (1976).

BEATRIX HAMBURG, M.D., born in 1923 in Jacksonville, Florida, is research psychiatrist in childhood and adolescent psychopathology at the Clinical Research Branch of the National Institutes of Mental Health. She has written several articles on the problems of the adolescent.

DAVID A. HAMBURG, M.D., born in 1925 in Evansville, Indiana, is president of the Institute of Medicine, National Academy of Sciences. He is the editor of *Psychiatry as a Behavioral Science* (1970), and co-editor of *Coping and Adaptation* (1974).

HERBERT E. KLARMAN, born in 1916 in Chmielnik, Poland, is professor of economics at the Graduate School of Public Administration of New York University. His published works include *Hospital Care in New York City* (1963), *The Economics of Health* (1965), and, as editor, *Empirical Studies in Health Economics* (1970).

JOHN H. KNOWLES, M.D., born in 1926 in Chicago, is president of the Rockefeller Foundation. He is the editor of *Hospitals, Doctors and the Public Interest* (1965) and *The Teaching Hospital: Evolution and Contemporary Issues* (1966), and the author of "The Struggle to Stay Healthy," a bicentennial essay for *Time* magazine (1976).

WALSH McDERMOTT, M.D., born in 1909 in New Haven, Connecticut, is emeritus professor of public health and medicine at Cornell University and special advisor to the president of the Robert Wood Johnson Foundation. He participated extensively in developing the present-day treatments for syphilis, typhus and typhoid fevers, bacterial pneumonias, and tuberculosis. He is co-editor of the Beeson-McDermott *Textbook of Medicine*.

STANLEY JOEL REISER, M.D., born in 1937 in New York City, is assistant professor and director of the Program in the History of Medicine at the Harvard Medical School, and co-director of the Kennedy Interfaculty Program in Medical Ethics at Harvard University. He is the author of the forthcoming *Medicine and the Reign of Technology*.

JULIUS B. RICHMOND, M.D., born in 1916 in Chicago, is professor of child psychiatry and human development at the Harvard Medical School. His publications include *Pediatric Diagnosis: Interpretation of Signs and Symptoms in Different Age Periods* (1962), *Currents in American Medicine* (1969), and other studies in pediatrics and child development.

DAVID E. ROGERS, M.D., born in 1926 in New York City, is president of the Robert Wood Johnson Foundation in Princeton, New Jersey. He is the author of many publications in the field of infectious disease and, more recently, in the field of medical education and problems in the delivery of medical care.

ERNEST W. SAWARD, M.D., born in 1914 in New York City, is associate dean and professor of medicine and social medicine at the University of Rochester School of Medicine and Dentistry. He has published several articles on health-care problems.

LEWIS THOMAS, M.D., born in 1913 in New York City, is president of the Memorial Sloan-Kettering Cancer Center in New York City. He is the author of *The Lives of a Cell* (1974), and of various scientific papers in the fields of experimental pathology and infectious disease.

AARON WILDAVSKY, born in 1930 in Brooklyn, New York, is president of the Russell Sage Foundation. He is the author of several books, the most recent of which are *Budgeting: A Comparative Theory of Budgetary Processes* (1975), and (with Nelson Polsby) *Presidential Elections* (1976).

Index